The Changing Face of Health Care Social Work

Sophia F. Dziegielewski, PhD, LCSW, is a professor in the School of Social Work at the University of Central Florida (UCF). She is the editor of the *Journal of Social Service Research* and has over 130 publications, including 7 textbooks, over 90 articles, and numerous book chapters. Ms. Dziegielewski is the recipient of several awards and has presented at numerous professional workshops and trainings on health, mental health, and preparation for social work licensing across the country. Throughout her academic, administrative, and practice career, she has been active in research and the protection of human subjects, specializing in the area of health and mental health. She has also been active in clinical practice, maintaining a current license in her field as well as serving as an expert witness in the courts.

The Changing Face of Health Care Social Work

Opportunities and Challenges for Professional Practice

Third Edition

Sophia F. Dziegielewski, PhD, LCSW

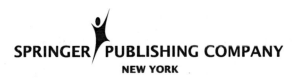

SPRINGER PUBLISHING COMPANY

NEW YORK

Springer Publishing Company, LLC
11 West 42nd Street
New York, NY 10036
www.springerpub.com

Acquisitions Editor: Stephanie Drew
Production Editor: Michael O'Connor
Composition: diacriTech

ISBN: 978-0-8261-1942-1
e-book ISBN: 978-0-8261-1943-8
Instructor's Manual ISBN: 978-0-8261-2972-7

Instructor's Manual: Qualified instructors may request this supplement by emailing textbook@springerpub.com

13 14 15 16/5 4 3 2 1

The author and the publisher of this Work have made every effort to use sources believed to be reliable to provide information that is accurate and compatible with the standards generally accepted at the time of publication. The author and publisher shall not be liable for any special, consequential, or exemplary damages resulting, in whole or in part, from the readers' use of, or reliance on, the information contained in this book. The publisher has no responsibility for the persistence or accuracy of URLs for external or third-party Internet websites referred to in this publication and does not guarantee that any content on such websites is, or will remain, accurate or appropriate.

Library of Congress Cataloging-in-Publication Data

Dziegielewski, Sophia F.
 The changing face of health care social work: opportunities and challenges for professional practice/
Sophia F. Dziegielewski, PhD, LCSW
—Third edition.
    pages cm
 Includes bibliographical references.
 ISBN 978-0-8261-1942-1
 1. Medical social work—United States—Methodology. 2. Managed care plans
(Medical care)—United States. 3. Hospitals—Case management
services—United States. 4. Hospitals—United States—Administration.
5. Social work administration—United States. 6. Medical care—Computer
network resources.
 I. Title.
 HV687.5.U5D95 2013
 362.1'0425—dc23

                                        2013002645

Special discounts on bulk quantities of our books are available to corporations, professional associations, pharmaceutical companies, health care organizations, and other qualifying groups. If you are interested in a custom book, including chapters from more than one of our titles, we can provide that service as well.
For details, please contact:
Special Sales Department, Springer Publishing Company, LLC
11 West 42nd Street, 15th Floor, New York, NY 10036-8002
Phone: 877-687-7476 or 212-431-4370; Fax: 212-941-7842
E-mail: sales@springerpub.com

In my life, I have grown to believe that intelligence consists of the knowledge that one acquires over a lifetime. Wisdom, however, is far greater. Wisdom requires having intelligence but realizing that it means nothing if it is not shared with others. In wisdom, there is a natural giving of the self to others, with no fear of loss. It means realizing that the knowledge we have is measured purely by what we can teach and share with others.

This book is dedicated to one of my earliest and wisest teachers, my "other" mother, Esther Mooney.

Contents

PART IV: CONCLUSION

Contributors

Diane C. Holliman, PhD, LCSW
Associate Professor
School of Social Work
Valdosta State University
Valdosta, Georgia

George A. Jacinto, PhD, LCSW, CPC
Associate Professor
School of Social Work
MSW Program Coordinator
University of Central Florida
Orlando, Florida

AnneMarie Jones, PhD, MSW
Associate Professor
Mississippi Valley State University
Itta Bena, Mississippi

Joshua Kirven, PhD, MSW
Lecturer
School of Social Work
University of Central Florida
Orlando, Florida

Preface

This third edition of *The Changing Face of Health Care Social Work* reviews the basic concepts related to the delivery of social work services in health care settings. When health care is responsive to those in need, the provision of services must be equitable, safe, timely, efficient, effective, evidence-based, and patient-centered while simultaneously exemplifying best practices for all. As pressure continues to increase, however, the equitable distribution and availability of affordable health care have changed. This has left many providers and patients alike filled with expectation and speculation as to what constitutes essential service delivery. Reflective of the title of this book, *The Changing Face of Health Care Social Work*, regardless of the face that emerges, the changes and system revisions will continue to be extensive and costly.

The importance of the contributions that social workers make in this constantly changing environment centers around providing responsive, direct, supportive services with patients and their families, whether it is in the home, the community, a hospital setting, a clinic, or other health care institutions. Social work has a long history of recognizing the importance of treating the whole person and linking that person and his or her needs to the situation or environment. This flexibility extends to the basic definition of those who are served and requires the use of terminology that allows for recognition and acceptance. For this reason, clients, throughout the book, will be referred to as patients and social workers will be presented as service providers to patients and their families in hospital settings, clinics, and institutions, with particular stress on their provision of supportive, transitional, and aftercare.

The Patient Protection and Affordable Care Act (ACA) is just one recent example (U.S. Department of Health and Human Services, 2012) of the extensive changes our health care system is experiencing. Replacing previous attempts related to managed care, this law, put into effect in 2010, is expected to reach full implementation by 2014. The ACA changes the way health care services are delivered and affects all types of care given, regardless of the setting. This Act, with its continual refinements, promises to hold insurance companies accountable by setting standards for reform. It provides the groundwork for controlling health care costs while guaranteeing more service choices that enhance the delivery of quality health care. To assist with providing access, this program supports the coverage of 32 million Americans who currently do not have health care coverage and is expected to open accessibility for affordable care to many more (Ofosu, 2011).

It is clear that as the face of health care changes, so do the challenges that social workers encounter in providing behavior-based outcomes and objectives that will lead to best practices. These challenges need to be embraced as opportunities, and social workers represent a profession rich with the understanding, awareness, and skills needed to provide services in the fluctuating and complex environment surrounding the provision of care.

Knowledge of how to navigate this complex environment helps social workers to remain flexible and accept this challenge while preparing for the changes needed. This knowledge supports the re-evaluation of current services with concomitant recommendations for updated changes. This flexibility allows social workers the opportunity to remain players in this era of competition among providers performing similar functions in developing best practices.

Social workers must continue to show that what they do is necessary and effective, with supportive services that go beyond just helping the patient. Patients cannot be treated as if they are in isolation, and for services to be effective significant others, family, support systems, and environmental–situational changes must always be considered. Effectiveness must also involve validation that the greatest reporting of concrete and identifiable therapeutic gain was achieved with the least amount of financial and professional support. This means that not only must the treatment that social workers provide be therapeutically effective, it must also be professionally competitive with other disciplines that claim similar treatment strategies and techniques. In health care, the importance of recognizing the person-in-situation has never been more important, and this needs to be balanced with the expectation that this will be accomplished with the least amount of resources possible.

Simply stated, health care social workers need to embrace these changes and become PROACTIVE at all levels of practice.

P: **Positive positioning**: Health care social workers need to *present* and *position* themselves as competent professionals with *positive* attitudes in all health care service settings, regardless of the type of health care practice being provided.

R: **Recognition of patient needs**: Health care social workers need to be aware of and well versed in assessment outlining the needs of the patient. Realizing that the patients cannot be viewed in isolation and that their support systems must all be considered in *recognition of patient need*.

O: **Organize and empower patients and providers**: The role of the health care social worker goes beyond simply providing concrete services to a client. Rather, it involves *organizing* and empowering patients, providers, and communities to help themselves receive safe, accessible, and affordable health care services. For providers, social workers need to gather and organize information supportive of the changes that are occurring, while encouraging the development of strategies to continue to provide safe, ethical, and cost-effective service.

A:	**Address service needs**: Health care social workers need to *address service needs* and identify the policies and issues that are relevant to providing ethical, effective, efficient, evidence-based, and cost-effective service.
C:	**Collaboration with other providers**: Embracing a team approach is essential for addressing client needs and concerns in a comprehensive way that leads to best practices. *Collaboration with other providers*, regardless of the type of team employed, will serve to complement orthodox medical practices and techniques. Utilization of a team approach supports the use of integrating traditional medical approaches with more holistic ones that increase health and wellness.
T:	**Teaching and empowering others**: Health care social workers are essential providers who assist with *teaching and empowering patients and significant others* on how to utilize their own self-support as well as support systems. They recognize that patients cannot be treated as if they are in isolation and know how to organize the social support system.
I:	**Investigation that leads to innovation**: *Investigate* and apply *innovative* approaches to current patient care problems and issues. *Involve* and assist providers, making all aware of the details most essential to a comprehensive assessment rich with change strategy and innovation.
V:	**Values and ethics**: Two cornerstones of health care practice are the *values and ethics* central to our profession. These are expectations strongly rooted in our practice skills, where each worker abides by a comprehensive ethical code.
E:	**Empower our patients and ourselves**: Most important is the expectation to *empower our patients and ourselves* by stressing the importance of *education* for self-betterment as well as strategies for individual and societal change.

As social workers face the many changes that are in store for all health care providers, we need to remember that in this era of cost cutting and cost containment, we can remain viable players. After all, social workers can provide unique treatments, and in some cases (to spur competition) similar treatments for less money. In the social workers' *Code of Ethics*, we are sworn to provide reasonable fees and base our charges on an ability to pay. This makes the fees social work professionals charge very competitive when compared to psychiatrists, psychologists, family therapists, psychiatric nurses, and mental health counselors who profess they can provide similar services.

This fact can provide enticement to coordinated care agencies to contract with social workers instead of with other professionals to provide services that traditionally have fallen in the social work domain. This book advocates a proactive stance for health care social workers and is designed to serve as a practical guide for understanding and addressing the philosophy of practice in our current health care environment. Suggestions are made for achieving ethical time-limited, evidence-based social work practice in these settings. At the end of each chapter, a "Summary and Future Directions" section is provided that will help social workers to understand what can be expected and how to prepare for the practice changes needed in order to remain viable clinical practitioners.

A Note To Instructors

An Instructor's Manual, complete with a test bank, activities to enhance learning, and a sample syllabus, is available for qualified faculty who adopt the book as a text for their course. Instructors can send an e-mail to textbook@springerpub.com to request these useful materials.

Sophia F. Dziegielewski

Acknowledgments

I am very grateful for all the help I have received from the many practitioners and educators in the field of health care social work across the United States. Thank you for providing me with your first-hand experiences in the area of health care and talking openly about the challenges and struggles that you face on a daily basis. These visionary social workers deal with the challenges of this changing environment as well as bear the burden of exploring and subsequently influencing how these changes will affect our future professional practice. In addition, I would like to thank my patients and the patients of these contributing social workers for helping us to see the effects of these health care strategies within an individualized "person-in-environment" framework. Furthermore, I would like to express my sincere thanks to the coauthors who helped to write chapters in the previous edition as well as several chapters in this latest edition of the book and all the individuals at Springer Publishing Company who helped in the production of this third edition of the book.

Finally, time and effort necessary to complete a book imposes burdens on those with whom we share our lives inside and outside the work environment. I would especially like to recognize Linden Siri, who for over 32 years has provided an environment rich with love, understanding, and support, as well as my family members, colleagues, and friends who understood and supported me when I said, "I can't, because I have to work on this book." It is through this type of encouragement and support that all things really are possible.

PART I

Understanding the Practice of Health Care Social Work

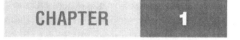

CHAPTER 1

Health Care Practice in Turbulent Times

This book reviews the basic concepts related to the delivery of social work services and the many roles of the social worker in health care settings. Whether we call patients *clients* or *consumers*, the efforts of the social worker generally involve assisting *patients/clients/consumers* (hereafter referred to as patients) and their families in hospital settings, clinics, and institutions as well as providing supportive transitional and aftercare. As pressure continues to increase the availability of affordable health care insurance for all, the changes and system revisions to make this happen will be extensive.

Recently, the Patient Protection and Affordable Care Act (ACA) is just one example (U.S. Department of Health and Human Services, 2012). This law, which was put into effect in 2010 with expectations of full implementation by 2014, seeks to hold insurance companies accountable by setting standards for reform that allow for lower health care costs and guarantee more choices that enhance quality of care. The ACA supports health care changes as well as improvements to health care access, quality, and service. This program clearly supports the coverage of 32 million Americans who currently do not have health care coverage and opens the doors for affordable care to many more (Ofosu, 2011). Advents such as this continue to evolve and require that all health care professionals be open to change while balancing quality of care and utilizing evidence-based practices that are effective and cost-efficient (Dziegielewski, 2010a).

Effectiveness in this area involves patient/client/consumer advocacy at the most basic level. In this system of care, health care professionals will ultimately decide, with the input of consumers, who will qualify and receive services. Therefore, efforts to shape service provision and the choices available have never been more important. With the influence of high-level

policies and interest groups, advocacy must extend beyond simply helping the patient. Effectiveness must also involve validation that the greatest
reporting of concrete and identifiable therapeutic gain was achieved with the
least amount of financial and professional support (DePoy & Gilson, 2003).
Social workers are trained to address the psychosocial needs of the patients
served and support an important continuum of care essential for linking the
person to the environment (Ofosu, 2011). This means that not only must the
interventions that social workers provide be socially acknowledged as necessary, they must also be therapeutically effective (Franklin, 2002). The time
has also come for social workers to embrace illness prevention that can assist
to minimize the effects of chronic illness on individuals, families, and their
support systems (Zabora, 2011).

In addition, the services social workers provide must be professionally competitive with other disciplines that claim similar treatment strategies
and techniques. This has led to the rebirth of all efforts for patient betterment to be evidence-based to be acknowledged as effective (Donald, 2002).
These efforts have been hailed as critical to tertiary prevention, which when
applied properly, can lead to the detection of psychological distress and how
these stressors can exemplify the medical symptoms experienced such as
pain and other somatic complaints (Zabora, 2011).

What is evidence-based health care?

Evidence-based health care practice is best understood as a systematic
framework for making decisions that takes into account the patient's
needs, values, and expectations while incorporating the best evidence
available in providing the services needed. In this type of practice, the
social worker must use his/or her own clinical expertise and support
all intervention methods with the best methods shown to be effective
through rigorous testing and research. Evidence-based practice involves
treatment or intervention options as well as risk management considerations for individuals, families, and groups.

Over the last 20 years, the battle continues in the health care arena
to do "more with less." This has never been more evident than in the current state of the economy where many Americans continue to struggle to
keep their homes and question the continuation of what was generally
accepted to be the American dream. Social workers are one group of players in this complex environment where the traditionally held notion that
"social workers can provide similar treatments for less money" can actually
remain strong.

In the social worker's code of ethics, all professionals are sworn to
provide reasonable fees and always take into account a patient's ability to
pay (National Association of Social Workers, 1996, with its latest revision

in 2008a). This makes the fees social work professionals charge competitive when compared with psychiatrists, psychologists, family therapists, psychiatric nurses, and mental health counselors who profess to provide similar services. This cost-saving emphasis can provide enticement to health and mental health agencies to contract with social workers instead of other professionals, especially in areas that traditionally have not been in the domain of social work practice (Dziegielewski, 2010a). With the right marketing, this cost-saving emphasis can help social workers gain additional ground, adding to their employment desirability.

Income, poverty, and health insurance data reported by the U.S. Census Bureau collected in 2011 indicates that the number of people without health insurance increased between 2009 and 2010, although the uninsured rate between 2009 and 2010 did not show any statistically different changes. When this information is coupled with a real median income decline between 2009 and 2010 and this was also accompanied by an increase in the poverty rate—providing affordable health care benefits to the American people remains a topic of intense debate (DeNavas-Walt, Proctor, Smith, & United States Census Bureau, 2011).

This book is designed as a practical guide to help social workers understand the roots of social work practice, stressing the importance of the person-in-environment and person-in-situation, and utilizing this information as a foundation for embracing the changes to come. As a skilled professional, the incorporation of evidence-based social work practice will need to serve as the cornerstone of all we do while always taking into account the uniqueness and situation-based strategy needed to help each individual patient/client/consumer. To prepare for the future, each chapter ends with discussing what the current state of affairs is and what can be expected in the future.

Case Study

The following case study example depicts a common practice situation that health care social workers often address.

Ms. Martha Edda had been living with her family for approximately a year. Before that, she had lived independently in her own apartment. Ms. Edda had to leave her apartment after she was found unconscious by a neighbor. The apartment was unsafe and filled with rotted food, urine, and feces throughout. On discovery, Ms. Edda was immediately admitted to the hospital. Originally, she was believed to have had a stroke. Later, she was formally diagnosed with a neurological condition called vascular dementia. Doctors believed that she was in the moderate to advanced stages, as Ms. Edda, at age 62, had pronounced "stroke-like" responses and memory difficulties.

After discussion with the hospital social worker, it became obvious that Ms. Edda needed a supervised living arrangement. Ms. Edda, however, refused placement and stated she was fine to live on her own if her daughter refused to take her home. Joan, Ms. Edda's daughter, admitted openly how guilty she felt about what had happened to her mother, but did not think she could handle her at home. To assist her daughter in the placement decision, the social worker reminded Joan that the family would be able to benefit from Ms. Edda's receiving services from a home health care agency and that a community day care program could be explored. After being convinced by the medical staff, Ms. Edda's family decided to give it a try and Joan took her mother home.

Once in the home, Ms. Edda did receive home health care services. However, much to her daughter's surprise, all services stopped after just 2 months. Although the services she received initially were limited, she had started to work out a routine to supplement the care offered. When she was told that even the limited services she received to help with the care of her mother were about to stop, she felt panic and did not know what she was going to do. Ms. Edda's daughter had relied heavily on these services, particularly the nurse aides who helped with Ms. Edda's baths. Ms. Edda weighed 170 pounds and could not get into or out of the tub by herself. To help address this problem, Joan recruited the help of her husband, who reluctantly agreed. Ms. Edda constantly complained when he helped that she was embarrassed and resented the fact that her son-in-law would see her naked as she was placed in the tub. Her daughter discounted these concerns saying that her physical care took preference over her emotional concerns related to his assistance.

This caregiving situation was further complicated because Ms. Edda could not get into the adult day care center in the area because there were no spots available. She was placed on a waiting list. Ms. Edda required help with all of her activities of daily living, and her daughter feared leaving her at home alone during the day. So, Joan quit her job to help care for her.

On the morning of January 12, Joan found her mother lying face down in her bed. She had become incontinent of bowel and bladder, was unable to speak, and her facial features appeared distorted on the left side of her face. When Joan could not arouse her, she began to panic and called an ambulance. Ms. Edda was immediately transported to the emergency department.

In the emergency department, numerous tests were run to see if Ms. Edda had had another stroke. Plans were made to admit her to the hospital, but there were no beds available. Based on the concern for supervised monitoring and possible bed availability in the morning, an agreement was made to keep her in the emergency department overnight. In the morning, she was admitted to the inpatient hospital. While in the hospital, Ms. Edda remained incontinent and refused to eat. She was so confused that the nurses feared she would get out of bed and hurt herself. Therefore, she was placed in restraints for periods throughout the day and monitored regularly.

After 2 days, most of the medical tests had been run and were determined to be negative. Ms. Edda's vital signs remained stable. The physician thought that her stay in the hospital could no longer be justified, and the social worker was notified of the pending discharge. When the call was placed to prepare Ms. Edda's family for her return home, the case manager was told that the family would not accept her and that they wanted her to be placed in a nursing home. The case manager, who was a nurse, referred the case immediately to the social worker for assistance. The social worker was concerned about this decision because she knew that Ms. Edda did not have private insurance to cover her nursing home stay and she was too young for Medicare eligibility. This meant that an application for Medicaid would have to be made. Although when approved eligibility was retroactive and when complete it provided more long-term and comprehensive coverage, this state-funded program had a lower reimbursement rate. Most of the privately run nursing homes drastically limited the numbers of patients they would accept to fill these beds. After calling around, the social worker was told no beds were available.

When the social worker related her discharge problem to the physician, he simply stated, "I am under pressure to get her out, and there is no medical reason for her to be here—discharge her home today." Because it was after 4:00 p.m. and the administrative offices had closed for the day, the social worker planned to try to secure an out-of-area placement the following day.

When the physician returned at 6:00 p.m., he wanted to know why the patient had not been discharged. The nurse on duty explained that a nursing home bed could not be found. The physician became frustrated and wrote an order for immediate discharge. The nurse case manager called Ms. Edda's family at 6:30 p.m. and told them about the discharge. Ms. Edda's family was angry and asked why she was not being placed in a nursing home. The nurse case manager explained to the family that discharge orders had been written, and she was only trying to do her job. Ms. Edda's daughter insisted on speaking to the discharge physician before picking up her mother. A message was left for him, and at 8:00 p.m. her call was returned. The physician sounded frustrated when he told the family that all medical emergencies had been addressed, and she no longer needed hospital services. Ms. Edda's daughter became furious and yelled, "If she is still incontinent and in restraints, how do you expect me to handle her?" Seeing how upset she was, the physician softened his voice and said, "I will put the nurse on the phone to update you on her condition. In addition, the social work case manager will call you in the morning to arrange home health care services."

When Ms. Edda's daughter arrived at the hospital, her mother was wearing a diaper. Pleased to see the patient's family member, the nurse sent for a wheelchair and helped place her in the chair for transport to the family's car.

Although this situation may sound unbelievable, unfortunately, situations similar to this one continue to occur. This case study is an accurate depiction of the events that occurred. With Joan's perseverance, she was eventually able (several months later) to get her mother placed in a nursing home. However, the strain was so great on Joan that she ended up requesting that she be placed on medication to combat depression. Joan also began to fight with her husband and children over numerous issues related to the time required for her mother's care and the loss of the second source of family income. Like most American families, her paycheck was used not only to supplement basic needs (e.g., rent and food), but also for any sources of family luxury (e.g., movies and dining out). It is clear that in situations such as this, the price of this seemingly "cost-effective" yet restrictive case management strategy far exceeded the dollar emphasis placed on it. Sadly, in this situation, the patient and her family become the *silent victims*.

For all professionals working in the health care area, these types of reports can be considered commonplace. There was a calm (possibly cold) desperation reflected in the tones of many professionals involved in this case. Feelings of desperation and frustration are not uncommon when many professionals, not only social workers, feel trapped within a system where patients trust the professionals to have power to intercede on their behalf (i.e., to heal and to help). For health care social workers, the belief continues that they are regulated and snared within a system that does not allow them to exercise what they believe is the best ethical course of action. It appears apparent that ethical conflicts will continue to become more acute as social workers will need to balance quality of care with service limitations. Originally, it was postulated that the concept of a health care delivery team (physicians, nurses, social workers, physical therapists, etc.) with specialized roles could best help the needs of each patient while in the health care setting. However, when professionals are feeling frustrated, this degree of specialization can also provide a barrier—creating patient/client/consumer–health care worker separation.

The emphasis placed on team member specialization (i.e., these are my specific job duties and responsibilities) can serve as a catalyst for individual members to avoid taking overall responsibility for patient welfare. This avoidance can create a type of shock absorber, affectionately known in the business as the patient "buff and turf." During "buff and turf," only surface concerns related to the patient are addressed. The real issue is left untouched, and the case is referred to the next professional on the health care delivery team. For example, in this case, the nurse avoided responsibility by stating that she was only doing her job. Later, the physician commented superficially and handed the telephone to the nurse for the problematic details. The original nurse case manager was quick to refer this more difficult case to the social worker and the social worker could feel her frustration rising when she was not sure how to help the patient to get the services she needed as these services were simply not available.

The social work case manager was expected by other professionals on the health care team to handle the "difficult placement services." For example, some nursing professionals believe that nurses involved in discharge planning should take more of an administrative role; others see the nurse's role as teaching patients and families complex postdischarge treatments, such as breathing treatments, decubitus and skin care, feeding tubes, and home injections (Penrod, Kane, & Kane, 2000). This leaves the responsibility to fall on the shoulders of the social work provider, ignoring the inadequacy of the placement limitations and available options. In cases like this, it is important to note that the reality of the situation is that none of these professionals had the power to take control over what was happening; however, the patient, the family, and possibly the community still believe they did or should have.

Cases like this force professionals to question whether the services available are sufficient, and this can lead to frustration and potential burnout. Many also question the system and what is happening to patient care as they knew it. The question remains: Is what is really happening now different from what would have occurred 20 years ago? The answer for many social workers is "yes." For example, 20 years ago, Ms. Edda (see the case study earlier) would have been kept in the hospital until a bed could be found. Although this alternative might be best to help the overall family situation, is it really an efficient and effective use of an expensive hospital stay?

One point remains evident—there are problems in the current system. However, this shadows only the major problems in what came before. Within this changing health care system, there does not appear to be an easy answer for this dilemma. Little emphasis is placed on community support (Meenaghan, 2001). Health care social workers can be assured that in these turbulent times, more changes in the delivery of health care services will result based on cost-containment, thus making advocacy an ethical imperative (Jansson, 2011).

Today's Health Care Social Worker

Name: Mary O. Norris, MSW, MPH, LCSW
List State of Practice: Florida
Professional Job Title: Clinical Social Worker

Duties in a Typical Day:
I am director of a department composed of over 40 clinicians who
provide services at two hospitals. Our department's goal is to
provide clinical interventions to both inpatients and outpatients.
Our department also has six discharge planners that are responsible for the discharge planning.

　　Arriving early in the mornings to work allows me to gather
my thoughts and set priorities for the day. The schedule is com-
prised of attending committee meetings, meeting with supervisors to strategize how to handle issues, and working on various
projects. There is also the usual complement of voice mails and
e-mails that need responses.

What do you like most about your position?
Developing our department as the mental health counselors has
always been considered a calculated risk. Thus, it is most rewarding now to witness the growth of line staff and watch them
flourish in the practice of their clinical skills. Equally satisfying
is seeing clinical social workers being recognized for the clinical
expertise they bring to the health care team.

What do you like least about your position?
Although I enjoy the coordination and sense of satisfaction I
get in team building, I miss providing direct patient and family care.

**What "words of wisdom" do you have for the new health care
social worker who is considering working in a similar position?**
It is essential to have sufficient "hands-on" experience. Com-
plementing this background should be additional education in
administration so as to have the requisite theoretical and ana-
lytical skills. For me, having the dual degree Master in Public
Health and Master in Social Work has been invaluable. Further
professional commitment is demonstrated by membership in
a professional organization such as the Society for Social Work
Leadership in Healthcare. Membership provides a wealth of networking opportunities and mentors to assist in the leadership of
a department.

(continued)

(continued)

What is your favorite social work story?
While working as a clinical social worker on a pediatric pulmonary team, I counseled a young man with cystic fibrosis. When we first met he was extremely shy and nonverbal. During these 3 years of clinical interventions, we worked on body-image, self-esteem, and sexuality issues. By the time I left this position, he had become verbal and self-disclosing regarding the many issues surrounding the impact of his chronic illness.

Several months after relocating to another city, the chief of pulmonology called me to notify me that the patient was hospitalized and was asking to see me. It seemed he was in the end stages of his disease and the team was uncertain if he truly comprehended the gravity of his situation. After having spent time at his bedside and with his family, I was preparing to leave. During the entire visit, he had never alluded to what issues were behind his request for my visit. Finally, he yelled out in a labored breathing, "Everyone out but Mary." He said he needed to ask me something but could not. Having then explored with him his impending death, he verbalized his comfort level with dying; however, he was still unable to explain why he wanted to speak with me. I proceeded to ask him several questions trying to understand his obviously intense issues. After verbalizing several possible concerns, I had hoped to "hit" upon the right topic. Finally, I suggested he write down his thoughts. He then handed me a written note on a piece of brown paper towel. The note simply said to my surprise, "Please ma'am, take off your shirt. Thank you." He said, "Mary you know I have never been with a woman. I know I am dying, and I just want to be with one before I die."

"I am so flattered to have you ask me this." I responded. "I am your social worker, not your girlfriend." We talked a little more, and I told him good bye. He died during the night. When I went back to the pulmonary team, they were all anxious to know whether he knew he was dying. My response was, "Believe me, he knows!"

Tomorrow's Health Care Social Worker

Name: Wanda Watson
List state of Practice: West Virginia
Professional Job Title: Insurance Agent

State why you want to become a health care social worker.
I want to be a social worker in health care because I feel this is where the greatest need is. I am especially interested in the clinical aspect

(continued)

Tomorrow's Health Care Social Worker (*continued*)

of the field. Knowing how the health care delivery system works and with my insurance knowledge I feel I can advocate for better service delivery methods in communities where such services in rural health is limited and social and economic problems exist. For these reasons I feel being a social worker in both a clinical setting or in a community setting where clinical social work services are available would allow more patients access to the services they need.

What do you think your previous experience will bring to the position?
My first experiences in social work began with my years working for Head Start and from there as a Child Protective Service worker. While still working as a CPS worker, I knew I wanted to broaden my education in the social work field, so I began pursuing my master's in social work. I soon found that trying to hold down a full-time job, especially one so demanding and with few flexibilities, and taking evening classes, working on class projects and internships, left me with having to make choices whether to quit my job or the MSW program. Well, I chose to continue with my MSW program and pursue a job that had more flexibility. The career option I chose was outside the realm of social work, but the hours were great and the flexibility was what I was looking for, which allowed me to go full throttle in pursuit of my master's.

The experience I have gained while working as an insurance agent has given me a broad view of both the health care side and the insurance industry side. The ever-changing health care needs, costs, and laws make it very challenging for both health care providers and insurance companies. As health care costs rise, so does the cost to have affordable health care coverage, making it more and more difficult for struggling families to afford health care coverage, especially for retirees with little or no health coverage, for disabled workers, and for the senior population needing coverage beyond what their Medicare will cover. Insurance companies also have to keep up with the constant rise in health care costs and at the same time be profitable, passing increased costs along to customers with increased premiums and higher deductibles and co-pays. Working with mostly the senior population and their families as an insurance agent has helped me to understand more of the struggles they face when it comes to health care and being on fixed incomes and a lot of times having to choose between getting prescriptions filled or meeting their daily needs such as nutritious foods and having enough to pay their monthly utility bills. With this situation being very common in the rural

(*continued*)

(continued)

communities where I provide services, I find myself referring patients to social service agencies for help.

Mental health needs can also be a struggle for patients and their families as most insurance companies limit what they will cover or will not cover certain mental diagnosis at all. Existing and preexisting conditions can also be a barrier in obtaining insurance coverage, making it almost impossible for patients to get the health care they need because in most cases companies will only insure healthy individuals. Long-term care is, and will continue to be, the costliest care, not only to the individual and their families but also to insurance companies. As medical advances will allow patients to live longer, baby boomers will be among the largest of the aging population, therefore making more of a burden on an already struggling health care system.

I believe the experiences I have gained in the five and a half years as an insurance agent will only help me to be more empathetic and understanding toward meeting the needs of patients that I serve and take a more proactive role as a social worker.

What area of health care social work interests you the most?
I am most interested in the clinical aspect of social work as I feel this will continue to be an area of social work that has a need for individuals who will advocate for as well as provide ongoing services to patients.

What words of wisdom or helpful hints do you have for other social workers looking to pursue a career in this area?
If you don't already have your master's in social work, get it. This will open up a world of opportunities and don't stop there. Seize every opportunity to learn from others, do volunteer work, get with an organization that will allow you to help organize community events and network with others to further your knowledge, and always be willing to help others, as this is where you get your greatest rewards. Social workers are always interested in helping other social workers.

What is your favorite social work story?
I have to say my favorite story was when I was a new CPS worker and we received a call that two small toddlers, one aged 2 and the other 3, were at risk. Their mother had been partying all night and had come home and then passed out cold and the children were outside all day alone without any supervision. So myself and another CPS worker went on the call. When we got there the little girls were outside crying their hearts out, wanting their mommy

(continued)

Tomorrow's Health Care Social Worker (*continued*)

to wake up. We went in and the mom was still passed out and would not respond to us, so we did what we called a "snatch and grab." We took the children and they told us they hadn't eaten or had anything to drink all day and they were filthy. The little 2-year-old girl seemed to settle down a little after we got them put in the car seat, but the 3-year-old was still crying for her mommy.

As we went down the road toward the office, we knew they hadn't eaten so we were discussing where to get them something to eat and I asked them if they wanted a "Happy Meal" from McDonalds and the 3-year-old stopped crying and said, "What is a Happy Meal?" I asked her if is she had ever had a Happy Meal before and she shook her head no. Well, that settled it, they had to have a Happy Meal. We pulled up to McDonalds and asked them if they wanted a cheeseburger or Chicken McNuggets and the 3-year-old wanted both for her and her sister, so we got them each a Happy Meal with side order each of McNuggets. The girls were so excited to get those meals and the little toy that came with it. This just made me realize how we can take the simplest of things for granted and for these little girls this was their first experience getting a Happy Meal and how happy it made them in the worst of times for them. This is how I knew I was in the right career and in the right place and what an impact social workers can make in the lives of children and their families in communities. This experience showed me how important social work is to all we serve.

EFFECT OF THE ENVIRONMENT ON HEALTH CARE DELIVERY

To understand the current practice of health care social work, we must first examine the environmental context of general health care delivery. This high-pressure health care environment requires that the following factors coexist,—as different and contradictory as they may be are expected to coexist (Table 1.1 lists and briefly describes the five factors).

The first factor to be considered is the public demand for quality service and expectations for the delivery of state-of-the-art care. When compared to other countries, the United States ranks high in how it employs technology and delivers state-of-the-art care to its recipients (Anderson & Frogner, 2008). Politicians, consumers, and consumer advocates all agree that the American health care system, although capable of delivering such care, is desperately in need of repair and reform. Programs such as the Patient Protection and Affordable Care Act of 2010 will help to mitigate this situation but can fall short in many areas if they are addressed at all (Jansson, 2011). Americans continue to watch this transition and the resulting provision of health care with hesitancy and

Table 1.1 Factors That Influence Health Care Delivery

Factors	Results
Quality of service and technological advances	Constant updating of training and equipment required to provide state-of-the-art care
	Constant updating for providers in terms of utilization of technology (e.g., computers and Internet)
Number and variety of professionals in competition	"Buff and turf" service delivery
Organizations that deliver services	Organizational competition Strive to survive and progress
Preserving quality of care	Pressure to provide "more for less"
Cost containment	Cost-based service delivery is given primary consideration rather than quality patient care

trepidation of ending up with "less for more." American people are demanding quality service, but as costs continue to skyrocket they are not willing to support increased costs in a system they believe is plagued by waste.

In addition to quality service, patients want to be able to make their own health care choices and want to gain access to state-of-the-art technology with clear links between medical knowledge and technology in the provision of quality service. Therefore, health care delivery systems are expected to hire and retain the most qualified personnel, as well as purchase the most sophisticated equipment. The pressure to secure these services is great because without these ingredients health care agencies cannot effectively compete for "covered" or "reimbursable" patient/client/consumer resources. This is expected at a time when there is also a movement to return to the climate of the 1990s with insurance companies facing more restricted choices of doctors and hospitals and access to specialized care.

The second factor related to the problems found in health care delivery is associated with (and among) the varied groups of professionals who actually deliver health care services and the desire for entrepreneurialism. This varied group of professionals may have complementary as well as competing goals for the provision of services, although all must agree on ensuring quality patient care. In the health care environment, the definition of what constitutes a health care provider is so broad it often can encompass any individual who provides services to health care consumers. When examined more closely, however, it becomes clear that physicians and nurses often take the lead in providing direct services and in the hospital setting are often considered essential providers. When using this strict definition of "essential" this distinction would make other health care providers ancillary. In addition, when physicians gravitate to high-paying medical specialties such as cardiology, obstetrics, oncology, and other specialties they will continue to compete with one another for services (Jansson, 2011).

The provision of services is further complicated by the sheer numbers of health care professionals in practice. The number of these professionals has increased dramatically over the years and as we continue to specialize and embrace entrepreneurship, this will only increase the competition among the disciplines for patients relative to the care provision they have available.

In addition, not only have the number and type of health care professionals increased, but so has their education level. In the 1990s, it was documented that 4.9 million individuals in health delivery required some type of professional training or a college degree. According to the U.S. Census Bureau (2012), 16,415,000 individuals are employed in the health care and social assistance industry as of 2010, as opposed to 9,296,000 in 1990. In addition, when compared to physicians' offices in particular, the number decreased considerably to 2,316,000 (U.S. Census Bureau, 2012, Table 162). It is no surprise that the number of social workers has grown along with physician assistants, nurse practitioners, multiskilled health workers, laboratory technicians, occupational therapists, and physical therapists. This can leave the position of the social worker to be viewed as just one of many "adjunct" professionals involved in health care delivery.

To compare salaries of **social workers in health care** with those in other professions such as

- clinical nurse specialist
- case manager
- staff nurse RN
- counselor
- recreational therapist
- physician family medicine

try this web address: www1.salary.com/Non-Profit-and-Social-Services-Salaries.html

---

After addressing the increased number of professionals providing health care service delivery, to avoid confusion, an examination of similar or duplicating functions that many of these professionals perform must be made (Buppert, 2002). This is particularly relevant for those directly providing services in the allied health fields, of which social work is part. Often the roles that social workers perform overlap with these other disciplines (Dziegielewski, 2010b). For example, today nurses are often asked to run therapeutic support groups in the health care setting. This invitation remains contradictory to the traditionally held belief that most group leadership was considered the realm of the social work professional. Based on the increased number of allied health care professionals, and the overlapping of skills, tasks, and roles, one point remains certain: all trained professionals will be forced to continue to compete and strive to locate a solid niche in the behavioral health care market where patients can shop for the best and most comprehensive coverage for their families.

The third factor that compounds the problems found within current health care delivery involves not only the individual providers but also the organizations of delivery. Insurers as well as patients/clients/consumers alike are seeking the best options available for their health care dollars. This pressure has clearly forced the market to embrace consumer choice, but it can also encourage recruitment and business strategy that can lead to false advertising and misleading claims. Since hospitals and other health care providers can compete for the same patients, the pressure to stand out or provide unique care that may or may not be state-of-the-art remains tempting. Previously, most health care organizations focused their recruitment and marketing strategies for expansion on services provided. However, today the ideal organization for health care delivery cannot ignore the pressure that is placed on service delivery as it relates directly back to insurance reimbursement. From a business point of view it comes as no surprise that each health care delivery organization must ensure its own survival. It also becomes clear why striving to survive and progress, embracing the retail aspects of health care, creates an air of competition that was originally designed to provide quality and competitive services for all (Malvey & Fottler, 2006).

To compete in a retail environment a variety of major strategies have been incorporated (Malvey & Fottler, 2006; Fottler & Malvey, 2010). Strategies include advertising the provision of low-cost traditional health services promising superior service through technology or patient service as well as specialization into certain areas of practice (i.e., centers of excellence) where there can be an emphasis on diversification outside of the traditional bounds of health care delivery (i.e., wellness centers). At times, this can lead to ingenious ways of re-labeling traditional services to be attractive to the American health care consumer. For example, recently under the influence of behavioral health care policies, many organizations have begun to look toward presenting their service in a new and different light. The shift toward wellness, although some believe somewhat limited in the United States when compared with other countries, has been a source of great attention (Jansson, 2011). The progression remains slow, but nonetheless in retail advertising and public attention an emphasis toward maintaining and promoting wellness is a societal and political paradigm shift that cannot be ignored.

As with all societal change, people or the culture are slow to respond; therefore, this paradigm shift will require changes be implemented at the most basic levels. For example, there is little debate that in the traditional medical model, the individual who receives the services has traditionally been referred to as the "patient." Based on this overriding philosophy and the prevalence of this term in the literature, this term is repeatedly used throughout this book. In health care social work, this has caused many social workers to stop using words such as "patient" when referring to the individuals served and to adopt the dominant label used in the medical environment.

This societal paradigm shift is consistently represented in the medical model where the receiver of services has traditionally been viewed as "sick."

However, today the use of the term "patient" has been modified and now incorporates the wellness, outcomes, and cost-effective approach reflected in the literature. Many health care professionals agree that referring to an individual service recipient as the "patient" still carries the older meaning of sickness and would still like to see it revised. These professionals feel that the term "patient" is in conflict with the wholeness and prevention strategy that is advocated by most organizations expected for increased marketability. To address this rift, terms often considered to replace the term patient include "patient" (a term familiar to social work professionals), "service consumers" or "patrons" (to represent those buying or purchasing a service), "product recipient" or "individual recipient" (those receiving a direct service), and "covered persons" (reflecting those who have some type of medical insurance coverage). Those in favor of the euphemism "covered persons" argue that it is not used just to indicate medical coverage but to be indicative of the universal care perspective and the assurance that comes with an individual having the security of medical coverage.

No matter what the final determination for the label for individuals who receive service—the influence it will have in enhancing the survival and progress of the organization, and the marketability, so to speak, most assuredly will be considered. As for social workers practicing in the health care arena, they will probably soon follow suit, and use the terms to identify the recipient defined by behavioral health care plans. After all, as one of the allied health care professionals providing service, conforming for uniformity can provide legitimacy and eligibility within the system. So don't be surprised if you see these terms pop-up in this book with an emphasis on the word "patient" as they abound in the literature and can at times be difficult to avoid.

The fourth and fifth factors involve trying to balance between preserving the quality of care delivered and maintaining cost control. Today, although these factors may be considered equal to political motivation, any discussion of health care delivery especially when surrounding capitation models and revenue schemes will end up assessing cost containment applying a retail entrepreneurial mentality (Fottler & Malvey, 2010). Many health care social workers also feel the pressure for cost containment. As a health care social worker, it is my expectation along with other providers that continued emphasis on cost containment will continually rise to the top at the sacrifice of maintaining quality of care (Dziegielewski, 2010a, 2010b). Therefore, the role of the social work professional needs to be rich in actively advocating for the provision of quality services (Colby & Dziegielewski, 2010; Franklin, 2002; Gibelman, 2002; Rock, 2002). However, Colby and Dziegielewski (2010) warn that social workers need to do more than simply ensure the provision of "micro" (individually based) or "mezzo" (environmentally based) quality services. They urge social work professionals to be active in the "macro" aspect of practice by monitoring policies and programs that will affect not only the patients they serve directly but also all Americans. Advocacy of this type means actively identifying and supporting state and federal legislation that provide basic standards of quality care. The provision of services allowing for universal accessibility, affordability, and service comprehensiveness needs to be endorsed while maintaining culturally sensitive practice (National Association of Social Workers, 2001).

HISTORY, FOUNDATIONS, AND FUTURE PERSPECTIVES IN HEALTH CARE

The need for cost containment, in health care can easily be traced back to the late 1970s and into the middle 1980s, where it was estimated that the number of individuals without health insurance in the United States increased from 28.7 million to 35.1 million (U.S. Census Bureau, 1984). This left millions of Americans who experienced health risks with an inability to afford needed health care (Roland, Lyons, Salganicoff, & Long, 1994). This fact particularly disturbed insurance companies that complained of bitter upsets, and in 1988, the nation's top 12 health insurers reported financial losses of $830 million (Edinburg & Cottler, 1995).

In review, the 1980s represented a time when the nation was in the midst of economic stagnation/recession (Mizrahi, 1995); the alternate health care reform strategies suggested to alleviate this unprecedented burden were all of a "solution-based" or "evidence-based" nature (Donald, 2002). To address this situation, a course of action was considered successful if it ultimately resulted in a decision-making framework that considered research and other forms of evidence in decision making supporting efforts toward cost control, containment, or reduction.

In the early 1990s, the message of concern was clear, and the social climate was rich with politicians' verbal responsiveness to the American peoples' concern for reform. This acknowledgment was reflected in the election strategy of many of the candidates seeking office. It was not uncommon for many of the campaign platforms to present possible solutions designed to address health care reform. In fact, President Bill Clinton in his 1992 election campaign speeches made health care reform his highest domestic priority (Mizrahi, 1995). Numerous proposals were considered for health care reform, from single-payer-system approaches to limited policies for universal health care coverage.

It is clear why in the early 1990s, the debate that secured its place in the forefront of the social and political agenda was health care. The cost of health care delivery was defined as a national crisis and the emphasis on implementing a managed care delivery system was hailed as one way to control this. Many thought that several of the key causes of this inflation of costs in health care delivery were beyond control and any attempt at doing so was doomed to failure. Yet, the managed care policies that were prominent in the 1990s did indeed limit health care costs. What they also did, however, was limit the choices of consumers and providers, causing dissatisfaction that later would develop into other alternate approaches (Mathews, 2012).

Some believed that managed care was doomed for failure because there were societal factors that could not be controlled by simply implementing a new type of service delivery. Among these concerns was the belief that health care costs were being pushed beyond control by the increasing number of Americans reaching "old age" that would require services. This population shift and the care that older adults would require simply could not be addressed by a change in health care policy. Other concerns centered on the continual technological advances within the society. New technological advances were happening so quickly it was not clear how providers could keep up with the latest equipment and services needed to maintain the competitive edge when providing services to consumers. The concern focused on whether the unregulated and the varied costs of the services provided would soon spin out of control if they were not clearly regulated (Edinburg & Cottler, 1995).

Other concerns supporting the implementation of managed care in the 1990s included: (a) the fact that many health care consumers were considered medically uneducated and unknowledgeable about medical services and could benefit from predetermined benefit plans; (b) Americans were sensitive to and resistant to paying more for the delivery of medical services; (c) the insurance industry was highly fragmented with managerial administrators and leaders who were trained based on a different environmental context that did not include "standardized cost-containment techniques"; (d) there were simply too many hospital inpatient beds with the pressure to have them filled; (e) there was a focus on acute illness rather than a more holistic, wellness, or preventive perspective; (f) there was insufficient medical outcomes-based data that focused the benefit as the end result of service; (g) there were difficulties separating quality-of-life issues from technological advances, causing heroic attempts to implement expensive procedures without regard to quality of continued life; and (h) the medical community had been rocked by numerous malpractice suits that resulted in fear and pressure making managed care a way to ensure fewer complaints (Edinburg & Cottler, 1995; Shortell & Kaluzny, 1994).

Even though many of these societal and technological factors were considered difficult to address and change, the 1990s were a time of great concern related to the future predictions of the cost of health care delivery. Cost-containment strategies remained strong: in 1990 health care costs were estimated at more than $640 billion (Shortell & Kaluzny, 1994), and it was estimated at that current rate, accrual was expected to reach $1 trillion (Hernandez, Fottler, & Joiner, 1994) to $1.5 trillion by the year 2000 (Skelton & Janosi, 1992).

In 2002, the National Institutes of Health could receive a funding increase of $3.7 billion for the fiscal year that began October 1, with an additional expectation to double the agency's funding over five years, under a bill approved by a U.S. Senate subcommittee (Reuters Health Information, 2002). To fuel the concern further, as the years progressed the baby boomers would reach their 70s and 80s and in the year 2030 would bring health spending to an astonishing peak at $16 trillion—or 30% of the gross domestic product (Burner, Waldo, & McKusick, 1992).

After the 1992 presidential election, the victor, democratic President Bill Clinton, proceeded to address his campaign goal by establishing a task force to complete a plan for health care reform. The model emphasized was different from the single-payer approach that he had originally supported early in his campaign. This later approach involved a type of managed competition in which purchasing alliances were formed that would have the power to certify health plans and negotiate premiums for certain benefit packages (The Health Security Act, 1993). Since employer–employee premiums would finance payment for these plans; the actual consumer out-of-pocket cost could vary based on the benefit package chosen. Title XVIII, Medicare, a federal entitlement program to pay for physician and hospital services for disabled individuals or others age 65 or older, remained a separate program. Title XIX, Medicaid, a means-tested program based on provision of medical services for low-income Americans, was included in the plan (Mizrahi, 1995). One possible economic reason for the attraction to include Medicaid in this reform process was that between 1990 and 1991, one-third of the increase in the total U.S. expenditures was based on states' use of this program (Letsch, 1993).

The future of most health care delivery (70% of all coverage) was to be provided by managed health care plans (Edinburg & Cottler, 1995). In this system, managed care plans covered preauthorization for service by qualified consumers; precertification for a given amount of care with concurrent review of the treatment and services rendered; continued determination of the need for hospitalization through a process of use review; and predischarge planning to ensure proper after-care services are identified and made available (Hiratsuka, 1990).

Five major types of managed care programs for health care delivery followed and all employed social work professionals (Wagner, 1993). The first were *managed indemnity plans*. In these plans, traditional coverage was offered; however, the cost of the plan was directly related to the usage needs and requirements of the subscriber. A second type of managed care plan included the *preferred provider organization* (PPO). Here employers or insurance carriers contracted with a select group of health care delivery providers to provide certain services at pre-established reimbursement rates. The consumer had the choice of who to contact to provide the service; however, if the option of using a provider not on the provider list was chosen, higher out-of-pocket expenses resulted.

A third type of managed care plan was the *exclusive provider organization*. This plan type was generally considered more restrictive than the PPO because the consumer did not have the choice to go elsewhere, and services had to be provided and received by the contracted organization or partnership. Employers often chose this type of health care delivery as a cost-saving measure. If a consumer did go outside of the system, reimbursement was generally not obtained (Wagner, 1993). Once a member, the use of these facilities is referred to as the only way to gain reimbursable access to specialty care services (surgery, etc.).

A fourth type of managed care program was the *point-of-service* plans. Usually at the initiation of coverage, a choice was made whether a PPO format or an indemnity/HMO format for delivery of services was requested. This allowed the consumer to have some ability not to forfeit the power to go outside of the provider system with minimal additional cost (Wagner, 1993).

The fifth type of managed care program was one of the oldest and the most commonly related to the idea of managed care plan—the *health maintenance organization* (HMO). These plans provided service for a prepaid fixed fee. These organizations provided both health insurance and health delivery in one package. If a consumer went beyond the traditional services offered by the HMO, the HMO determined where these covered services could be obtained. Five common types of HMO models for service delivery were staff models where the physicians were employed directly by the HMO (i.e., a type of closed model); group models where contracts are held with multi-specialty groups of physicians (i.e., a type of closed model); network models, which resulted in a greater choice of physicians because any specialty physician who had the proper credentials could join (i.e., an open panel plan because enrollment was not limited to a contracted staff or group); individual practice association models where the physician became a member, but still could retain his or her own professional office; and direct contract models where physicians were contracted to provide services on an individual basis (Edinburg & Cottler, 1995). The concept of using managed care plans through the use of health care organizational providers was not a new one. This type of delivery was originally formulated to provide efficient, comprehensive, and high-quality health care services (Shortell & Kaluzny, 1983).

Now that managed care plans have been around long enough to assess, some interesting trends have been noted. The first rests in the possibility of increased efforts toward prevention. It was originally hoped that managed care would provide more preventive services than the traditional system of care it was replacing. It was hoped that the controlled access point to the system of care from a primary care physician and the economic incentive to focus on wellness would stand paramount in service provision efforts. Unfortunately, some professionals feel strongly this has not been the case and that these managed-care physicians are no more likely to offer these services than other physicians operating in a traditional setting (Pham, Schrag, Hargraves, & Bach, 2005).

The pluralistic delivery of current health care needs has opened the doors to embracing a type of *coordinated care* that connects primary care physicians and specialists, technology enhancing diagnostic centers, hospitals and acute and long-term care facilities, home care agencies, emergency receiving centers, and pharmacies. Care coordination involves focused attempts to assist the patient/client/consumer to utilize independent providers integrating the receiving patient care services and activities. Coordinated care attempts to eliminate health care fragmentation of services (Bodenheimer, 2008).

In presenting this history related to managed care one thing remains clear—today, health care expenses continue to rise at inconceivable rates. As of 2012, these earlier fears have indeed come to fruition as health care spending continues to grow at 1.5 percent the rate of the gross national product and is already 20% of the economy (Hixon, 2012). This continues to be of such serious concern that Hixon (2012) and others believe that in the United States, the primary source of debt is health care costs. Critics are quick to point out that the United States continues to spend far more on health care than any other country in the world (Hofschire, 2012).

Once again, similar to the 1990s, we are facing a pivotal decision. If the rising cost of health care is not controlled, it will indeed create a significant threat to the U.S. economy. This threat is so pronounced it will extend far beyond health care provision affecting all aspects of government fiscal stability (Hofschire, 2012).

As the reality of our current situation and the budget implications continue to grow, managed care philosophies appear to once again be gaining in popularity. The supporters, however, say that in coordinated behavioral health care management there is one primary difference— technology is at the forefront of improving care, and all efforts are viewed as being in partnership with cost-cutting strategies (Mathews, 2012). In addition, insurers are responding to pressures from the public and employee organizations, and costs for health care are shifting more to the employee with the promise that this shift will result in lower premiums. For example, in managed care, the emphasis has been on the use of HMOs with prescribed provider panels and hospitals within the HMO system. In coordinated care networks, the services are often categorized so that providers in the top categories can still be accessed; they just cost the employee/ consumer more when utilized. In health care the new buzz word is "care coordination" or coordinated care, which is different from managed care as it does not require specific preclearances before treatment.

At the same time, as momentum for coordinated care continues to grow, so too does the public outcry for immediate answers to effective and affordable health care. Supporters have returned to the call for a national health care plan that will address the needs of all Americans and provide health care to our most needy populations. This was indeed the original intent of the 2010 federal passing of the Affordable Care Act (ACA). This act created near universal health care coverage and set minimum standards for health care insurance and mandated that employers offer health care insurance or that individuals have access to it with a type of exchange program. Since approval of this legislation is so new the jury is still out on its success, but without more specific controls in place related to access and need, fears are that health care spending will grow significantly. Furthermore, the debate continues to rage as to what role the government should have in the scope of health insurance coverage and provision of services resting in the government sector as opposed to the private one. As for managed care, it is quite possible it is indeed subtly moving back to the forefront with advances in technology providing the fundamental difference between what was and what will be (Mathews, 2012).

FUTURE CONSIDERATIONS FOR PRACTICE

In summary, the complexity and diversity required to define the current structure and financing of coordinated care in our health care delivery system can be daunting. In the American health care system, special interest groups and the specialists who provide the service have extraordinary power. Unfortunately, to further complicate our system of health care delivery, attempts at a standard definition continue to change and what needs to be included to constitute coordinated care has expanded and broadened in complexity. The introduction of the Affordable Care Act has brought about tremendous opportunities for many Americans in securing health and behavioral health needs (Ofosu, 2011). Affordable health care is a right that many believe belongs to all U.S. citizens. For social workers, the time is right for not only supporting health care but becoming active in prevention and advocacy, thereby supporting programs that reduce health care spending while maintaining quality care (Zabora, 2011).

Generally speaking, one characteristic remains consistent across all evidence-based health care provision strategies, and that is the need to provide an array of features that will ultimately balance new technologies and quality of care with cost containment (Donald, 2002).

In addition, directives and principles originally supported by the traditional methods of managed care have been extended, and coordinated care principles have taken up the slack. Coordinated care involves evidence-based practice principles, brief goal-directed treatment, outcomes that are measureable, primary and preventive care, and the importance of case management (Rock, 2002; Zabora, 2011). Social workers need to continue their practice emphasis in this area and become more proficient in addressing the person as a whole, integrating health and mental health as well as mixing mind and body influences toward the achievement of comprehensive patient/client/consumer care (Dziegielewski, 2010a, 2010b).

For health care social workers, practice expertise will be dependent on the use and development of the most modern technology-based principles. This requires that intervention strategies continue to incorporate the use of computer-based data systems, telephone audio and visual counseling, multimedia educational tools as well as the Internet. In health care practice, computers are now essential tools used for assessments, progress notes, routine correspondence, and reports. Social workers, similar to other health care professionals, will need to master the utilization of this technology employing these techniques to assist patients to record data, develop treatment and plans, and secure the services they need.

In closing, the intention of this first chapter is to set the stage for what was central to health care delivery in the 1990s and the subtle and not so subtle changes that will take place in the coming years. Enlightenment regarding some of the macro concepts, ethical dilemmas, and resulting problems that a health care social worker can confront while ensuring service delivery is outlined. Health care social workers need to be aware of the implications that societal, philosophical, and technological trends have had on the delivery system and how the history of runaway health care expenses continues to directly influence current expectations for service delivery.

The ACA has brought many questions forth in terms of its strengths and limitations (Gorin, 2011). Efforts to improve quality and control costs such as ACA combined with requirements for evidence-based practice have truly transformed health care service provision. Changes relevant to controlling health care costs have required that social workers be flexible while embarking on new and varied expectations of what they will be required to perform. For today's health care social work professional, issues and problems similar to those experienced by Ms. Edda (see the case study earlier) are not unusual; unfortunately, unless health care social workers strive to understand and anticipate current and future trends in service delivery—cases like the one presented will become more common.

Glossary

Coordinated care   Patient care strategies that follow a management philosophy designed to improve patient care outcomes.

Exclusive provider organization   This form of a managed care plan is generally considered more restricted than the PPO. Consumers do not have the choice to go elsewhere. Services must be provided and received by the contracted organization or partnership. Many times this plan is referred to as the "gatekeeper" because its use of the services provided is the only way to gain reimbursable access to specialty care services.

Health care delivery organizations   In today's health care environment, these organizations are considered responsible for providing low-cost traditional and specialized health services; incorporation of technology into the service provided; diversification outside of the traditional bounds of health care delivery (i.e., wellness centers); and creating new ways to re-label traditional service to be more reflective of the environmental demands.

Health maintenance organization (HMO) plans   These plans provide service for a prepaid fixed fee. These organizations provide both health insurance and health delivery in one package. If a consumer must go beyond the traditional services offered by the HMO, the HMO determines where these covered services will be obtained. Five common types of HMO models for service delivery include staff models (physicians are employed directly by the HMO), group models (contracts are held with multispecialty groups of physicians), network models (where enrollment is not limited to contracted staff or group providers), individual practice association models (physicians become members, but can still retain his or her own office and consumers), and direct contract models (physicians are contracted to provide services on an individual basis).

Length of stay   This is the actual time used or allotted (usually specified in number of days) that a consumer uses or receives a needed health care service.

Managed care   An organized system of care that attempts to balance access, quality, and cost-effectiveness of care.

Managed care programs   The Programs designed to provide an array of features that balance quality of care with cost-containment strategies that allow them to survive and progress.

Managed indemnity plans   A type of managed care program where generally traditional coverage is offered; however, the cost of the plan is directly related to the usage needs and requirements of the subscriber.

Patients/clients/consumers   These are the most common terms used to describe the individual that is considered the point of contact or focus for providing care benefits. In this text, the word "patient" will be primarily used as it is most consistently used in the health care literature.

Preferred provider organizations (PPOs)   Here employers or insurance carriers contract with a select group of health care delivery providers or service organizations to provide certain services at pre-established reimbursement rates. The consumer has the choice of who to contact to provide the service; however, if the option of using a provider not on the provider list is chosen, higher out-of-pocket expenses will result.

Primary and preventive care   Where patient/client/consumer care is focused on ambulatory and community-based care approaches as well as physicians' offices and health maintenance organizations.

Prospective payment system   This is a system of reimbursement for what is determined the average length of stay or duration of care for an individual with a certain medical or psychiatric diagnosis.

Questions for Further Study

1. What changes do you predict for the field of health care social work based on the pressures to balance cost containment with quality of care?

2. What do you see as some of the strengths and weaknesses of ACA? What do you see as the role of social work in supporting and or refuting this legislation?

3. Based on what you know of the social work profession, what new areas of practice "marketability" would you suggest for social work professionals to consider?

4. What do you believe is critical information to allow social workers to balance social work ethics with the reality of the practice environment?

Selected Websites Related to Health Care for the Consumer

Guide to Health Care Quality: Consumer Guide
www.ahrq.gov/consumer/guidetoq/

Health Care Ratings Insurance: Consumer Reports
www.consumerreports.org/health/insurance/health-insurance.htm

Consumer Guide to Health Care Providers
www.dca.ca.gov/publications/healthcare_providers.pdf

CHAPTER 2

The Evolution of the "New" Health Care Social Work

No text on health care social work practice would be complete without a review of the profession's struggle to define the historical and current role of the health care social worker. What is most disturbing in today's practice environment is the fact that many individuals outside the social work discipline continue to remain unsure of what it is the health care social worker does. In addition, social workers themselves often battle over what constitutes "health care" social work. Establishing and agreeing upon a unified definition of health care social work remains critical for survival in today's service delivery environment influenced greatly by the Patient Protection and Affordable Care Act (ACA) (U.S. Department of Health and Human Services, 2012).

The current practice of health care social work is reflective of the environment where change and constant restructure are the usual state of affairs. Today, health care practice can present challenging times for all health care professionals (Jansson, 2011), not just social workers. Changes in the scope of practice, the roles social workers assume, and the expectations of both patients/clients/consumers (hereafter referred to as patients) and practitioners have occurred quickly; and many times professionals feel trapped and lost in this whirlwind of activity.

In this turbulent, ever-changing environment, professional social workers must constantly balance "quality-of-care" issues versus "cost-containment" measures for the patients they serve (Dziegielewski, 2010a, 2010b). This delicate balance must also be addressed in a time when the social worker's role and current position in the health care setting are tenuous at best. As social workers, many of us continue to remain skeptical as to whether quality of care and cost containment can ever reach an equitable balance that will benefit all, whether we refer to those served as patients, clients, or consumers.

The most important aspect of the profession of social work that makes it unusual when compared with other disciplines is the perspective of helping individuals, families, and groups and taking into account the situation and environment. This unique perspective, stated in its most simplistic form, is that of recognizing the importance of the "individual in situation" or the "person-in-environment" stance (Hepworth, Rooney, Rooney, Strom-Gottfried, & Larsen, 2010). Today, however, for the health care social worker, recognizing the cultural uniqueness of an individual or person within an environmental context or situation can be considered to be much more complicated than what was traditionally perceived (Lum, 2003).

This perspective requires that the health care social worker go beyond the traditional confines of the health care institution and consider the needs of the individual, family, group, or community regarding their unique situations or environments. In the turbulent health care environment, the practice of the health care social worker must not only concentrate on providing important concrete services that patients need to function effectively within their environments but also try to anticipate future changes in those environments to ensure that services remain effective and helpful to the patient served. Advocacy which rests at the heart of the services performed for patients cannot lose sight of the fact that it is indeed more than helping the patient, as it also involves empowering the patient to help him- or herself. This requires utilizing as much as possible the patient's own resources. In addition, the health care social worker, also affected by the environment, must ensure that he or she continues to be able to maintain his or her own position as a service provider.

DEFINING HEALTH CARE SOCIAL WORK PRACTICE

Recently, I consulted with a colleague who has been a health care social worker for 20 years. She had been asked to justify her position and the health services she rendered in the home health care environment—a job she had been doing for the last 12 years. She knew the services she provided, but thought that these tasks needed to be presented in a perspective that made her duties different and marketable when compared with the nurses and other professionals working with patients. She feared if she could not do this, budget cuts would force her duties to be turned over to the nurses and physical therapists, and she would lose her job. She also believed that as of late she was receiving fewer referrals and thus was unable to provide adequate care to patients in need. Although nurses often visited patients, they were generating fewer social work consults. When my social worker friend asked the nurses why this was happening, she was told that no clear need for a social work assessment could be established, based on the nurses' increased role in determining service use criteria. Her concern escalated when one of the agency's patients attempted suicide in response to the recent death of his wife. Although the patient was being seen regularly by the nursing service for medication injections, no referral was made to the social worker—even after his wife's death.

This social worker's concern is real, as the competition for professional legitimacy increases, and social workers are forced to compete for a place in the health care arena. Questions that seek to establish what social workers do, different from the services of other professionals, are becoming more common. Developing an answer to satisfy these questions is now necessary. This social worker, like many others, is being forced to justify his or her current and continued role as a vital member of the health care delivery team. The traditionally held belief that what social workers do is different, necessary, and unique from other counseling professionals continues to be questioned; the environmental climate of maintaining quality of care and cost containment is demanding that it be answered.

To help address this issue and the unique contributions that social work brings to the practice of health care, a clear linkage between social work and the other related disciplines needs to be established. Traditionally, the role of social work has been to advocate for the poor, the disadvantaged, the disenfranchised, and the oppressed (Hepworth et al., 2010; National Association of Social Workers [NASW], 2008a). Historically, this has been accomplished by promoting and enhancing patient well-being in a societal or environmental context. In this book, as in most of the health care literature, the term "patient" is considered inclusive of the patient/client/consumer, and when the term "patient" is used, it may involve individuals, groups, families, organizations, or communities.

According to the National Association of Social Workers (NASW) (2008a) as stated in the revised *Code of Ethics*, the social work profession needs to strive to enhance human well-through empowerment while assisting those that are vulnerable and unable to assist themselves. All helping efforts need to take into account the social context while addressing problems in living. The activities for completion of the helping process can include direct practice, community organizing, supervision, consultation, administration, advocacy, social and political action, policy development and implementation, education, and research and evaluation.

Considering this definition, it becomes obvious that the general role of the social work professional in dealing primarily with the poor and the disadvantaged has expanded over time. For the health care social worker, in particular, it now involves working with a diverse population that can include those who are homeless, suicidal, homicidal, divorced, unemployed, mentally ill, medically ill, drug abusing, and delinquent, just to mention a few. In addition, the health care social worker must always strive to achieve restoration, enhanced wellness, the provision of concrete services, and prevention. Strategies to assist patients must address all these areas, because many times these factors are considered to be intertwined and interdependent (Colby & Dziegielewski, 2010).

UNIQUENESS OF HEALTH CARE SOCIAL WORK SERVICE PROVISION CONTINUING EDUCATION

Given their understanding of the human condition, most social work health care professionals agree that, in general, the profession of social work is different from most of the other helping professions. Today, however, this assumption has come under direct attack. There are two important reasons for this attack: (a) in our current system of health care delivery, the number of practicing health care professionals has risen dramatically (Jansson, 2011) and (b) these professionals often perform the same or similar tasks that overlap with practitioners from other disciplines (Ellingson, 2002).

This will continue to make survival in the health care arena difficult for health care social workers, especially if we do not openly acknowledge and embrace the competition created by the circumstances noted earlier. For example, in discussion at a NASWs branch meeting, the issue of providing health care social work professionals with an ongoing series for continuing education was addressed. Many of the social workers at this meeting thought that if the state was going to require continuing education, then social workers should be able to obtain these hours through "related" workshops or seminars that were available. In principle, this would make it easier for social work professionals to expand their choices of workshops and allow them to learn from other professionals.

As the task of establishing speakers and exploring topics for presentation began, a statement was made by one of the members and rapidly escalated into a heated discussion. Simply stated, the member asked, "How can we truly say that what we do as health care social workers is different from these other disciplines when we choose to receive most of our continued educational training from them?" This comment caused a lengthy debate. Some social work members stated that they appreciated this "additional" information, whereas others said it was not "additional" at all; it was "required" for effective practice. Regardless of what side was taken, most would agree that as social workers battle for a place in the health care delivery system, this "lack of uniqueness" concerning the skills and techniques often employed could be used against them. This makes the argument that social workers provide services not provided by other professionals a complicated one.

The disagreement and mixed emotions shared in this small meeting are not uncommon. Many states continue to struggle with continuing education requirements for social workers in general. How much is needed? Who should be eligible to provide programs? Also, if social workers work as a part of a health care team, doesn't collaborative education increase awareness of the types of activities that all on the team can help with to better serve the patient?

In this meeting, although many questions were left unanswered, a resolution was reached; however, it was not unanimous. These social workers recommended that continuing education should be required for all social work professionals, and this education could be provided by social workers or "other professionals." Thirty hours were recommended, with a minimum of 15 hours being provided by social work professionals only. Although this policy recommendation was made for all areas of social work practice, most workshop presenters and topics under consideration were from the health care area.

For health care social workers, in particular, the issue of the "uniqueness of social work services" remains a problem that we are forced to address. The competition for service delivery is fierce, and health care social workers must clearly establish that (a) what they do works; (b) they can do it quickly and in the most cost-effective way possible; and (c) what they do is different, contributing uniquely to the health and well-being of the patients served (Dziegielewski, 1997a).

In the educational setting, Peleg-Oren, Aran, Even-Zahav, Molina, and Stanger (2008) stress the importance of including specific information related to different health care settings. These authors believe that to remain competitive, educational learning objectives need to focus directly on increasing social work skills in mediation and team building. These two elements are such an important aspect of practice that they need to be emphasized in the classroom and also applied directly in healthcare settings. In social work, this can be applied in the course information provided and in field work experience. The authors present a model called the Supplementary Education Model as an option to supplement educational knowledge with skill building.

In summary, all education strategies whether through continuing education or in the traditional classroom need to highlight the importance of collaborative efforts. These partnerships rest firmly with the social worker's views on the importance of the person-in-situation stance. Social workers are in an excellent position to assist other team members to recognize the importance of treating the whole person and how he or she relates to his or her environment. Social workers are also keenly aware and can assist to point out the importance of patient situations involving mental distress, as well as family, economic, and social factors. As advocates they can play an important role utilizing a biopsychosocial approach to address patient need and provide environmentally sensitive care (Gehlert, 2006).

RELATED HELPING DISCIPLINES

As stated in Chapter 1, many other disciplines in the health care arena are doing the tasks that have traditionally been considered the role of the social worker. These individuals have varying degrees and types of education (See Table 2.1). In turn, social workers are also doing some of the tasks that have traditionally belonged to other disciplines. This complicates the ability to establish clearly a definition of what the health care social worker does as being different and unique from the other related disciplines.

This is further complicated by the fact that so much of what is done is from a team perspective where communication, treatment strategy, and care

Table 2.1 Training of Different Disciplines in Primary Care

MD, Psychiatry—4 years of college, 4 years of medical school, 4 years of residency (paid and practicing while in supervised learning).

MD, Internal Medicine—4 years of college, 4 years of medical school, 3 years of residency, unless they specialize in med/peds (4) or med/psych (5).

MD, Family Practice—4 years of college, 4 years of medical school, 3 years of residency. DO.

MD, Pediatricians—4 years of college, 4 years of medical school, 3 years of residency.

PhD or PsyD, Psychologists—4 years of college, 3–4 years of doctoral work, 1 year internship, dissertation, licensing examination.

MS Psychologists—4 years of college, 2 years of graduate school, licensing examination, requires ongoing supervision by a doctoral level psychologist for 2 years, then an examination.

MSW Social Workers—Can bill for services in FQHCs. MSW requires 4-year degree plus 2–3 years of graduate work that includes one or usually two supervised field placements.

MA/MS/LPC Counselors: Requires 4 years of college, 1½–2 years of graduate school, placement. Cannot bill for services in FQHCs.

Nurse Practitioners—4 years of college, examination, work as an RN, 2 years Master's degree with internship, sometimes additional work in a specialty certification, restricted prescribing.

Physician Assistants—4 years of college for most, some experience in the medical field for most before school, 2 years of medical training, restricted prescribing, supervision by an MD.

Nurses—RN, LPN.

Medical Assistants—Career School or Junior College, take subjects such as anatomy, physiology, medical terminology, surgical instruments, medical law, lab safety.

List compiled by Betsy Kent, West Virginia, Social Worker

management can overlap. Staff from multiple disciplines work together under the auspices of multidisciplinary, interdisciplinary, transdisciplinary, and pan-disciplinary teams (see "Types of Teamwork" Box). Once working in this team environment, the level of coordination can vary from working together as a cohesive unit to role and boundary blurring where an overlapping of functions can confuse all including those on the team and the patient served.

This discussion of the type of teams that can be utilized in service delivery provides fertile ground for understanding how service delivery can be unsuccessful when fragmentation occurs (Bunger, 2010). See "Types of Teamwork" Box, for a description of types of teamwork. When professionals see their roles as being separate and do not talk or share with other professions,

Types of Teamwork

Multidisciplinary Teams	A group of professionals working together for a common purpose, working independently while sharing information through formal lines of communication to better assist the patient/client/consumer.
Interdisciplinary Teams	A group of health care professionals who work together for a common purpose, working interdependently where some degree of sharing roles, tasks, and duties can overlap with both formal and informal lines of communication to better assist the patient/client/consumer.
Transdisciplinary Teams	A group of health care professionals and the patient/client/consumer and identified members of his/her support system freely share ideas and work together as a synergistic whole where ideas and sharing of responsibilities are common place in routine care.
Pandisciplinary Teams	A group of health care professionals who work together in a specialized area where each member of the team is seen as equal in the delivery of care with similar skills for assisting the patient. There are no distinctions, and the professional is considered an expert in an area not necessarily a professional discipline. For example, if it is working in geriatrics, all individuals would be considered a skilled professional listed by subject area rather profession.

Some ideas for the table definitions were modified from *Communication Research Trends* (2002), Volume 21 (3). Retrieved from cscc.scu.edu/trends/v21/v21_3.pdf

many patients can fall through the cracks. Regardless of the type of teamwork highlighted, the human factor in cooperation cannot be overlooked.

For example, most individuals know the difference between nursing and the role of the nurse and the role of the social worker; however, in today's health care environment, this distinction is no longer clear. Not only is there a blurring of roles between these two professions, regarding the delivery of health care services, but there is also overlap. Many nurses are now delivering services that were traditionally the role of the social work professional.

The role of the nursing professional is also rapidly changing. In the past, nurses generally focused on the direct provision of medical and health-related services from the medical model perspective. Traditionally defined, a nurse was a person formally educated and trained in the care of the sick and infirm (dictionary.reference.com/browse/nurse). It is this traditional role that secured them a place in health care along with physicians. When looking at service delivery, physicians and nurses are referred to as *essential* personnel. In terms of patient care, this title may assist to support their role in the team process, but it can also cause confusion when nontraditional roles are assumed. In the past, most of the psychosocial issues regarding patient care were either consulted with the social worker or left directly for the social worker to address. Today, however, this simplistic definition of the role of the nurse, and role of the social worker, has clearly changed. No longer can the roles and tasks performed by social workers and nurses be so clearly differentiated. Nurses are now doing much more varied tasks than what would have been previously considered as "unusual nursing methods" of practice.

For example, for over a century, "discharge planning" has been a part of the practice of health care social work and nursing. Historically, both disciplines recognize the need for formalized services that reflect discharge planning and have often worked together to provide subsequent aftercare activities. To date, studies (Holliman, Dziegielewski, & Datta, 2001) have looked at the differences between social work and nursing and the overlap of activities that often occur. This role sharing has recently been noted as prospective payment systems have assigned discharge planning activities increased status, and overlapping and convergence of social work and nursing tasks have led to turf battles. The overlap and sharing between the two disciplines have led to the question of the exact role of the social worker and the nurse and what exactly does the social worker contribute to this area of practice.

For the most part, nurses and social workers agree that social workers are better qualified to provide concrete services such as setting up home equipment, arranging nursing home placement, and helping patients understand insurance and finances. However, both social workers and nurses have seen themselves as qualified to perform the tasks of supportive counseling (Holliman et al., 2003). Both disciplines also agree that discharge planning efforts need to be individualized as the needs of the patient can be complex, diverse, and need dynamic interventions (Watts, Gardner, & Pierson, 2005). This need is more acute given that the time to prepare patients for discharge has all but vanished given decreasing lengths of hospital stays and the push to move patients out quickly (Maramba, Richards, Meyers, & Larrabee, 2004).

In addition, there have been studies focusing on systematic differences between the two groups. For example, Sheppard (1992) studied the communication styles of social workers and nurses during their interactions with physicians. Sheppard found that nurses contacted physicians more frequently than social workers, and the reason for contact often differed. Nurses generally contacted physicians about the patient's condition and treatment. Social workers contacted physicians less frequently; and when they did, they addressed the case's outcome, the final treatment plan, or family issues.

Bennett and Beckerman (1986) believed that the 1970s brought a change of status regarding the professionals who performed discharge planning. These authors pointed out that the "drudges of yesteryear" (i.e., those social workers who did not avoid assignments to medical and surgical services) had been transformed into major players. Carlton (1989) and Ross (1993) commended social workers for their ability to work with elaborate systems and claimed that social workers were the best-qualified professionals to do discharge planning. Cox (1996) in a study of discharge planning with patients suffering from dementia found that social workers were the team members most involved and influential with discharge decisions and nursing home placements. Atkatz (1995) found that social workers were commonly involved in discharges with the homeless because of the problematic placement issues with this group. Social workers were also frequently involved in cases of discharge planning with HIV/AIDS patients (Fahs & Wade, 1996; Marder & Linsk, 1995), the mentally ill (Gantt, Cohen, & Sainz, 1999; Tuzman, 1993), and infants with special care needs (Gentry, 1993). These earlier studies support the importance of including social workers in discharge planning, especially when multiproblem cases occur and there is a lack of available community resources.

From the nursing perspective, several sources have claimed that nurses are qualified discharge planners because their medical training allows them to complete physical assessments, assist with aspects of care, complete care plans, provide medical information with referrals, and assess the quality of health care resources and facilities (Ward, 2012).

Discharge planning remains a priority in nursing; however, the perceptions of what this requires vary. It has also been linked with case management where in its most simplistic form, discharge planning is simply defined as making sure the patient leaves the hospital as soon as possible. Some nursing professionals believe that nurses involved in discharge planning should take more of an administrative role; and others see nurses' role as teaching patients and their families complex postdischarge treatments such as breathing treatments, decubitus and skin care, feeding tubes, and home injections (Penrod, Kane, & Kane, 2000).

The primary debate in the area of discharge planning focuses on who should be doing it and what should be done? Turf battles between social work and nursing have increased over the last decade, as health care resources have become more limited. In summary, despite the continuous debates about who should do discharge planning, there is no empirical evidence that one group is more qualified than the other. Social work and nursing alike have a long history in discharge planning and case management dating back to the 19th century (Cawthorn, 2005). Holliman et al., (2003) concluded that despite role conflict and overlap, both social workers and nurses are able to make unique and substantial contributions in health care. The importance of including the family and interdisciplinary communications along with ongoing support is essential, especially in high-risk discharges involving some of our most vulnerable populations (Bauer, Fitzgerald, Haesler, & Manfrin, 2009).

In addition, a more recent article by the Ontario Association of Social Workers in 2009 clearly outlined the contributions of the health care social worker, and when participating as the lead member of the discharge planning or community outreach teams, they are invaluable in reducing duplication and rushed placements while creating a supportive environment for patients and their families.

In addition to health care, many nursing and other professionals have been encouraged to recognize the importance of the biopsychosocial framework for practice. As an advocate, awareness of the complete person is highlighted strongly advocating for more awareness of the mental health aspects of practice and advocating for a new holistic approach to practice that includes taking into account mental health (Jansson, 2011). These professionals believe that nursing and other professionals need to expand and actively reach for a more comprehensive stance from which to base practice intervention strategy. According to these professionals, the aspect of care that individuals are more than the sum of their parts must be incorporated into every aspect of professional nursing service. Whether it is the sheer numbers of nurses available to practice or the significant shifts in ideological thought among nurses practicing in the field, the profession of nursing is changing. Many of these changes have and will continue to affect the field of social work and the health care social work provider. In health care delivery, nurses and physicians who are referred to as critical providers of medical services have a great deal of power in establishing a firm place in providing services. Social workers, as many other allied professionals, are not considered essential. Therefore, nurses, in particular, can and often do compete for jobs or direct services that were usually done by social work professionals.

This means that nurse professionals are now, in addition to their traditional medical duties, initiating individual therapy, group therapy, crisis therapy, family therapy, mind–spirit therapies, health counseling and therapy, social work supervision, administrative services, and numerous other services that were usually considered the role of the health care social worker.

After reviewing the services provided by helping professionals in the health care area, there is a great deal of overlap of roles and functions. There is also a new trend to include lay individuals referred to as *market assisters* where these trained nonprofessionals will be available to assist people in the enrollment and care delivery process among those eligible to receive services from ACA-supported agencies. With all the overlap, it is easy to see where confusion can originate as to the actual differences between the services these professionals provide regarding the human condition. However, on careful examination, one ingredient remains conspicuously weak in the professions described, but prominent within social work. It is assistance to better the human condition, with the primary emphasis being placed on the environment that influences, surrounds, and reinforces it.

In summary, the greatest single factor that makes the health care social worker unique is the long, uncontested professional stance of *person-in-situation* or *person-in-environment*. This stance remains our heritage or more practically stated our guiding light for practice and intervention. Many of our basic texts describe the importance of including this concept, and application in the classroom setting remains central to all practice activity (Hepworth et al., 2010).

However, social workers are not the only professionals aware of the importance of addressing a patient within the environmental context. Other disciplines have also recognized the importance of including a person–environment stance. Therefore, many of the traditional premises central to the field of social work such as understanding that the patient equals more than the sum of the parts have been adopted by other health-related helping professionals. These professionals now use many of the same principles and ideas of social work, and this overlap serves to further blur the differences between the disciplines and the uniqueness of the roles that each professional provides.

DEFINING CLINICAL HEALTH CARE SOCIAL WORK

Clinical social work in the health care setting is an area of practice that has sometimes been referred to as *medical social work*; it is not uncommon to see these terms used interchangeably. The *Social Work Dictionary* defines medical social work as a form of practice that occurs in hospitals and other health care settings that facilitates good health, prevention of illness, and aids physically ill patients and their families to resolve the social and psychological problems related to disease and illness (Barker, 2003). To highlight the concept of facilitating good health further, wellness with its emphasis on promoting and maintaining a sense of patient well-being has recently gained in popularity. In this definition, it is also important to acknowledge the role of the medical social worker in sensitizing other health care professionals to the social-psychological aspects of illness (Barker, 2003). In practice, the health care social worker addresses the psychosocial aspects of the patient, alerts other team members to these needs, and facilitates service provision. In addition, not only does the social worker represent the interests of the patient but also is expected to be reflective of the "moral conscience" for the health care delivery team.

As defined in this book, clinical health care social work practice includes a full range of social work services. These services include social work assessment or diagnosis, goal establishment, interventive foci, methods, and referral. However, it is important to note that whenever possible, brief or time-limited intervention methods are strongly recommended as the state of art in health care practice and necessary for future practice survival

(Dziegielewski, 2010a, 2010b). When using time-limited interventions, no single theory or standard for practice application should govern a social worker's attempts to help an individual, group, family, or community resolve the problem being addressed. Furthermore, application of time-limited techniques may also be difficult to implement in the health care setting due to the limited contact time available. Many times the health care social worker is forced to see a patient only briefly and this short time span can only provide concrete service provision.

Today's health care social worker must remain aware of time-limited treatment standards and techniques but must also be flexible and open to change. In summary, what Carlton (1989) stated still remains relevant:

"clinical social work in the health field is a mutual process of face-to-face interventions in which the professional social worker provides social work services to patients, including services on behalf of those patients, who use them to resolve mutually identified and defined problems in patient social functioning precipitated by actual or potential physical illness, disability or injury" (Carlton, 1984, p. 6).

Keeping this traditional definition in mind, one caveat is suggested to address the changing environment and that involves meeting face-to-face. With electronic technology, interactions can be quite successful with contact that is not considered the traditional face-to-face as this earlier definition describes. As electronic communication, telemedicine, video calling, and so forth continue to gain in popularity, these types of communications will become more common, and recognition and acceptance to daily practice are expected. In telemedicine, clinical healthcare is provided from a distance. Hailey, Ohinmaa, and Roine (2004) completed a systematic review of the benefits, and after reviewing 605 publications on the topic with varying degrees of quality articles, the jury is still out although it does show promise.

Regardless of the advent of new technology, the struggles that social workers must face in the health care area today should not be underestimated. Oftentimes the health care social work professional is viewed as "just" one of many providers. This makes striving for purpose justification regarding service provision a daily struggle. Yet, it has become obvious that a clear statement of purpose and clarity of role performance are expected to compete for and maintain a seat at the health care delivery table.

Establishing a clear definition of health care social work practice, either today or in our past, has not been an easy task. Health care social workers must remain flexible in the delivery of services. As a profession, this flexibility needs to be maintained not only to help our patients but also to adjust to the environment in which our patients exist and need to be served. Our responsibility is clear in applying these skills in the current health care environment providing a clearer understanding for all what it is social workers can do (Power, 2009).

ROLE OF THE HEALTH CARE SOCIAL WORKER

The current state of social work practice in the health care setting mirrors the turbulence found in the general health care environment. The current economic downturns have massive ripple effects, and social workers are experiencing this first hand. For those working in the hospital setting, referrals from the emergency department are growing rapidly (Ellis, 2009). Medical social workers, like other health care professionals, are being forced to deal with numerous issues that include declining hospital admissions, reduced lengths of stay, and numerous other restrictions and methods of cost containment. Struggling to solve these issues has become necessary based on the inception of prospective payment systems, restrictive behavioral care plans, and other changes in the provision and funding of health care (Jansson, 2011). Previous research has linked not receiving services to higher rates of high-risk patient relapse (Coulton, 1985). Social workers are being forced to discharge patients from services more quickly, and patients are being returned to the community in a weaker state of rehabilitation than ever before (Bywaters, 1991).

With so many changes in the social environment, there is little consistency in the delivery of health care social work with a high emphasis placed on cost containment (Davis & Meier, 2001). When health care administrators are forced to justify each dollar billed for services, there is little emphasis placed on the provision of what some term as "expendable services," such as mental health and well-being services, thorough discharge planning, and so on.

Unfortunately, the services that social workers perform are often placed in this category, and, as a result, they often feel the brunt of initial dollar-line savings attempts (Dziegielewski, 1996, 2010a). As discussed earlier, just the sheer numbers of allied health care professionals who are moderately paid provide an excellent hunting ground for administrators pressured to cut costs. These administrators may see the role of the social worker as adjunct to the delivery of care and may decide to cut back or replace them with concretely trained nonprofessionals simply to cut costs. These substitute professionals do not have either the depth or breadth of training that the social work professional has, which can result in substandard professional care. For example, a trained paraprofessional in hospital discharge planning may simply facilitate a placement order. Issues such as the individual's sense of personal well-being, ability for self-care, or family and environmental support may not be considered. Therefore, the employment of this type of paraprofessional can be cost effective but not quality care driven. If personal/social and environmental issues are not effectively addressed, patients may be put at risk for harm.

The patient who is discharged home to a family that does not want him or her is more at risk of abuse and neglect (Kemp, 1998). A patient who has a negative view of self and a hopeless and hapless view of his or her condition is more likely to try to commit suicide. Many paraprofessionals or members of other professional disciplines can differ from social work professionals because they do not recognize the importance of culture and environmental factors as paramount to efficient and effective practice. The de-emphasis or denial of this consideration can result in the delivery of "cheap" but substandard care.

As administrators strive to cut costs by eliminating professional social work services, the overall philosophy of wellness has been sacrificed for a concentration on cost cutting. However, it is important to note that many times these types of staff reductions are not personal attacks on social work professionals. Actually, oftentimes, changes and cutbacks in the delivery of services and those who provide them are done to address an immediate need—cost reduction. The fluctuating and downsizing of social work professionals, as with other allied health professionals, may simply reflect the fluctuating demands of the current market (Falck, 1990, 1997).

Ross (1993) points out that health care employees who are at the greatest risk of being subjected to losing their place in the delivery of health care services (a) are those who do not create direct hospital revenues; (b) are not self-supporting parts of the health care delivery team; (c) hold jobs where productivity is not easily measured or questionable; (d) provide service where the long-term benefit for cost of service is not measured; and (e) engage in a service where the professional's role is often misunderstood, challenged, and underrated in the system. Unfortunately, social workers, along with other allied professionals who participate in the health care delivery system, often meet these criteria. Therefore, it is important for social work professionals to be viewed as an essential part of the health care delivery team providing both needed direct clinical services and fiscal support for the agency setting.

In closing, it is important not to confuse the social worker who works in a restrictive care environment with the concept of providing case management in the health care setting (Davis & Meier, 2001). In the traditional provision of case management services, the goal is to get the patient the best and most cost-effective treatment based on patient need. However, Frankel and Gelman (2012) remind us that there is one common goal that case management shares with social work and that is stressing the importance of systems theory. From this perspective, systems theory provides the underpinnings of this activity and is clearly linked to our historical roots. The premise remains simple everything that a person experiences is related to what is in his or her surroundings. Simply stated it is influenced by the environment. The combination of many events has brought the individual and his or her significant other, family, friends, or community to this point. This cannot be ignored, and treatment of the system from a holistic framework will always yield the best and most lasting problem resolutions.

CHAPTER SUMMARY AND FUTURE DIRECTIONS

The problem of developing and exposing a definition of health care social work as described in the beginning of this chapter is not an uncommon one. With changes in technology and the introduction of new electronic ways of communication, it seems as if more changes are to be expected. Originally, the roots of the health care social worker, similar to those of the social work profession, were generally linked to serving the poor and the disenfranchised. However, over the years, the role of the health care social worker has expanded tremendously. This makes defining exactly what social workers do a difficult task. Clarity of definition has been further complicated by changes in scope of practice, the diverse roles of social work, technological advances, and the expectations within the patient–practitioner relationship. This turbulent environment requires that social work professionals constantly battle "quality-of-care" issues versus "cost-containment" measures for patients, while securing a firm place as professional providers in the health care environment. Some social workers continue to express concern that accountability requirements can distract from what is most important quality patient/client/consumer care (Aronson, Sammon, & Smith, 2009). These concerns are well placed and should not be taken lightly.

In this chapter, a general definition of the role of the health care social worker was presented along with a discussion of the issue of role ambiguity and confusion. Some of the differences between health care social workers and the other related disciplines were outlined. The major distinguishing factor found was the practice-based environmental stance that has historically reflected the roots of social work practice. Therefore, health care social work needs to be viewed as the professional "bridge" that links the patient; the multidisciplinary, interdisciplinary, transdisciplinary, and pandisciplinary teams; and the environment (see Chapter 5 for a more detailed definition of these terms). Now, more than at any time in the past, it is important to define clearly the similarities and differences between the professions. The numbers of health care professionals in practice have risen dramatically; and these professionals who often perform similar or duplicating functions are competing for limited health care jobs.

For future marketability and competition, it is believed that social workers need to move beyond the traditional definition and subsequent role of the health care social worker. In the area of clinical practice, new or refined methods of service delivery need to be established and used. Social workers are encouraged to assume positions such as managers, owners of companies, staff, administrators, supervisors, clinical directors, and case managers where they can help influence specific agency policy and procedure. They also need to make themselves aware of basic programs beyond their own individual practice that can affect health care service delivery. The specific recommendations, techniques, and guidelines discussed in the following chapters will be useful in helping health care social workers to equip themselves with the tools in practice, administration, and supervision that they will need to secure a seat at today's table for health care delivery.

In closing, several steps are suggested for social work professionals to help the profession survive the numerous changes presented with behavioral health plans that offer more restricted choices of doctors and hospitals and limited reimbursement schemes.

First, social workers need to market the services they provide and link them to cost effectiveness. Social work is an old profession in the competition scheme when compared with many of the newer health care delivery professionals. The profession's traditional roots have been linked to the poor and disenfranchised (Hepworth et al., 2010), both of which are not considered desirable patient populations in behavioral health care. This is not to suggest that social workers abandon our roots simply to appear more marketable in the scheme of budget-conscious coverage. Rather, we should consider professional self-marketing and emphasize the myriad services that we actually do provide.

It is essential to link the provision of each service the health care social worker provides with the cost saving it provokes. For example, traditional services, such as provision of hospital discharge planning, should emphasize dollars saved in the overall prospective payment reimbursement system. Dollar amounts should be calculated for presentation of justification of overall savings because of service provision. A second example regarding saving costs through prevention can involve the home health care social worker. The home visits provided can serve as a means to assist families and patients in the home to acquire needed counseling to defuse stressed situations, provide needed social support, and access to services to maintain community placement. The cost-cutting feature of living in the community is phenomenal when compared with institutionalized care of patients. Options like these are facilitated by the provision of effective social work services.

A new mind-set needs to be established with service provision. Each service needs to be competitive and emphasis placed on income generated or cost savings incurred. Many times, even without direct income being generated, services can be valued based on the costs they can save the organization.

A second concept necessary for health care social workers to compete successfully in the health care environment is to present our professional roles as essential ingredients to the success of the health care interdisciplinary team. For this to happen, the process must start with the individual social work professional. Each social worker, with each service provided, be it discharge planning, referrals, or direct clinical work, needs to make the patient aware that the service being provided or coordinated is being done by a social work professional. Because some services can be completed by the social worker, a nurse, case manager, or other professional, it is important to know the social worker is providing the service. Laypeople may mistake social workers for nurses, teachers, or even call them counselors. Many times we become so task oriented that we forget this simple but essential point. Be sure to tell all you serve that you are a social worker.

As you work with the health care team, you also must make them aware of the importance of your role in the overall success of the team. Helping to think of the services you provide in a cost-saving prevention perspective will also help with gaining professional recognition. You help the other team members to be able to complete their jobs; and in addition, help to save them time and money.

A third aspect for the survival of social work in the health care delivery scene rests in advocacy and social change. Here, social workers need to support and lobby for political and social recognition of the value of social work services from both a quality-of-care and cost-effectiveness basis. In this constantly changing environment, it is important for social work representation to be visible and ready to secure its current position and additional positions that may come open. Lobbyists, well aware of social work's goals and missions, need to be strategically placed as these insurers seek to reduce costs and what providers will be maintained. Insurers need to be made aware of and enticed to include the services that social workers can provide.

Finally, the role of the social worker in behavioral health care needs to continue to grow beyond what is considered traditional. Social workers need to continue to market themselves and let others know when they occupy positions, such as managers, owners of companies, employees, administrators, supervisors, clinical directors, and case managers. Once in these positions, social workers will have power to help influence specific agency policy and procedure. They also need to make themselves aware of basic programs and services available beyond their own individual practice that can affect overall health wellness and service delivery. The profession of social work is strong enough to compete, but there is no time for hesitancy. The plans for tomorrow are being outlined today. These plans outline the delivery of services in which health care social workers can and need to remain an integral part.

Glossary

Allied health care workers   Professionals involved in health care delivery to the individual, group, family, or community that is the focus of intervention.

Clinical social work practice   Often referred to as medical social work (see *medical social work*).

Family counseling   A practice methodology that centers on the "family" as the patient/client/consumer or unit of attention.

Health care practice   The activities that are conducted that are designed to enhance physical and psychological well-being.

Health care social work   The practice of social work that deals with the aspects of general health, specifically in the areas of wellness, illness, or disability. The social work professional can address these issues through working directly with either individuals, groups, families, or communities, or through the auspice of broader social change.

Health care social worker   Is seen as the professional "bridge" that links the patient/client/consumer, the multidisciplinary or interdisciplinary team, and the environment.

Hospital social work   Historically defined as the provision of social services in a medical setting. Currently, refers to the delivery of social work services in hospitals and related health care facilities.

Market assisters   These are trained lay individuals who are paid to assist patients/clients/consumers in the enrollment process determining Affordable Care Act (ACA) eligibility.

Medical social work   A form of social work practice that occurs in health care settings with the goal of assisting those who are physically ill, facilitating good health, and prevention of illness.

Nursing   A field of practice versed in medical matters and entrusted with caring for the sick.

Practice of social work   The application of social work knowledge, theories, methods, and skills to provide professional sound, ethically bound, culturally sensitive social services to individuals, groups, families, organizations, and communities.

Psychology   The profession and science concerned with the behavior of humans, and related mental and physiological processes.

Public health   Tasked with prevention of disease and maintenance of health in the population.

Telemedicine   This avenue of delivery for patient care utilizes telecommunication technology to deliver patient care. This involves real-time interactive video capabilities.

Questions for Further Study

1. In your own words, state several concrete differences between the services that nurses provide and social workers provide in the health care setting.

2. What do you believe can make health care social work practice an integral part of health care delivery?

3. What characteristic of social work practice makes it the most marketable in today's health care practice arena?

4. What do you see as the greatest obstacles to the use of telemedicine when serving patients/clients/consumers as opposed to traditional face-to-face approaches?

5. How do you believe health care social work will be defined in the future?

Websites Related to Health Care Social Work

Health care research and policy information
www.ahcpr.gov

Open Arms Patient Advocacy Society
www.openarmsadvocacy.com

International Websites

These websites provide international information to practice, policy, and research with publications offered in all health-related realms, i.e. public health issues related to medical conditions, mental health, substance abuse, targeting childhood through geriatric populations, in various populations, and within environmental impacts.

The World Health Organization
www.who.int/en/

The Royal Society for Public Health
www.rsph.org.uk

National Websites

These websites are produced from academic institutions within the United States and provide information in practice, police, and research within the United States but also in the international realm.

Information for Practice
ifp.nyu.edu/

An online resource for bibliometrics tools, the website provides news and journals that inform practice from within the field of social work and related allied health profession on trends relating to public health, including mental health and substance abuse.

NASW-New York Chapter: Social Work in Health Care
www.naswnycarchives.net/SocialWorkinHealthCare.html

This website is provided by NASW-New York Chapter. The content varies and is updated regularly. It outlines the areas many social workers are active in health care and presents links to related articles and other information that would be helpful to health care social workers.

The Society for Social Work Leadership in HealthCare-Texas Chapter
www.sswlhc-tx.org/

This website provides information related to this organization dedicated to helping social workers advance knowledge in the area of health practice and policy settings.

Today's Health Care Social Worker

Name:	Christopher L. Getz, MSW, PA
List State of Practice:	Washington
Professional Job Title:	Clinical Social Worker/Physician Assistant

Duties in a Typical Day
I deal with people who have suffered a major tragedy surrounding a disease. I provide educational training to the patient and his or her family members on the medical aspects of the disease and how to learn to live and cope with the disease process. I often act as an advocate to help the patient get the necessary supports to improve the quality of his or her life.

What do you like most about your position?
I really enjoy working with the wide diversity of patient problems and issues. I enjoy helping patients learn how to best cope with the disease process, encouraging empowerment each step of the way.

What do you like least about your position?
I often work long hours. At the end of the day, although I feel satisfied with what I have accomplished, I sometimes wish I could have done more.

(continued)

(continued)

> **What "words of wisdom" do you have for the new health care social worker considering work in a similar position?**
> In the area of medical social work, it is important to completely understand the process of the disease, from both a medical and psychosocial point of view. It is critical for the social worker to help the patient to adjust and work through his or her feelings. Social workers need to help patients anticipate and prepare for the future. In terms of a progressive disease, acceptance and preparation are critical factors leading toward patient/client/consumer empowerment and change.

CHAPTER 3

The Evolution of Social Work Practice in Health Care

Interest in health care social work is generally linked to the social factors that link health and mental health in illness and disease. The practice of social work that deals with the aspects of general health, specifically in the areas of wellness, illness, or disability, is known today as health care social work. Looking at the influence of creating an environment that favors general health and wellness, medical social work can be viewed as one of the oldest and well-established fields of professional social work practice. Throughout history, clinical health care social work has often been called medical social work. Even today, these terms can still be used interchangeably. In addition, the social worker today skilled in health care must also have expertise and a keen awareness of health policy issues and how to use this information to best address the needs of the patient/client/consumer (hereafter referred to as patient). It is not uncommon for social workers to assist eligibility for health services as well as application procedures (Darnell & Lawlor, 2012).

ALMSHOUSES

The general premises, resulting in the roots of health care social work, can be traced back as far as the 1700s to the almshouses, which were considered places of refuge for society's poor, medically sick, and mentally ill patients of all ages. The almshouse was often referred to as the "poorhouse" or place of death. These philanthropic institutional settings were often scarcely funded. They primarily housed only society's outcasts, particularly, those who were poor, incapacitated, and suffered from contagious diseases. In society, individuals who had any form of family support were cared for at home. In these early days, health care was considered a private matter, and individuals and their families were expected to take care of themselves. Therefore, the alm-shouse was used as an "option of last resort," providing a type of indoor shelter and relief for the destitute. The almshouse, and the workers who staffed them, can be noted as one of the earliest practice areas for health care providers. The health care workers who provided caretaking services in the almshouses often became ill. These workers, similar to the occupants of the almshouse, were subjected to poor sanitary conditions and numerous conta-gious diseases.

In 1713, William Penn founded the first almshouse in Philadelphia; in 1736, a second one was founded at Bellevue Hospital in New York City. The almshouse in Bellevue usually housed the mentally ill and later became one of the most famous mental health hospitals in the state of New York. Throughout history, the almshouse has been noted as a community-based institution, often viewed as the forerunner of today's hospital (Nacman, 1977). The development of these institution-based services is considered important to create the basis for institutionalization of health care for the first time in this country. Service within these institutional settings remained standard until the 1800s when slowly the services needed for sick individu-als began to be viewed separately from services needed to house the poor (Colby & Dziegielewski, 2010).

Individuals who could afford medical care did not want service from these institutions, and philanthropic gifts were used to start new and more proficient facilities for providing care (Nacman, 1977). The poor were even-tually separated out, and although "indoor" relief was still provided, they were expected to live and work in special facilities. In many cases, the gov-ernment actually contracted with private individuals to feed and provide shelter and clothing for these individuals in exchange of contracted labor services. Soon children were also removed from the almshouses by the efforts of the Children's Aid Society. These children were later placed in orphan-ages. In 1851, the mentally ill were also removed and sent to improved facilities primarily through the crusading efforts of Dorthea Lynde Dix. Basically, the "holding tank" nature of the almshouse was replaced with a more segregated form of institutionalized care such as the orphanage and other residential facilities.

When the Revolutionary War began, soldiers needed to receive ade-quate medical care in order to return to battle. To facilitate this need, New York Hospital, designed to treat the military, was the first hospital to actu-ally begin to provide systematized training to medical students. By 1840, hospitals originally founded by philanthropy were now beginning to spe-cialize and provide care to certain populations or for particular diseases (Nacman, 1977).

It was around this time that "indoor" forms of social welfare relief, where the individual had to live within the institution to get services, were replaced by "outdoor" forms of relief in which the poor were pro-vided with concrete supplies, goods, and services while living in their own homes.

CHARITY ORGANIZATION SOCIETIES

With the emphasis on the provision of health care service to be delivered outside of the institution came the emergence of Charity Organization Societies. The first American Charity Organization Society was in Buffalo, New York, in 1877. These groups are considered important in the historical development of health care social work, because they provided the basis for the modern social service agencies of today. The workers they employed are often considered to be some of the first to deliver these social services in the home setting to poor and disenfranchised individuals. These early visitors to homes are believed to have helped start the foundation for the home health care social worker of today. These service workers were referred to as friendly visitors.

The charity organizations and the workers who represented them, however, were not considered objective. Many times, these workers defined who was worthy of assistance and who was not. For example, children and older adults were believed to be unable to control their situations, whereas younger adults could. The ideology subscribed to here was primarily one of social Darwinism where only the strongest and best people would survive. The friendly visitors were usually upper-class individuals whose mission was to reform or redeem the poor with whom they came in contact. There were specific plans that had been predetermined to fix the problems they encountered. Each organization set its own limits and parameters and handled situations as they saw fit.

Weaknesses in this form of health delivery included (a) no systematized way of delivering services and duplication of the services often occurred; (b) most services delivered were on a "one-time" basis, and no education or teaching was provided to negate future problems, and (c) the service workers were not professionally trained and many times approached individuals' predetermined notions of patient worth and aptitude. Often these early health care workers believed that the patients they served were at fault. In many cases, the patient was seen as responsible for the problem, because it was believed that the problem originated "within the patient," not within the system. In turn, little advocacy for the improvement of public health standards was noted, although some referrals for direct medical intervention did occur.

HOSPITAL SOCIAL WORK

Hospital-based social work practice has been in existence since the late 19th century, when early social service professionals were sought to help bridge the patient's environmental system with the hospital where care was rendered. These early social workers extended beyond the traditional bounds of the hospital to educate the patient and the general public about environmental factors that influence health (Cabot, 1915). This theme of connecting the institution, the person, and the environment represents a generalist perspective common throughout the history of hospital social work.

Johns Hopkins Hospital established its first social work program in 1907; the first social worker to be employed there was Helen B. Pendleton (Nacman, 1977). Because of internal conflicts at the hospital, Ms. Pendleton did not stay in this position long, and another social worker soon took her place. At the same time, Ida Cannon, working closely with Dr. Richard Cabot, became the Director of the Social Service Department at Massachusetts General Hospital (Rehr & Rosenberg, 2006). Among other leadership responsibilities, Ida Cannon, often termed the mother of medical social work, was influential in conducting educational training that made others aware of social services and its important contribution to the comprehensive care of the patients served (Sedgwick, 2012). Through his chronological account, Sedgwick (2012) also reminds us of the work of Janet Thornton who was paramount in establishing the presence and relevance of social work in the hospital setting, contributing to both clinical practice and professional and community education. With this early recognition and contribution, it is no surprise that approximately 4 years later in 1910, New York State began to support after-care programs for discharged patients.

The inclusion of these early health care social workers is important as they highlighted the need and laid the groundwork for the addition of professional social work services. These early social workers were often responsible for the care, maintenance, storage, and return of the medical record as well as for determining who was eligible to receive indigent care. Generally, medical records were not treated as confidential, and information regarding content was distributed on a need-to-know basis. Often these social workers were considered moralistic and paternalistic regarding worker–patient interactions.

In these early days, health care social work services were generally assigned to and performed by hospital nurses. These nurses were often considered convenient choices for employment, because they were easily accessible, already knew agency procedure, and were aware of community resources. Later, however, it was established that more specialized training in understanding social conditions was needed, with an emphasis on employing social work professionals. To address this need for specialized training in social work, the School of Philanthropy was developed in 1898. This organization was designed to outline rules and guidelines for the profession; however, it did not actually influence formal social work education until 1932 when the schools that formally taught social work joined together to establish curriculum rules.

In 1918, the National Conference of Social Work in Kansas City helped to form the American Association of Hospital Social Workers. This was the first professional social work organization in the United States (Carlton, 1984). The formation of this association clearly established the acceptance of health care social work as a legitimate form of social work services. As the role of health care social work expanded beyond the traditional bounds of the hospital, a name change for the organization was initiated that would be more inclusive. To reflect this expansion in 1934, the name of this organization was changed to the American Association of Medical Social Workers. Actually, it was the American Association of Medical Social Workers that constituted one of the seven professional social work associations that merged together in 1955 to form the National Association of Social Workers.

In the 1920s, the debate as to whether social work was a profession was highlighted by Flexner's proposition that it was not. This debate prompted social workers to make attempts to clearly define what they did and the role they played among the helping professions (Austin, 2001; Thyer, 2002). In the 1930s, "removing patients" or discharge planning was devalued and described as an administrative or clerical function (Bartlett, 1940). Therefore, from 1920 to 1970, the trend was for social workers with the least formal education to provide concrete services and discharge patients, whereas those with more skill would focus on more abstract and presumably more difficult and more specialized functions such as counseling (Davidson, 1978; Kadushin & Kulys, 1994).

In 1928, the American College of Surgeons developed and included a minimum standard of service provision for social service departments. In the 1920s and 1930s, the United States military started to add social workers to their ranks. Regardless of theoretical orientation or exact role performed, once the formative years were established, social workers and the services they provide have been considered necessary. Reflected throughout the years and in service commitment through the National Association of Social Workers, as well as other professional groups (e.g., the Association of Health Care Social Workers, the Association of Clinical Social Workers, and the Council on Social Work Education), health care social workers have maintained an active role in the policies, procedures, and service delivery required by today's demanding health care environment.

During this time period from 1920 to 1980, rising health care costs caused great concern, and different ways to address and reduce these costs were explored. As the role of the hospital expanded so did the need for hospital social work, and departments headed and staffed by professional social workers emerged within hospital administrative structures.

In 1983, diagnosis-related groups (DRGs) were introduced into hospitals as a prospective reimbursement system where hospitals billed according to diagnosis rather than the costs of services. With these specific treatment guidelines and expected time limits, pressure increased for hospitals to discharge patients as expediently as possible. Actually, it was during this time that discharge planning became recognized as a vital function within the hospital. Therefore, the professionals who performed the tasks that facilitated timely discharge were considered essential to the health care delivery team (Holliman et al., 2003). With the pressure to reduce costs, however, attempts to eliminate what might be considered nonessential professional staff also emerged. This fear of job loss helped to increase the competition among disciplines already serving as part of the patient-care team. The competition between social work and nursing amplified, and nurses started to show an increased interest in discharge planning activities. Unfortunately, in the 1990s, downsizing to reduce costs caused many services that were considered nonessential to be eliminated, and in some cases, hospital social work departments were eliminated (Dziegielewski & Holliman, 2001; Holliman et al., 2001). Hospital social workers were generally recognized for their supportive interventions (i.e., counseling and adjustment), rather than for direct placement. This cost-saving administrative decision had many ripple effects in the social work profession including limiting the availability of social work supervision and continuing education for social worker discharge planners (Holliman et al., 2001).

PULLING IT ALL TOGETHER

Having first explored the history and development of professional health care social work practice, the foundation for what it is that social workers do in this field is outlined. Although this role has changed throughout time, social work has remained strong with its commitment to direct service and advocacy. Therefore, health care social work is always more than just basic clinical practice. Although the concentration in this book is primarily on the clinical practice of health care social work, it is important to note that the concept of health care social work is much broader. It always needs to include an awareness of the person in his or her situation or environmental context. This awareness always involves taking into account how any intervention attempt will affect the individual, the family, the group, and the community. From an advocacy standpoint, awareness of institutional, community, state, and federal health policy and program planning and administration is essential to comprehensive patient care within an environment that is constantly changing.

Difficulty in trying to define this branch of social work is not new, and problems with establishing exactly what the health care social worker does has long since been a thorn in the side of health care administrators who justify funding. Based on the varied and situation-dependent circumstances each social worker must deal with, it becomes easy to understand how difficult it really is to understand and predict exactly what a health care social worker will do in practice. Health care social workers in particular are known for their ability to "fix what is broken" and to do this with an incredible sense of urgency and competence in the most cost-effective manner possible. Given the complexity of the human situation, sometimes this task is not as simple as it might sound. Therefore, it remains difficult to say exactly what health care social workers do. Now, imagine having to "do it" in a constantly changing environment (Davis & Meier, 2001). Unfortunately, this is the world in which the health care social worker often struggles to best meet the needs of the patients they serve.

ROLES OF THE HEALTH CARE SOCIAL WORKER

The Social Work Dictionary (Barker, 2003) describes the role of the "health care worker" as "a generic name for all the professional, paraprofessional, technical and general employees of a system or facility that provides for the diagnosis, treatment and overall wellbeing of patients" (p. 164). This dictionary definition, however, makes a clear distinction between the terms "health care worker" and "allied health care worker". To distinguish between the two terms, clearly one must remember that (a) health care workers usually refers to nonprofessional staff involved in health care delivery, and (b) allied health care workers refers to the professionals involved in health care delivery. The health care workers are generally those nonprofessionals who work in health care, such as home health aides, medical records personnel, nurses' aides, orderlies, and attendants (Barker, 2003). The allied health professional, conversely, excludes physicians and nurses but does include professional personnel of hospitals and other health care facilities. Physicians and nurses are not considered allied service providers, because their service is considered essential and necessary to any basic medical care provided. Allied health care providers include audiologists, dietitians, occupational therapists, optometrists, pharmacists, physical therapists, psychologists, social workers, speech pathologists, and others.

It is here under the auspices of the *allied health professional* that the health care social worker generally performs most of his or her duties in the health care arena. It is believed that health care social workers serve this area well because of their broad-based training on the biological, psychological, and social factors (i.e., the biopsychosocial approach) that can affect a patient's environmental situation.

PROVISION OF CORE CLINICAL SERVICES

Today, the role of health care professionals has been clearly established. Social workers can now be found in every area of our health care delivery system. Core services provided to individuals, families, and groups include (a) case finding and outreach, which primarily relates to helping patients and their families not only to identify the health care services that they need but also how to obtain them; (b) preservice or preadmission planning that is designed to anticipate barriers to accessing care; (c) assessment ability, especially about the need for the provision of social work services and planning for continued health and well-being; (d) concrete service provision as in admission and discharge from service planning; (e) psychosocial evaluations, assessing patients from a biopsychosocial perspective with cultural considerations appropriately highlighted; (f) the identification of clear goals and specific objectives that need to be accomplished during health care service delivery; (g) direct clinical counseling that reflects the therapeutic intervention strategy for individuals, families, and groups that considers the biopsychosocial perspective; (h) assistance with short- or long-term planning, where patients and their families are helped to anticipate their current and future service needs; (i) direct assistance with service provision of preventive remedial and rehabilitative measures; (j) provide information and education through instruction on significant health issues and problems that will assist patients, their families, and significant others; (k) provide training and support for continued health and wellness program development and participation; (l) referral service, which includes helping patients to gain access and learn how to use these services; (m) ensure continuity of care for the patient as connections are made to other health care service providers; and (n) patient advocacy, which means teaching patients how to obtain needed resources or on a larger scale, advocating for changes in policy or procedure that can have a direct or indirect benefit for the patient.

As can be seen in the boxed-text example, "Voices From the Field," the core clinical skills and the services provided by health care social workers can involve more than what has traditionally been called "discharge planning." Health care is a changing environment where even the classic definition of discharge planning has been altered. Social workers are not only coordinating discharges and services; they are also providing oversight for the multidisciplinary or interdisciplinary teams to be sure that patients are getting the services they need. Furthermore, once the team agrees that a patient is ready for discharge, it is often the social worker who is held responsible for ensuring that transfer forms are completed, patient and family education has been done, and the records that support continued care are ready for transfer.

VOICES FROM THE FIELD: WORKING WITH CHILDREN AND CHRONIC ILLNESS

Special thanks to Breanne Anderson for gathering and formulating this information.

To find out the opinions of health care social workers in the field, six practitioners from a large hospital in the Southeast were interviewed. This large southeastern hospital is equipped to service the everyday medical needs of children, with units specializing in HIV and AIDS care, infectious disease, children's cardiology, critical care, trauma, neonatal intensive care, oncology/hematology, sexual trauma, and urgent care. The six subjects were members of a psychosocial team that worked primarily with children suffering from a chronic life-threatening illness and their families.

The subjects were asked about the services they provide to pediatric patients with chronic or life-threatening illnesses and their families. The interviews lasted approximately 30 minutes and were conducted

(continued)

(continued)

over a 2-week time period at the availability of the professional. Each participant agreed to participate and have the interviews recorded for review. The participants ranged in age from 27 to 42. Five participants were female and one was male, four were Caucasian, one was African American, and one was Hispanic. They have been in practice from 2 to 23 years, and in their current positions between 1 and 17 years. One individual worked with infectious disease, one with oncology, one in the cardiology unit, two float throughout the hospital and cover the ICU and special care units, and one works at an outpatient, infectious disease clinic. Five of the participants also spend time working at an outpatient pediatric behavioral and therapeutic clinic provided by the hospital. They were each asked seven questions related to patient services:

1. What services are you providing to clients/patients and their families?
2. What services are most important to the patients and families you serve?
3. What services had the lowest utilization rate?
4. What additional services do you feel need to be offered?
5. Are the services you provide generally short-term or long-term?
6. Do you believe adequate services are available to children and families?
7. How do the patients and families you serve find out about the services that are available to them?

1. **What services are you providing to patients and their families?**
   On the first question, subjects provided a wide variety of responses with little consistency between how often these services were provided. See below for a list of services. The services reported by these social workers are considered areas of need and benefit for these children and their families.

   List of services provided
   Coping skills, bereavement, behavioral adjustments, community referrals, assistance with adjustment to diagnosis, education, Department of Children and Families liaison, discharge planning, patient counseling, outpatient counseling, assessment, crisis counseling, play therapy, assistance disclosing diagnosis to the child and family, and working with groups.

2. **What services were most important to your patients and the families you serve?**
   Again, the social workers differed on exactly what services were most important. Most agreed that some consistency in reporting back to patients with follow-up information is crucial. They also reported that the use of therapy or counseling sessions, inpatient services, and education services were requested most often by the patients they served. These social workers felt counseling and education services were the most important services for patients and their families (see the list below).

(continued)

VOICES FROM THE FIELD: WORKING WITH CHILDREN AND CHRONIC ILLNESS (continued)

List of most important services
All services are important; inpatient services, support groups, crisis counseling, therapy and other counseling services, education services, coping skills.

3. **What services had the lowest utilization rate by patients and their families?**
In response to this question, five of the six respondents stated that patients did not often seek out the social worker to see what outpatient referrals were available. They also reported that oftentimes patients failed to follow through or schedule second appointments. This worried some of the social workers, because they felt that even though many patients and families did not seek them out for these services, they were still needed (see the list below).

List of least utilized services
Behavioral services, outpatient, referrals, education, and assistance in disclosing diagnosis to child.

4. **What additional services do you feel need to be offered?**
Palliative or end-of-life care and bereavement support for families and patients were given as the most important service that needed to be offered. The social workers felt that many of the families and friends of these patients needed support to help deal with the loss of friends and loved ones. In addition, as a supportive measure, groups to address the loss issues were suggested helping family members to adjust to the serious illness or death of their loved one.

List of additional services
Bereavement, long-term mental health, government program assistance, specific diagnosis group counseling, parent support groups, sibling support groups, psychiatrist on staff, and palliative care.

5. **Are the services you provide generally short-term or long-term?**
The response to this question was spilt as three social workers reported that services were generally provided on a short-term inpatient basis, and the other three stated that services were available on a long-term basis. All the social workers agreed that it could be provided, but support and time to engage in this activity was what prompted three of the social workers to say that they did not provide this service. In addition, all the six social workers agreed that services could be available a lot longer to patients after discharge from the hospital if the patient and family follow-up improved. For these social workers, all agreed that although long-term services were available, utilization rates were low.

(continued)

(*continued*)

---

6. **Do you believe adequate services are available to children and families?**

   All the social workers believed that for the most part, the services provided were adequate to meet the needs of the patients and their family members. Two social workers reported that services were not available to the families, because their workload demands were prohibitive in this area. The primary concern the social workers voiced was that they wished that all services did not have to be tied to the patient. For example, a social worker could not assist a family to meet needs that were not related to the patient such as budget problems that were disruptive to the entire family structure. See below for a list of specific comments.

   Parents and siblings services
   - Available to siblings as long as it is related to the patient ($n = 1$)
   - Referrals are provided to family members ($n = 6$)
   - Family therapy sessions are provided ($n = 2$)
   - Counseling services are available to all members of the child's family ($n = 4$)
   - Services are not available to family members ($n = 2$)

7. **How do the patients and families you serve find out about the services that are available to them?**

   The social workers stated that there were certain patients they were required to visit, and this is how and when services were explained. These patients included all those in ICU, who suffer from *failure to thrive*; those who have been in the hospital for more than 6 days; those who are younger than 3 months of age; or any child who has experienced severe trauma or abuse as designated by the hospital on returned visits. The most common reason to see patients was because a physician referred them, and five of the six social workers listed that as their primary reason. It is during these visits that patients and their families were informed about the services that the social worker could offer (see the list below).

   Knowledge of services
   - Required visits
   - Referrals provided by doctors
   - Contact if they see signs of needing assistance
   - Open door policy
   - Services are offered at patient discharge

   It is hoped that presenting the opinions of social workers actually working in the field will help the reader create a greater understanding of what the social workers in this health care setting are actually doing. One of the subjective comments that these social workers acknowledged was that there was a desperate need for supportive services with this population. Yet overall, all six reported that there were not enough available resources to address the problems that

---

VOICES FROM THE FIELD: WORKING WITH CHILDREN AND CHRONIC ILLNESS (continued)

these patients and their families encounter from a micro, mezzo, or macro level. To add to this discontent, the social workers acknowledged that they often found difficulties in providing services along with patient's and family reluctance for utilization or follow-through on services provided. It is recommended that further research and study be done to investigate both the needs of these patients and the benefits from services currently provided. For these social workers, it is not clear why families are not keeping second appointments or utilizing referrals as given. To address this issue, more research in the area is needed. In turn, more information is needed as to what can be done to better educate psychosocial providers in the best methods for serving this rapidly growing population. It appears that the number of patients suffering from chronic conditions and life-threatening illnesses is continuing to grow. This unprecedented growth makes it absolutely necessary that an effective system of providing the needed mental health services, and additional needed supports services be developed.

Today's Health Care Social Worker

Name:	Yuhsin Lee, MA, LCSW
List State of Practice:	Florida
Professional Job Title:	Licensed Clinical Social Worker

Duties in a typical day

I am a social worker at a Homeless Program of a VA Medical Center. My job is to provide intensive case management service to chronic homeless veterans and to house them. My colleagues and I share direct outreach efforts to bring veterans who are in the shelters or on the street to the program. We also collaborate with local homeless shelters, transitional houses, community agencies, and the county legal system to identify homeless veterans. After a thorough assessment, depending on the needs and functional levels of the veterans, we make referrals for medical, mental health, or substance abuse treatment and/or provide affordable housing information, assistant living information, and transitional housing services. I also assist veterans to apply for Section 8 housing at the local Housing Authority, provide on-going

(continued)

(continued)

monthly home visits, and provide referrals for assistance with security and/or utility deposits, rent, utilities, employment, and other related services.

What do you like most about your position?
This position and the services we offer help to provide some stability to veterans and their families. Maslow's hierarchy identified food and shelter as fundamental needs of human beings and only when a patient's physiological needs are met will they start to deal with other issues in their life such as security, employment, love/relationships, mental health, and substance abuse and develop a deeper sense of self-pride. The program helps many veterans to transition into the community supporting them to go from transient and drifting to stable and productive. Many homeless veterans struggle with physical illnesses, mental health illnesses, substance abuse, and unemployment. In my position, I am able to help provide the services needed to help veterans meet fundamental needs while getting them ready for other tasks to better their lives.

What do you like least about your position?
There are a few veterans who are not happy with the services offered and show a sense of entitlement. These veterans feel that the VA needs to take care of all their problems because they served our country and refuse to believe that resources are limited within the VA. These individuals become very upset when they learn that they are not eligible for certain programs or service assistance. Also, the case management for these veterans, although essential to help them settle into the community, can be tedious and at times unrewarding work.

What "words of wisdom" do you have for the new health care social worker who is considering working in a similar position?
Working with this population can be difficult and may seem hard at times, but if you stay with it, I am sure you will find it to be extremely rewarding.

What is your favorite social work story?
A veteran went through 17 foster homes through his childhood, and over the years, he lost all contact with his family. He did not do well in school because of all the transitions and changes related to his experiences in different foster homes. He failed three different grades and never obtained his High School Diploma or GED. All he wanted was to join the Army as a way to

(continued)

Today's Health Care Social Worker (*continued*)

achieve stability in life. When he turned 18, he joined the Army and served 8 years during the Vietnam War in a combat zone. After his military service, he had several different jobs that forced him to stay mobile, and so he never really settled into a place of his own.

He started drinking alcohol at age 16 and has been struggling with a substance abuse problem for over 50 years. To date, he has completed five different substance abuse treatment programs. Owing to the nature of his jobs, he has stayed at hotels when traveling and has not had a permanent residence. When he did not have money to pay for hotels, he would stay at the local homeless shelters. In 2010, he rented an apartment in West Virginia, but after a few months, he went back to homeless shelters, because he "drank his rent money away."

Our team encountered this veteran through one of the outreach efforts at a local homeless shelter in 2011. We were able to provide this veteran a transitional house and subsequently were able to assist him to apply for Section 8 housing. He has been living at his own apartment since February 2012. At the most recent home visit, the veteran stated, "I had a very hard life and never would have thought I would end up with the great life that I have now. I am very happy and have everything I need. I am very grateful for what I have and there is nothing better than to have a home to come to at the end of the day. It is home sweet home." For the past 20 months, this veteran has been able to maintain his sobriety with a few relapses. He is also very close to quitting cigarette smoking and openly states that he finally has the stability he always wanted. It feels good on a professional level to see his success.

The role of the clinical social worker in the health care setting is a complex one. The responsibilities are often varied, and health care social workers must be willing to assume the roles needed plus remain flexible enough to advocate for change strategy that represents the best interest of the patient (see Table 3.1).

Supervisory, administrative, and community-based services go beyond the role of what is generally considered the core of health care social work, and remaining aware of this concept is essential for comprehensive practice.

Table 3.1 Core Services Provided by Health Care Social Workers

Service	Description
Case finding and outreach	Identify and assist patients to secure services they need
Preservice and planning	Identify and subsequently help patient/family to plan and gain access to health care services
Assessment	Identify patients in need of service, screening to identify health, and wellness issues
Concrete service provision	Assist patient/family to secure concrete services to assist with current and post health service needs, such as admission, discharge, and after-care planning and services
Psychosocial evaluations	Gather information on patient biopsychosocial, cultural, financial, and situational factors for a formal psychosocial assessment plan or report
Identification of goals and objectives	Establish mutually negotiated goals with specific objectives to address patient health and wellness issues
Direct clinical counseling	Help patient/family to deal with situation and problems related to health intervention needed or received
Assistance with short- or long-term planning	Help patient understand, anticipate, and plan for services needed based on current or expected health status
Information and health education	Direct provision of knowledge through instruction on areas of concern regarding patient/family health and wellness
Assistance with wellness training	Help patients to establish a plan to secure continued or improved health status based on a holistic prevention model
Referral services	Provide information regarding services available and direct connection when warranted
Continuity of care	Assist patient/family to be sure that proper connections are made with the linking of all services needed considering the issue of multiple health care providers
Patient advocacy	Teach and assist patients how to obtain needed resources or, on a larger scale, advocate for changes in policy or procedure that can have the direct or indirect benefit of assisting the patient

PROVISION OF SUPERVISION

Supervision in the field of social work has a long, rich history. Kadushin (1976) provided a basic definition of supervision:

An agency administrative staff member who is given authority to direct, coordinate, enhance, and evaluate on-the-job performance of supervisees for whose work he [or she] is held accountable.

> In implementing this role the supervisor performs administrative, educational, and supportive functions in interaction with the supervisee in the context of a positive relationship. The supervisor's ultimate objective is to deliver to agency patients the best possible service, both quantitatively and qualitatively, in accordance with agency policies and procedures. (p. 21)

This general definition of social work supervision applies well to the field of health care social work, with the addition of "flexibility" that is based on the reality of many ongoing changes in health care and how these changes can affect the health care practice environment. In the health care field, so many programs are under cost-containment restraints. This can lead to reorganization, cutbacks, and ultimately reductions within the workforce. Davis and Meier (2001) warn that this can be a particular problem for health and mental health workers, because they are continually forced to modify practice provisions based on third-party payers who refuse to cover services regarding what needs to be provided or issues with length of stay. This makes the role of the social worker and thus the supervisor difficult, because "whatever these programs are called, they all involve reductions in funding that can result in fewer programs or resources, more restrictive service policies, closing and reorganization of physical offices, and loss of jobs by attrition or firing" (p. 269). Therefore, no matter what the program or service to be delivered, training for successful health care social work in today's environment must emphasize a clear focus on controlling the rising costs of health care.

It is believed that the allied health professionals trained in this way will clearly reap the greatest rewards in coordinated health care. The flexibility and the changes required for practice survival that deviate from the traditional delivery of social work services often create a stressful environment for the supervisor, the supervisee, the organization, and the patient or family being served.

Scaife (2010) believes that *supportive supervision* in human service organizations cannot be underestimated. This type of supervision can help to address areas such as staff morale and work-related anxiety. If these factors are left unaddressed, they can lead to decreased job satisfaction and commitment to the agency. Supportive supervision can help to build worker self-esteem and emotional well-being. In social work, this is important as it can help to reduce the connection between high levels of stress and job satisfaction, which can ultimately result in employee burnout (Dziegielewski, Turnage, & Roest-Marti, 2004).

The National Association of Social Workers (2003) recommends that supervision be a combination of case presentations and education about these cases in a protected environment. The role of the supervisee is to provide information to the supervisor about assessment, diagnosis, and proper treatment of the patient. Supervision therefore has two primary objectives: (1) case management where the patient's needs are addressed, recognizing his or her situation and planning intervention strategy, and (2) to develop the knowledge and skills of the supervisee (NASW, 2003b).

The role of the supervisor, in turn, is to engage in a reciprocal dialogue where oversight, guidance, direction in assessing, diagnosing, and treating patients are provided, while doing so in a nonthreatening environment that is conducive to learning. In a survey completed by Kadushin (1992), supervisees identified the need for uninterrupted time allocated to supervisory sessions as essential and one of the greatest problems in current supervisory settings. This is particularly problematic in the health care area, where frequent changes based on program cutbacks can lead to organizational stress and forced decisions that may not be based on the best interests of the patient or his or her family being treated.

Clear goals and guidelines about what constitutes the tasks of medical social workers at the MSW and the BSW level are needed as both often provide services in the health care setting (Holliman et al., 2003). This lack of a clear definition means that supervisors need to be careful in assigning cases and tasks to be performed. When clear definitions do not exist, it is possible to assign tasks that are beyond the competence of the social worker and that can compromise patient care and worker stress.

In today's health care environment, the health care social worker is often called on to serve in a reflective role in mediation (Scaife, 2010). Here the social work supervisor does not invest into the opinion of any side; however, he or she takes a stand of neutrality of conviction (Shulman, 2002). Advice and direction need to be given about how best to handle patient care issues for the supervisee, the multidisciplinary, interdisciplinary, intradisciplinary, and the pandisciplinary professional teams (see Chapter 2 for definitions of these terms), the agency, and community. This may mean that the supervisor must be able to recognize conflicts that are not overt and help the supervisee to address them in the most professionally ethical and moral way possible. As an advocate, the supervisor must be willing to assist with the development of needed services to patients, their families, and significant others, while not losing sight of the common ground that links the supervisee to administration (Shulman, 2002). The supervisor must also serve as liaison to the community on behalf of the patient. This last role will help to ensure that connections are made and contacts initiated.

The last area in which supervision in the health care setting is essential is in health education and health promotion programs. This is not a new area for social work; however, counseling that focuses on this perspective alone is. Based on the importance of this function for health care social workers, other areas of this book have been devoted to the specifics of teaching health and wellness issues in the medical setting. Supervisors need to be aware that this type of counseling is not generally stressed in the practice arena of most social work training programs. Attention to learning how to conduct this type of treatment and, in turn, help those who are being supervised to use it cannot be underestimated (see Table 3.2).

Table 3.2 Core Health Practice Supervisory Skills

Service	Description
Direct social work supervision	Provision of direct professional social work supervision through direction, guidance, and education on case service delivery and counseling
Direct supervision	Provision of direct professional supervision through direction, guidance, and education in case service delivery as a contributor to the interdisciplinary or multidisciplinary team
Administrative supervision	Education and advice for social work supervisee on policy and program issues
Consultation	Provision of consultation services to other social workers and to multidisciplinary and interdisciplinary professionals
Education	Assistance and participation in training professionals to administer health education and health promotion programs

ADMINISTRATION AS A CORE SERVICE

Generally, administrative duties are not considered in the core practice area of health care social work. It is not the scope of this chapter to be all-inclusive of what is involved in this role. However, health care social workers who serve as administrators have a direct relationship to service provision that cannot be overlooked. For social work administrators, similar to other health care administrators, there have been competing management philosophies and issues that must be addressed. On one side, administrators have been told to increase the participation of professional staff members in agency decision-making processes as well as to improve psychological commitment and involvement with the organization. This is evidenced in recent literature that introduces and emphasizes the use of quality circles and total-quality-management principles for building a corporate culture that reflects the incorporation of individual and management goals for the good of a corporate culture.

On the other side, financial and economic pressures have caused health care agencies to become concerned about securing adequate numbers of patients to justify service. This means increasing competitiveness and maximizing reimbursement potential. This often forces workers to be terminated while increasing the workloads for those who stay. A "more-with-less" mentality prevails that is not conducive to increased quality of life for employees. Often employee development and other "services" considered fringes are curtailed.

Given this paradoxical situation, social work health care administrators often feel trapped. Administration and funding agencies often send double messages to the administrator. This leaves the health care administrator with

Table 3.3 Core Administrative Services

Service	Description
Agency consultation	Provide consultation to agency administrators on how to enhance service delivery to patients and organizations
Program development	Assist the agency to refine and develop new and improved programs to service patient needs
Quality improvement	Assist the agency to be sure that continuous quality services are provided that meet professional and efficient standards
Service advocacy	Assist the agency in recognizing the needs of patients and help to develop new or needed services
Agency liaison	Serve as liaison to the agency on behalf of the patient, ensuring connections are made between the patient, the supervisor, and the community

limited power that is often not viewed that way. Professionals and other service employees often believe that the administrator is capable of and responsible for sorting and balancing the true "reality" of the situation, and administrators feel trapped in the middle and unable to base their decision primarily on provision of quality patient care.

Noting that human service administrators do not operate in a vacuum is important. They are often forced to respond to pressures in the environment that can influence the decisions they make and the guidance they provide about formation and implementation of policy and procedure. Although administrators provide consultation to agency boards and funding bodies on how to enhance service delivery to patients and organizations, they are limited. Often it is the boards and organizational personnel that oversee them that have the power to replace them. This is why it is essential that administrators work to develop procedures for ensuring procedural justice, due process, and ethical decision making. To help the administrator refine and develop new and improved programs to service patient needs, quality assurance, or continuous quality improvement activity is recommended. This is one way that an administration can assure that services provided are meeting professional and efficient standards. Administrators need to advocate and serve as liaisons to help with the development of needed services for patients, their families, and significant others (see Table 3.3).

PROVISION OF COMMUNITY OUTREACH

Health care social work services from a community perspective are considered the third area of nontraditional core health care social work services often provided. Simply defined, community organization involves an

Table 3.4 Core Community Services

Service	Description
Service outreach	Identify unmet needs and services that are not available to patients; advocate for programs and services
At-risk service outreach	Identify patients who are at risk of decreased health or illness; advocate to secure services for them
Community consultation	Provide consultation services to communities to assist with the development of community-based services
Health education	Participate and instruct communities on developing and implementing health education programs
Policy and program planning	Assist in formulation and implementation of health care policies and programs that will help to meet patient need
Liaison to the community	Serve as a contact or connection person between the patient and his or her family and the community

intervention process to help with social problems and to enhance social well-being through planned collective action. The health care community organizer strives to help address community problems or areas where quality of life can be enhanced (Jackson, 2001; Morales, Sheafor, & Scott, 2009). Services addressed from a community perspective include (a) service outreach with the identification of unmet needs, with emphasis placed on creating programs to service patients in underserved areas; (b) the identification of the service needs for at-risk populations; (c) to provide consultation services to other social workers, multidisciplinary, and interdisciplinary professionals; (d) participation and instruction in health education and health promotion programs to serve the community better; (e) policy and program planning issues to ensure that the needs of our patients are addressed; and (f) to serve as liaison to the community on the behalf of the patient. This last role will help to ensure that connections are made and contacts initiated (see Table 3.4). From a community perspective, health primarily involves availability and access to quality care. For health care social workers, community practice involves acknowledging whether hospitals and clinics and the services they provide are available to the patients in the area, as well as advocating for patients in terms of prevention and wellness (Kirst-Ashman, 2000).

CHAPTER SUMMARY AND FUTURE DIRECTIONS

Social workers, whether in the role of clinical practitioner, supervisor, administrator, or community organizer, are challenged to understand and anticipate the trend within our current health care system and the effects this propensity will have on their current and future practice. Incrementalism, which is often reflective of current health care planning, involves compromising and engaging in agreements based on the needs/wishes of various political forces. The essential outcome that is often used to measure success, regardless of the type of service delivered to individuals, couples, families, or communities, is cost containment. It is essential that every health care social worker comprehend that control of rising health care costs will ultimately be considered his or her responsibility, whether he or she has the ultimate power to control this trend or not. Often, quality-of-care issues will be surrounded and ultimately influenced by cost-containment strategy. This is not to reduce the importance of professional practice placed on quality control; however, to survive, all health care social workers will be expected to help contain costs regardless of the role they are expected to perform.

This emphasis on cost containment increases the importance of the focus on two primary aspects of health care social work practice. First, there must be an increased emphasis in the area of the macro–health care practice perspective. This perspective calls for greater social action and social change. To accomplish this, social workers must understand the nature of the problem being addressed. Evidence-based practice principles can help in collecting the data needed to analyze trends. Once gathered, sharing these data in a clear, concise, and understandable way is essential for future progress.

With this format in mind, social workers must work actively to make society understand its responsibility to create and regulate the health care industry. Believing that the health care system will eventually solve its own problems is ludicrous. Health care social workers, no matter what role they choose for practice delivery, must help to develop and present a format for approaching the problems in our current system and for establishing means for addressing them.

The second area that must be ingrained into all areas of health care social work practice is *advocacy* that leads to patient empowerment. It is important for health care social workers to release the mind-set that service delivery and cost containment and the policies dictated by it are all bad (Jansson, 2011). The benefits of managing health care costs can be pronounced for both patients and providers. The changes needed in health care policy are substantive (Miller, 2008). Implementing fiscal controls can help to capture what some have termed our runaway health care system. These controls can help in providing more accountable health and mental health treatment by forcing clear documentation on the need for service outlined with specific targeted goals and objectives for brief therapeutic treatment (Dziegielewski, 2008a).

Within these stated benefits of behavioral health care, there are also many pitfalls. As a health care social worker, advocating for patients' needs to include helping health care agencies recognize the person in environment and the complete needs of the patient being served. Emphasis on helping to develop new, more comprehensive services within a coordinated health care framework cannot be underestimated. Advocacy that leads to empowerment requires that the health care social worker teach and assist patients how to obtain needed resources. In addition, on a larger scale, it requires that he or she advocates for changes in policy or procedure that can have the direct or indirect benefit of assisting the patient to receive the services needed.

Glossary

Advocacy   When professional activities are aimed at educating, informing, or directly defending or representing the needs and desires of individuals, families, or communities through direct intervention or empowerment.

After-care   Continued treatment or social and physical support of patient/client/consumer convalescence.

Allied health care providers   These professionals are often considered adjunct in the delivery of medical services. Professionals in this area include audiologists, dietitians, occupational therapists, optometrists, pharmacists, physical therapists, psychologists, social workers, and speech pathologists.

Allied health care workers   Professionals involved in health care delivery.

Almshouses   Places of refuge for society's poor, medically sick, and mentally ill patients of all ages. Historically, referred to as the "poorhouse" or place of death. Considered the forerunner of the hospital.

Charity organization societies   Privately or philanthropically funded agencies that delivered social services to the needy. Often considered the forerunner of today's nonprofit social service agencies.

Patients   The individual, group, or family or community that is the focus of intervention.

Clinical social work practice   Often referred to as medical social work (see *medical social work*). In this book, the term "patient" is used to represent the patient/client/consumer.

Continuing education   Training provided to professionals to update or enhance their skills and knowledge in the field.

Family counseling   A practice methodology that centers on the "family" as the patient or unit of attention.

Friendly visitors   General workers and health care workers who represented the charity organization societies.

De-evaluation   A director attributes exaggerated negative qualities to an employee.

Health care practice   The activities conducted that are designed to enhance physical and psychological well-being.

Health care social work   The practice of social work that deals with the aspects of general health, specifically in the areas of wellness, illness, or disability. The social work professional can address these issues by working directly with individuals, groups, families, communities, or through the auspices of broader social change.

Health care social worker   The professional "bridge" that links the patient, the multidisciplinary or interdisciplinary team, and the environment.

Hospital social work   Historically defined as the provision of social services in medical setting. Currently, it refers to the delivery of social work services in hospitals and related health care facilities.

Medical social work   A form of social work practice in health care settings with the goal of assisting those who are physically ill, facilitating good health, and preventing illness.

Nursing   A field of practice versed in medical matters and entrusted with caring for the sick.

Practice of social work   The application of social work knowledge, theories, methods, and skills to provide professionally sound, ethically bound, culturally sensitive social services to individuals, groups, families, organizations, and communities.

Public health   Tasked with prevention of disease and maintenance of health in the population.

Quality care   Quality care reflects the degree of excellence required in service provision. Excellence achieved is directly related to the degree of consensus and conformity that can be reached in the society providing the service.

Questions for Further Study

1. What are the primary differences between what health care social workers see as their role as opposed to other professionals?

2. How have the historical roots of health care practice influenced social work practice as we know it today?

3. What do you believe can make health care social work practice an integral part of health care delivery?

4. What characteristic of social work practice makes it the most marketable in today's health care practice arena?

5. How do you believe health care social work will be defined in the future?

6. How has the role of the supervisor changed over the years?

7. What makes the role of the supervisor in the health care setting unique to other areas of social work practice?

8. What changes can social work professionals expect regarding the provision of core clinical skills?

Websites

Clinical Social Work Association: The Voice of Clinical Social Work
www.clinicalsocialworkassociation.org

The National Association of Social Workers
Considered the premier organization for social workers.
www.naswdc.org

Health Care and Social Work Jobs
Job openings in the field.
www.quintcareers.com/healthcare_jobs.html

Social Work in Health Care
www.tandfonline.com/action/aboutThisJournal?journalCode=wshc20

CHAPTER 4

Standards, Values, and Ethics in Clinical Health Care Practice

PROFESSIONAL STANDARDS IN THE HEALTH CARE SETTING

Social work, similar to other practice professions is established and coordinated under a professional set of standards, often referred to as a "code of conduct." This code is designed to govern the moral behavior of those in the field. In social work, the National Association of Social Workers (NASW) through the National Delegate Assembly is tasked with maintaining and updating this document for the profession. It has been said that the social work *Code of Ethics* is one of the most comprehensive ever written and is often used as a model for comparison by related professions (Colby & Dziegielewski, 2010). The latest revision to the NASW *Code of Ethics* was approved by the Delegate Assembly and published in 2008. You will find that most state licensing and registration boards for social work practice also have a specified code of ethics that social workers must abide by.

In addition to outlining a code of conduct for the profession, another primary function of the NASW is to help establish, define, and describe standards for professional practice. In 1977, NASW and the Joint Committee of the American Hospital Association, in a joint effort, published a standard for hospital social workers. Later, in 2005, the NASW published a more refined and revised set of criteria reflecting all health care settings, the *NASW Standards for Social Work Practice in Health Care Settings* (NASW, 2005). With today's rapid changes and growth within the health care field, it is expected that further revision of these standards will soon be completed. Although NASW publishes these standards, they openly admit that the application of these standards is a voluntary process. Use of these standards can only improve practice and service delivery—if they are adopted and carried out by health care social workers and their employers.

According to the *NASW Standards* the primary principle that must be considered in service delivery is that social work services need to be an integral part of every health care organization. Furthermore, it is essential that these services be made available to the population groups that social workers generally serve, which include patients/clients/consumers (hereafter most often referred to as "patients") as well as other individuals, families, significant others, special population groups, communities, health-related programs, and educational systems.

To provide continuity of care within a comprehensive format, all social workers employed in the health care arena are strongly encouraged to follow these guidelines established by NASW for health care professionals. These standards include the following: (a) promotion and maintenance of physical and psychosocial well-being, taking into account a biopsychosocial perspective; (b) promotion of conditions essential to assuring maximum benefit from case or care management in the delivery of services; (c) addressing both the medical care and other related service needs of the patient; (d) ensuring continuity of care that addresses a smooth transition for services needs while addressing gaps in existing services; (e) promotion and enhancement of physical and psychosocial functioning, taking into account any temporary or permanent disabling condition that leads to an inability for the patient/client/consumer to perform certain activities and tasks; and (f) cultural recognition and awareness as well as the promotion of ethical responses when clarifying patient desires and wishes in terms of the health care received.

WRITTEN PLANS THAT DOCUMENT SERVICE PROVISION

According to the *NASW Standards for Social Work in Health Care Settings* (NASW, 2005), several core standards are recommended to ensure professional service provision. To start the process every health care organization needs to incorporate these suggestions and create a comprehensive written plan for providing social work services. This written plan should clearly identify the expectations of the health care social worker. When treatment is being offered it is always best for these services to be carried out by a graduate-level social worker experienced in health care. When available, professional licensure of the social work professional is recommended. This individual should track not only health conditions but also functional status of the patient's activities which relates directly to the patient's abilities to complete basic activities and participate in life situations (Saleeby, 2011).

The written plan should have a clear explanation of agency policy and procedures, and how they can affect the health care social worker–patient relationship. The written plan should also stipulate the types of services offered and how the delivery of organized services will be completed. Patient confidentiality should always be ensured. Outreach services and patient advocacy needs to be made in an attempt to identify patients and families that could potentially require treatment. Specific decisions regarding the types of items needed in each proposed plan will depend on the health care facility employed and the specific circumstances of the case (Kagle, 2002).

SUPERVISION AND DIRECTION BY A GRADUATE-LEVEL SOCIAL WORKER

The second factor to be considered is that the provision of social work services should be administered under the direction of a graduate-level social worker from a school accredited by the Council on Social Work Education. Here, the social work professional who is assigned the directorship of the social work program will ultimately be considered accountable to the chief executive officer of the administration. Although it may happen on occasion in today's practice environment, supervision by another allied professional (e.g., a public health coordinator) or related discipline (e.g., nursing) has been traditionally discouraged. If supervision is provided by a professional other than a social worker, a firm awareness of the *Code of Ethics* of the social work profession is recommended. Since different professions may have a different set of practice and ethical standards, awareness of social work expectations is essential.

The director of social work in a health care program will have varied responsibilities within the agency setting. However, generally these responsibilities can be broken down into two areas: administrative and agency responsibilities and clinical and supervisory duties (Munson, 2002).

As a health care administrator, the social worker will be responsible for administration and agency responsibilities such as agency planning, including the assurance that there is adequate space, budget, and deployment of social work personnel to cover the needs of the program being serviced. Social workers often need to advocate for adequate space, especially to ensure privacy when working with and advocating for the patients we serve (Gelman, 2002). Patient rights are always held at the highest regard and ensuring patient privacy is essential for service provision. In budgeting, social workers must become familiar with the technique of *line item budgeting*. This financial planning technique will allow the social work administrator to estimate a proposed expense for a given year as identified and compare it with the year before. For the deployment of social work personnel and resources, there continues to be a constant struggle to balance need with cost containment and this could leave social workers vulnerable in terms of eliminating positions for the sake of cost savings.

When working within a bureaucracy with specific tasks and goals and a clearly defined hierarchy, social workers may feel trapped. When positions are at risk of being cut, all members of the team, including social workers, may be hesitant to suggest new and innovative changes. These changes may involve additional work which may be perceived as unnecessary in an already over-burdened system. In times of change and flux, the bureaucracy and expectations for service may become more arduous. Policies and procedures may be adhered to more rigidly and may become a particular frustration for social work directors and administrators. The desire for new and innovative programs that result in more comprehensive service delivery plans could be ignored.

Since the social work director is often responsible for the recruitment, selection, and retention of program personnel, the director needs to strive to recruit and select work force personnel that are respectful and reflective of diversity. The ethical underpinnings of the profession along with the standards set out by Title VII in the provision of the 1964 Civil Rights Act prohibit discrimination in hiring, placement, and so on, on the basis of race, color, religion, sex, or national origin. The social work director will need to always respect these standards, giving them the highest priority. Ensuring the best selections are made may require additional time and resources. In a rushed and pressured environment, however, efforts to hire for the position as soon as possible and a surplus of potential candidates can make this difficult to address.

With numerous cultural and demographic shifts, inclusion of women and persons of color in recruitment and retention efforts is essential. With reliance on equal opportunity and performance profiles, incorporation of these individuals into the management-success process is further encouraged. For social workers ensuring quality of care while respecting cultural differences and encouraging diversity is always a top priority. This will also mean taking into account racial and ethnic health disparities as well as issues related to the lesbian, gay, bisexual, transgender, and queer population (LGBTQ) (Wheeler & Dodd, 2011).

Once an employee has been hired, it is the role of the health care social work director to ensure that an adequate employee orientation is provided. This orientation needs to help the employee to recognize clearly and understand what is expected of him or her in the job setting. The probable changing status of service, and the flexibility required of the employee, should be openly introduced into discussion. Providing the employee with an orientation checklist that the employee completes and signs will document in writing that the employee has fulfilled the requirements of the orientation process.

Today, in the health care work environment, it is common for *employment contracts or agreements* to be used. The actual form and content of these contracts can vary, but they provide either verbal or written communication regarding expectation of the job requirements and basic employer and employee rights. The director's dual role begins with assisting the employee to better understand what will be expected of him/her and how performance will be measured. In the social service agency, the roles and functions the social worker completes always coincide with the ethical responsibilities of professional conduct outlined in our professional *Code of Ethics*.

Second, the director has the duty to safeguard the health care agency by updating and modifying contract inclusions, and clarify any misleading or ambiguous agency policy or procedures that could be misconceived.

Furthermore, to help in this clarification effort, it is generally the social work director who is responsible for an outline of social work procedures and documentation of what is expected of the employees under his or her charge. All efforts to clarify employee contracts, agency policy and procedure, and any related documentation, will lead to reduced claims that promises made during recruitment or hiring were not made or kept.

After the employee has joined the staff, evaluation by the social work director will be conducted. This evaluation often includes the creation of *professional supervisory profiles* and should be conducted on a regular basis. It is helpful to structure both summative and formative evaluations of the employee. The formative evaluation provides the opportunity to provide ongoing informal feedback and correction with regard to the employee's performance. This affords the supervisor an opportunity to provide assistance in skill-building and assimilation into the culture of the work environment. The summative evaluation that commonly takes place at the end of the first 6 months is a more global look at the employee's work during that period of time and documents the employee's progress in meeting the details of the position description. In reality, it should be noted that often the director may or may not have direct responsibility for this task. The director may be involved in the evaluation of members of the interdisciplinary team; however, input from a social work professional, particularly in the job evaluation and rating of another health care social worker, is strongly encouraged.

Social work administrators are warned against engaging in the practice of *assimilation*, especially regarding diversity. In this process of assimilation, differences among employees are acknowledged to exist, but avoided by trying to steer away from diversity issues altogether, ignoring how they can affect job performance. In addition, social work directors must also be aware of and try to avoid a process referred to as the *halo effect*. Here, the director allows personal influences of one or more notable traits to influence the overall rating given (Barker, 2003).

This can result in an unfair *devaluation* (attributing exaggerated negative qualities) or *idealization* (overestimating individual attributes) of the employee. In evaluating employees, the *Hawthorne effect* that involves reactivity should also be considered. The term *reactivity* describes the actions of an employee and how he/she acts in a certain way due to his or her knowledge of being watched. The employee's subsequent behavior change due to his/her awareness of being watched may not be relevant to job innovation or changes.

Besides the administrative and supervisory responsibilities of the health care social worker, the clinical and professional supervisory duties cannot be forgotten. All social workers must maintain high-quality record-keeping services (Kagle, 2002) and clearly set standards for the evaluation of work (Reamer, 2002a, b). Because these topic areas are beyond the scope of this chapter, the reader is referred to Chapter 7 on record-keeping for more detailed information. Other clinical services include professional supervision, provision of continuing education, and patient liaison services (see Tables 4.1 and 4.2).

Table 4.1 Administrative or Agency Director Responsibilities and Tasks

Responsibility	Task to be performed
Planning	List budget, space, and use patterns of social work personnel
Selection of program personnel	Hire social work professionals considering diversity as well as professional performance issues
Employee orientation	Ensure that the social work employee is oriented to agency policy, procedure, and services and how this can relate to the profession's *Code of Ethics*
Evaluation of program personnel	Complete supervisory job evaluations that have clear objectives and performance measures
Procedural documentation	List social work–related policies and procedures
Assuring quality	Participate in continuous quality improvement and service-monitoring activities
Continuing education	Provide or make available updated training opportunities for the social work employee as well as assist related disciplines in securing information on the role of the social work professional and provide direct training for other disciplines
Community education and training	Assist other disciplines and the public by providing education regarding health and wellness issues
Student education	Assist in the training and supervision of social work students
Agency–community liaison	Assist the agency to provide support and education within the community setting
Support and development of patient-centered research projects	Evaluate and develop research proposals that address the needs of patients served, ensuring efforts for the worth and dignity of each individual

Note. These standards have been modified from those originally presented by the NASW (2005).

Table 4.2 Clinical And Supervisory Director Responsibilities and Tasks

Responsibility	Task to be performed
Clinical documentation	Maintain and oversee quality record keeping for services delivered
Clinical evaluation/revision and research	Use evidence-based practice measures to ensure practice efficiency and effectiveness Evaluate current methods of practice
Professional supervision	Ensure quality professional supervision is either provided directly or made available
Continuing education	Ensure that adequate educational opportunities (e.g., workshops, seminars, etc.) are made available to employees
Patient liaison services	Ensure that adequate linkages are made for patients within and outside the agency

Note. These standards have been modified from those originally presented by the NASW (2005).

ENSURING EFFICIENT AND EFFECTIVE SERVICES: QUALITY ASSURANCE OR CONTINUOUS QUALITY IMPROVEMENT

Job-specific knowledge for the director of social work service programs as well as direct health care social work providers. In most health care organizations, this requires participating in either a voluntary or mandated effort to improve and assure that the quality and cost-effectiveness of services are provided. Generally, one or more programs to ensure that this continues to occur is implemented through some type of use-review process often referred to as *utilization review*. With the increased emphasis on quality of care and quality of life, the utilization of the *case mix system* method provides a venue for improving service quality. As part of the efforts of a health care agency to manage *quality improvement* (*QI*) or *continuous quality improvement* (*CQI*), data on clinical outcomes are gathered and integrated in a problem-solving format. Once this structure for maintaining quality care is in place, the development of quality indicators is stressed, as it allows for the comparing of outcomes and best practice efforts. See Figure 4.1 for important factors for social workers' in the utilization review process.

According to Heeschen (2000), the use of clearly defined quality indicators can improve the quality of many aspects of health care delivery. Opportunities for utilizing these types of systems include improved survey outcomes, increased reliability, allowance for verification, and utilization of

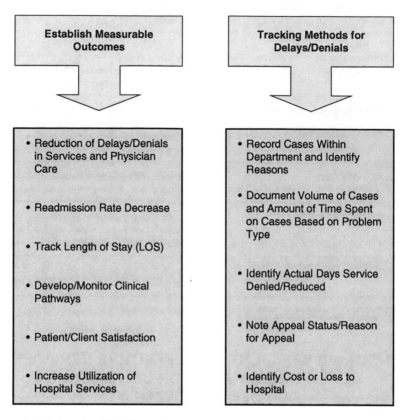

Figure 4.1 Factors in utilization review.

existing data sources for reporting. Also, standardization increases efforts for everyone, helping initiatives across numerous health care facilities to become more consistent in approaches to care. Health care social workers are often mandated to participate in and be responsible for a wide array of quality-assurance activities. These activities can include *patient* satisfaction measurements, use of services, reimbursement reviews, risk management, and due-process procedures.

No matter which activity or combinations of activities are used for conducting assessment for quality of services, it is clearly not an easy task. Furthermore, professionals and consumers may not necessarily agree on what constitutes "quality" care. Clearly defined quality indicators can help with this problem (Heeschen, 2000). Therefore, clarification is necessary on what constitutes quality of care, and at what level the society wishes it to be obtained and available to the people served. Today, this is further complicated by the realization that wellness or preventive services (which may have initial dollar costs associated with them) can head off problems that could be of future high cost to the provider.

Often health care social workers are asked to help with measurement of patient satisfaction. These measures can be obtained through interviews or questionnaires. Social workers need to be active in the creation of these measures to ensure that the patient being served perceives such measurements as nonthreatening and understandable. It is also important to note that, at times, funding bodies do not like receiving data regarding negative perceptions from patients served. The desire to satisfy funding bodies may cause reluctance to report accurate and clear reflections of the patient's perceptions when they are of a negative nature. The role of the health care social worker is important in helping to document and convey information about patient satisfaction as accurately as possible; in order to assist the agency in implementing changes and strategy to address the problematic areas identified (NASW, 2005).

In most health care institutions, such as hospitals, the process of quality assurance and use review procedures are often combined. Generally, controls for use review specifically address services provided to monitor and provide appropriate incentives to enhance the delivery of health care services. Services monitored generally include examining admission rates, providers, and services delivered; determining the appropriateness of inpatient admissions and usual length of stay; and the frequency of providing certain diagnostic and other therapeutic procedures. Often use review procedures can also be done across institutions to decide the appropriateness of the practice patterns at the agency (Heeschen, 2000).

Health care social workers need to be aware and remain active participants during quality-assurance activities. In this process, their role to serve as advocates for patient needs, to identify policies and procedures that are in need of changing, and program and service needs that are going unmet is essential. Social workers must maintain an active role in this process to ensure that they continue to be viable players and service providers in the health care environment.

Today's Health Care Social Worker

Name: Julie Gray, MSW, LICSW
Current Position: Supervisor, Senior Health Specialists,
                         Evergreen Hospital Medical Center
City, State: Kirkland, Washington

Duties in a typical day:
I manage and direct the daily operations of a geriatric medical practice owned by Evergreen Hospital. This includes providing supervision for physicians, a physician assistant, social workers, nurses, medical assistants, and support staff. I develop and manage the clinic budget. Additionally, I am responsible for process improvement projects in the clinic and ensuring that the clinic meets all JCAHO and Washington State Department of Health standards.

(*continued*)

Today's Health Care Social Worker (*continued*)

What do you find most enjoyable about your position?
The most enjoyable aspect of my job is helping our team develop an innovative model of geriatric medicine. One of our biggest challenges is to make certain the care we provide is cost effective, while at the same time, ensuring that the quality of care is not compromised. The obstacles seem enormous at times; yet, the rewards are great. Our stellar patient satisfaction scores keep me going on the rough days.

What do you find least enjoyable about your position?
The least enjoyable aspect of being a clinic manager/supervisor is dealing with various facility problems like plumbing disasters and broken fax machines.

What "words of wisdom" do you have for the new health care social worker who is considering working in a similar position?
I highly recommend completing a practicum in a hospital setting as a discharge planner or emergency department social worker. I also suggest that students take a course in medical terminology. Medicine has its own language and system of abbreviations; it is imperative that social workers have a solid grasp of the terminology so they can communicate with the team. If you aren't a student but want to enter the field of medical social work, experience in areas such as domestic violence, crisis services, and long-term care creates a basic foundation that will help you get your foot in the door. Be prepared to work weekends and holidays! For those wanting to manage a medical clinic, it is essential to have experience working in a clinic setting at some point in your career. Also, you must be able to demonstrate a career path where you took on progressive leadership responsibilities. Social workers can capitalize on their people skills and their extensive experience working as part of a multidisciplinary team.

What is your favorite social work story?
I enjoy telling the story about walking one of our patients out to the waiting room. She was in her late 80's and talked a mile a minute about her adventures volunteering at the local senior center. "My friends at the senior center say I talk too much," she suddenly announced in the middle of a complicated tale. Eventually, I was able to ask if I could call anyone to drive her home. She waved me off, smiled, and said, "Don't worry honey, I have my cell phone." Then, she sat down, pulled out a phone from her large purse and proudly called the taxi service. She died several months after my encounter with her. Whenever I am faced with a new challenge and start resisting change, I think about her energy and zest for life. She was frail; yet, she lived life to its fullest and never feared embracing new technology.

PROVISION OF PATIENT EDUCATION

Education is another important area for health care social workers to develop. Not only is providing continuing education important for social work and related disciplines, but it also is important for health care social workers to help in providing direct training for other multidisciplinary and interdisciplinary team members. Health care social workers can help inform or educate individuals and fellow professionals regarding the seriousness of a problem, or how serious it might become if left unattended (Kirst-Ashman & Hull, 2011). Often in this process, education is only the first step in persuading, thus creating a dialogue toward advocacy for your patient, the agency, and the community. Education as staff development can benefit both the employee and the parent organization.

All professionals need continuing enrichment and education. It is the responsibility of the employing agency not only to allow professionals to attend training, but to make it accessible to attend and sometimes cover the cost. When training is provided, having documentation of completion placed in the employee's file for future reference is important.

Important roles for health care social workers include serving as providers and facilitators of community education and training. If there is a concern to increase wellness behavior, providing education can increase awareness, leading to preventive care such as general physicals, immunizations, tests, and other procedures. In the health care setting, it is important to also consider providing educational services to student social workers as it is through mentoring and training that those students will prepare for their careers.

PROVISION OF RESEARCH SUPPORT

The final responsibility of the health care directors and providers is to participate in research studies and projects that will help to better address the needs of the patient. This area will be addressed in greater depth throughout the application chapters; however, the social worker with practice expertise is an excellent contributor to the establishment and implementation of research to measure both program and practice effectiveness.

VALUES, ETHICAL DILEMMAS, ROLE CONFLICTS, SELF-DETERMINATION, AND CONFIDENTIALITY

Most people in this country highly value a person's right to self-determination, privacy, and maintaining confidentiality. *NASW Standards for Social Work practice in Health Care Settings* (2005) is clear in stating that it is the responsibility of the social worker "… to be familiar and comply with local, state and federal mandates related to…" the use of confidential information (p. 18). In fact, not just social workers but all health care professionals need to maintain appropriate safeguards for ensuring the privacy of all patient information.

For social workers, ensuring confidentiality is a cornerstone of all intervention efforts. Each person has the right to determine to what extent personal information can be shared with others. Maintaining confidentiality requires an awareness of what and when information can be revealed, ensuring that patient privacy is held to the highest standards possible (Reamer, 2002a, b).

The Health Insurance Portability and Accountability Act (HIPAA) constitutes U.S. law and is designed to protect the privacy of a patient's medical records and other health information. For social workers in health care, familiarity with HIPAA is essential as this law covers the release of patient information to health plans, doctors, hospitals, and other health care providers. Having knowledge of how a patient's medical information is used empowers the individual to decide how and what information will be shared, used, and disclosed. Becoming familiar with this regulation is essential as HIPAA is specific on what information can be released and the protections necessary to his new rule.

Social workers should always check state regulations as some states differ in interpretation, but regardless, *NASW Law Notes* (2011) is clear in that if there is some confusion in terms of which one to follow—state confidentiality standards or HIPAA—always choose the one that is *most* protective of patient privacy (NASW, 2011).

Overall, protecting confidential information and ensuring patient privacy can be a complicated process, since there are certain circumstances in which breaching it is sanctioned by both state laws and professional standards. For example, in social work practice confidentiality may be breached with or without the patient's consent to report incidences of neglect and abuse (NASW, 2011). Other circumstances include when a patient may be a danger or harm to self or others, or when other compelling reasons exist, such as imminent harm to a patient, or when laws require disclosure (NASW, 2011). In the health care arena, most professionals agree that there are situations in which breach of confidentiality is certainly justifiable and expected. Yet, the principals that surround maintaining confidentiality are important for gaining patient trust and support. For the health care social worker, this can be a complex issue with many factors that must be considered in order for sound ethical decision making.

One of the dilemmas encountered by social workers is the question of the *duty to warn*. To understand duty to warn, the Tarasoff case is often cited (*Tarasoff v. Regents of the University of California*, 1976). Unfortunately, because interpretations of this case differ in regard to the therapist obligations for reporting, the exact course of action can be complicated. In practice today, the exact definition of what constitutes duty to warn can vary from state to state. Some states require that there is a duty to warn the person who may be an intended victim of a violent crime, whereas other states do not. In some states, there is a requirement for the disclosure of confidential information, but this information can only be given to medical or law enforcement professionals when there is imminent danger of injury to the patient or to others by the patient. Be sure you are aware of the laws in the state in which you practice and remember that these interpretations can differ across states (NASW, 2011).

Generally, the most common assumption is the belief that if the patient presents a danger to self or others that the practitioner must take reasonable steps to avert the expected harm. Since laws and expectations differ from state to state it is advisable to investigate alternatives in order to select the best course of action. It also may be helpful to consult with an attorney and make sure that the health care social worker is always covered under some type of malpractice insurance. Be sure to contact the malpractice insurance provider and ask for information concerning duty to warn. And, to verify the applicability to the state where the health care social worker is practicing, don't forget to check with the state licensing board. Furthermore, consult a mental health professional for advice or direction that is knowledgeable about the ethics of the mental health profession.

Regardless of what the exact policy is in the practicing state, appropriate deliberation and consultation with other professionals must be carefully documented. This is especially important when there has been disclosure by a patient to the social worker of a serious threat. Also, one question that often comes up is related to past criminal acts and whether these should be reported. In general, most states do not require reporting of prior criminal acts unless it involves a child or an elderly or vulnerable adult (NASW, 2011). However, it is important to always be familiar with the rules and reporting procedures in the state in which you practice.

For the field, maintaining ethical practice (including confidentiality) has been at the forefront in social work; so important, in fact, that in 2008, the NASW ratified and modified the existing version of the *Code of Ethics*. The importance and complexity of privacy and confidentiality is evident from the fact that an entire standard in the health care standards (Standard 4) is devoted to these issues.

The 2008 NASW *Code of Ethics* also provides lengthy standards with regard to privacy and confidentiality, clearly stating that social workers should "respect patients' right to privacy ... and ... should protect the confidentiality of all information obtained in the course of professional service, except for compelling professional reasons. A social worker should make every attempt possible to adhere to the rules of confidentiality and promoting self-determination, but as outlined above should also be aware when this is not possible and another action must be taken. In most cases where maintaining confidentiality is an issue, careful consideration is needed to determine what is sufficiently compelling to warrant a breach.

In health care social work, similar to all of social work practice, ethical decisions are not usually simple, right-or-wrong choices made without a great deal of thought. Instead, they generally involve choosing between two undesirable actions; and neither choice may appear to be the correct one, yet

NASW *Code of Ethics,* Standard 1.07, Privacy, and Confidentiality

(a)   Social workers should respect patients' right to privacy. Social workers should not solicit private information from patients unless it is essential to providing services or conducting social work evaluation or research. Once private information is shared, standards of confidentiality apply.

(b)   Social workers may disclose confidential information when appropriate with valid consent from a patient or a person legally authorized to consent on behalf of a patient.

(c)   Social workers should protect the confidentiality of all information obtained in the course of professional service, except for compelling professional reasons. The general expectation that social workers will keep information confidential does not apply when disclosure is necessary to prevent serious foreseeable and imminent harm to a patient or other identifiable person, or when laws or regulations require disclosure without a patient's consent. In all instances, social workers should disclose the least amount of confidential information necessary to achieve the desired purpose; only information that is directly relevant to the purpose for which the disclosure is made should be revealed.

(d)   Social workers should inform patients, to the extent possible, about the disclosure of confidential information and the potential consequences, when feasible before the disclosure is made. This applies whether social workers disclose confidential information on the basis of a legal requirement or patient consent.

(e)   Social workers should discuss with patients and other interested parties the nature of confidentiality and limitations of patients' right to confidentiality. Social workers should review with patients circumstances where confidential information may be requested and where disclosure of confidential information may be legally required. This discussion should occur as soon as possible in the social worker–patient relationship and as needed throughout the course of the relationship.

(f)   When social workers provide counseling services to families, couples, or groups, social workers should seek agreement among the parties involved concerning each individual's right to confidentiality and obligation to preserve the confidentiality of information shared by others. Social workers should inform participants in family, couples, or group counseling that social workers cannot guarantee that all participants will honor such agreements.

(g)   Social workers should inform patients involved in family, couples, marital, or group counseling of the social worker's, employer's, and agency's policy concerning the social worker's disclosure of confidential information among the parties involved in the counseling.

(continued)

(continued)

(h)   Social workers should not disclose confidential information to third-party payers unless patients have authorized such disclosure.

(i)   Social workers should not discuss confidential information in any setting unless privacy can be ensured. Social workers should not discuss confidential information in public or semi-public areas such as hallways, waiting rooms, elevators, and restaurants.

(j)   Social workers should protect the confidentiality of patients during legal proceedings to the extent permitted by law. When a court of law or other legally authorized body orders social workers to disclose confidential or privileged information without a patient's consent and such disclosure could cause harm to the patient, social workers should require that the court withdraw the order or limit the order as narrowly as possible or maintain the records under seal, unavailable for public inspection.

(k)   Social workers should protect the confidentiality of patients when responding to requests from members of the media.

(l)   Social workers should protect the confidentiality of patients' written and electronic records and other sensitive information. Social workers should take reasonable steps to ensure that patients' records are stored in a secure location and that patients' records are not available to others who are not authorized to have access.

(m)   Social workers should take precautions to ensure and maintain the confidentiality of information transmitted to other parties through the use of computers, electronic mail, facsimile machines, telephones and telephone answering machines and other electronic or computer technology. Disclosure of identifying information should be avoided whenever possible.

(n)   Social workers should transfer or dispose of patients' records in a manner that protects patients' confidentiality and is consistent with state statutes governing records and social work licensure.

(o)   Social workers should take reasonable precautions to protect patient confidentiality in the event of the social worker's termination of practice, incapacitation, or death.

(p)   Social workers should not disclose identifying information when discussing patients for teaching or training purposes unless the patient has consented to disclosure of confidential information.

(q)   Social workers should not disclose identifying information when discussing patients with consultants unless the patient has consented to disclosure of confidential information or there is a compelling need for such disclosure.

(r)   Social workers should protect the confidentiality of deceased patients consistent with the preceding standards.

Extracted from NASW Code of Ethics, Approved 1996, Revised 2008, Standard 1-1.07, p.10.

some considerations will outweigh others. For example, in practice, it is not uncommon for a social worker to have to make decisions related to maintaining the patient's right to self-determination and how this may actually cause him or her harm. In social work practice, ethical decisions often must be made quickly, but with sufficient thought and attention to assure the right decision is made (Loewenberg, Dolgoff, & Harrington, 2000). Furthermore, although helpful as a guideline, the NASW *Code of Ethics* does not provide specific direction when professional values clash.

The declared purposes for the *Code of Ethics* are to espouse ethical conduct and to control ethical violations by establishing guidelines of professional behavior (NASW, 2008a). The *Code states* clearly that, "Ethical decision making is a process" (p. 2). It recognizes that the decisions that need to be made will not always be easy or straightforward and will need to take into account all values, standards, and ethical concerns rank ordering them appropriately in forming an ethical course of action. These values, principles, and standards to which social workers aspire will place them in a position where, when they are judged, it will be done by a jury of their peers.

To further examine confidentiality in the practice setting, two studies in the area exemplify how ethical dilemmas arise in the field of social work with both individuals and groups.

A study by Holland and Kilpatrick (1991), conducted in Atlanta and the surrounding area in 1989, attempted to identify "dimensions of ethical judgment" used by 27 social workers (p. 138). All of the social workers held master degrees in social work and each had a different amount of experience in the field. Most of the social workers were female, and all were directly involved with patients. Holland and Kilpatrick (1991) contend that, to appropriately consider ethical dilemmas, social workers should be aware of, and not discount, their own and the patients' current circumstances. When ethical issues arise (e.g., fair distribution of resources or restrictions on divulging patient information) "information and skill are not sufficient to solve them. These issues require thoughtful analysis in the context of participants' values and commitments" (Holland & Kilpatrick, 1991, p. 138).

Their study focused on analyzing various ethical issues to which social workers are regularly exposed in their duties. In addition to defining, addressing, and resolving the issues, the participant's background and associations were analyzed, as well as any professional happenings that might have affected the respondent. An interview format was used to explore how practicing social workers comprehend and handle ethical issues, and their responses were examined in an attempt to recognize "common themes and differences regarding these issues" (Holland & Kilpatrick, 1991, p. 139).

The results of this study identified three dimensions that seemed to be fundamental to the ways that social workers managed ethical dilemmas. First, decisions were often based on a continuum ranging from "an emphasis on means to an emphasis on ends" (Holland & Kilpatrick, 1991,

p. 139). Reasons given for decisions made ranged from acknowledging laws and procedures to focusing on gaining positive outcomes for patients. In the second dimension, social workers made decisions based on interpersonal orientations that ranged from emphasizing patient autonomy and freedom to stressing the importance of mutuality. For example, many respondents emphasized patient self-determination over patient safety, while others justified denial of patient self-determination to protect the patient from hurting him or herself (Holland & Kilpatrick, 1991). In the third dimension, authority for ethical decisions was explored. In this area responses varied from "reliance on internal or individual judgment to compliance with external rules, norms, or laws" (Holland & Kilpatrick, 1991, p. 140). Many respondents based their decisions on personal self-direction rather than agency policy, and other respondents were more likely to follow the policies and laws (Holland & Kilpatrick, 1991).

Holland and Kilpatrick (1991) concluded that decisions made regarding ethical issues are most likely affected by prior experience, degree of professional developmental and situational factors that include the immediate organizational or professional context, the characteristics of their work roles, and the overall organizational culture. In closing, the authors observed that of the 27 respondents participating in their study, not one participant referenced the NASW *Code of Ethics* as a resource in helping make an ethical decision (Holland & Kilpatrick, 1991).

In a second study, Dolgoff and Skolnik (1996) investigated how 147 social workers made ethical decisions in the group setting. A survey instrument was used, which consisted of background information and seven vignettes with competing ethical issues. Each vignette was followed by an open-ended question, allowing for an explanation of the action needed to resolve the dilemma. The seven vignettes consisted of ethical dilemmas involving group self-determination, primary responsibility to patient, confidentiality, self-determination, informed consent, and authenticity. Also included was a list of sources that the participant would use to assist with the decision making. The choices included practice wisdom, *Code of Ethics,* another professional code, a particular philosopher or religious teaching, book or journal article, or other sources.

These authors concluded that the primary method used by social workers in the group setting for making ethical decisions was practice wisdom, which was highly influenced by contextual elements and personal values. In addition, the majority of the respondents sought compromise solutions rather than a specific "yes" or "no" type of answer. Similar to Holland and Kilpatrick (1991), Dolgoff and Skolnik (1996) showed limited use of the NASW Code of Ethics to assist with making ethical decisions, and additional instruction on the Code was suggested to better prepare students for ethical decision making. Although the two studies mentioned above do not specifically address confidentiality and self-determination, these previous studies do address ethical dilemmas in social work practice, and how decisions are made.

In a third, more recent study, Saxon, Dziegielewski, and Jacinto (2006) sought to further clarify the ambiguous nature of two of social work's most important values: self-determination and confidentiality. These authors created and distributed an open-ended survey instrument to 80 social work students after these students completed the required practice classes. The participants were asked whether they would break confidentiality based on a specific vignette and describe what decision was made and why. The results indicated that education (MSW versus BSW) and practice experience played a significant factor in the decision-making process and whether the respondent would break confidentiality. The respondents looked carefully at two factors in making their decisions: ensuring patient safety and self-determination. Regardless of the decision made, as supported in the Code of Ethics, it was clear that all social workers considered the outcome as part of a decision-making process that was not done haphazardly. Furthermore, the participants in this study recognized the ambiguous nature of problem solving in this area.

In closing, when looking specifically at issues of patient self-determination and confidentiality, managed health care has clearly affected the practitioner–patient relationship (Loewenberg et al., 2000). At times contractors may require patient information be reported back that could be considered in conflict with professional standards of confidentiality. Social workers may be placed in a dilemma regarding the NASW Code of Ethics and the contradiction encountered with information disclosure procedures of managed health care organizations (Loewenberg et al., 2000). In addition, technological advances utilized in current practice that stress the increased use of electronic data collection and storage may also put the confidentiality of patient information at risk.

Regardless of the exact impact of the managed behavioral health care practices coupled with the technological advances often employed, the professional decisions made by social workers are never easy and straightforward. This can create a new dimension that needs to be factored into an already ambiguous decision-making process where social workers cannot help but be influenced by either organizational or managerial expectations. These requirements add a number of complex elements to decisions about releasing confidential information regarding patients. It is not surprising that social workers would vary their approaches to maintaining confidentiality as they will continually need to adjust to the practice setting as well as the legal requirements established.

In the health care setting, there are no simple answers or clear guidelines that address ethical dilemmas with regard to decisions that violate patient self-determination or confidentiality. Maintaining patient self-determination and autonomy is an issue that must be considered with the primary importance being placed on avoiding self-harm when a patient is unable to meet his or her own care needs without assistance (Corey, Corey, & Callanan, 2003). For the health care social worker, it is important to remember that each individual and situation is unique and deserves careful ethical decision making (Saxon et al., 2006). Furthermore, the question remains unanswered as to whether the current process of ethical decision making is more representative of the "art" within the field of social work, rather than the "science."

As stated earlier, all social workers are expected to regularly make difficult decisions that in many cases have no "right" or "wrong" answer. Previous studies show that important social work values such as patient self-determination, ensuring patient safety and maintaining confidentiality can constitute an ambiguous process where there may not be a "correct" answer. This information reminds all educators and practitioners, particularly those who serve as supervisors, of the importance of including analysis of personal values and life experiences as well as social work ethics, laws, or agency policies (Loewenberg et al., 2000). If schools of social work and clinical supervisors spend little time on ethical content and decision making, social work students may be led to believe that learning about social work ethics on their own is necessary. Lack of information and training in this area can create a disservice to practitioners that will have ramifications in terms of decisions and resulting consequences.

In addition, there needs to be more discussion regarding the NASW Code of Ethics, focusing on how the code can serve as a universal resource for practitioners facing ethical dilemmas. The dearth of empirical literature regarding the issue of confidentiality suggests more research is needed. Since practice decisions are rarely based on dichotomous principles ("yes" or "no" answers), future research should involve a number of choices over a continuum spanning from least to most desirable. The continuum fits well with the principle of self-determination because most individuals prefer selection from two or more choices when solving complex problems. In this turbulent environment patient issues are often complex and multidimensional, and the greater knowledge and skill a practitioner is able to acquire in ethical decision making the better.

CASE EXEMPLAR

Marg, a medical social worker, could barely hold back frustration as the nurse called her to facilitate the discharge of her patient. The patient, a 14-year-old girl, was admitted the previous night. She had taken an overdose of aspirin and was kept in the hospital overnight for observation. The only thing holding up the discharge was Marg's signature on the discharge summary sheet. The patient had been medically cleared, and all members of the team were expected to sign off on the order for proper discharge procedure to be implemented.

Marg thought about her day and the five other patients for whom she had to find placement. She thought about the 45 patients on her unit, many she had not even seen yet. It would be so easy to sign the discharge summary and move on to the next patient. The nurse noticed Marg's hesitancy as she stood waiting for her to sign. "Her parents are in the waiting room; is there a problem?" asked the nurse. Marg knew what she wanted to ask, but she also knew what asking these questions involved.

> "Was it a suicide attempt?" asked Marg.
> "Yes, we think so," said the nurse.
> "Has anyone talked to the patient about it?" asked Marg.
> "Yes, the physician did," said the nurse.
> "Has anyone talked to the parents?" asked Marg.
> "Yes, the physician explained that she is now fine medically and suggested that they get some type of counseling. Do you want to talk to them about it?" asked the nurse.

Marg knew what answering this question meant. She had not had time to talk with her patient or the family. The hospital did not make a referral to social work or psychiatry for an evaluation; and even if they had, the quick and abrupt discharge would not have given them enough time to complete an assessment. Marg had been trained to deal with issues of suicide, and she knew that a rushed or avoidant approach to the matter would never be enough. Marg was familiar with patients who had attempted suicide and others who had succeeded. Marg knew what needed to be done to get the counseling prevention process started. She was also realistic and knew the time involved and the pressure she was facing to release a medically cleared patient. After thinking it over, her ethical and professional choice was made as Marg asked, "I really think I need to talk to the patient and the family before they go. Can you give me some time?"

ADDRESSING ETHICAL DILEMMAS

In the case example, direct application to the health care setting is made, making it easy to see how complicated such ethical decision making can be, even by the most experienced clinicians. For health care social workers, awareness and skill in formulating ethical decisions is critical.

The situation Marg faced is common, and similar to numerous quick and minimally planned discharges this hospital social worker was forced to make. The ethical and professional responsibility Marg felt to advocate for and assist her patient conflicted with the time demands placed by insurance reimbursement and use review standards. The approach of the other professionals on the team further complicated the situation. Many professionals, similar to social workers, also feel this pressure, and a type of role blurring occurs (Davidson, 1990; Dziegielewski, 1996; Netting & Williams, 1996). Situations like this often result in a "buff and turf" of responsibility. The process of buff and turf occurs when professionals do not accept responsibility for solving aspects of the patient's problem and either address them on the surface or simply pass the problem to another professional on the team (Dziegielewski, 2008b).

Although this case specifically involved a hospital social worker, ethical dilemmas such as this one are not unusual. All health care social workers need to realize and openly discuss the actual role of the health care social worker regarding performance expectations.

What social workers believe is their roles in the health care setting does not always match what other members of the team believe. Stated simply, often social workers and other professionals simply do not agree on the role of the health care social worker.

Often other health care professionals see the role of the social worker primarily as (a) an environmental manipulator helping the patient to adjust into the environment they will be entering after service discontinuance; (b) performing instrumental tasks (e.g., provide assistance for transportation and location of nursing homes, etc.); (c) being active in concrete service provision; (d) focusing on the discharge of patients and on creating outcomes beneficial to reducing lengths of stay (Berkman, 1996); and (e) assisting in problem solving to include assessing patient problems, examining possible solutions, informing and linking of community resources, and assisting with applications to obtain additional concrete services.

Based on these expectations by other professionals, it follows that social workers often feel misunderstood in the health care setting, especially because they see their role as (a) providing general counseling skills to patients and their families; (b) confronting psychosocial problems and identifying and addressing behavioral or emotional factors; (c) assisting patients and families around ethical decision-making issues; and (d) assessing, treating, referring, and gathering resources. Therefore, social workers can and often do perceive their role differently from the other members of the health care delivery team and when these interdisciplinary boundaries are crossed a lack of coordination can occur and increasing collaboration can only benefit this relationship (McLeod & Poole, 2010).

Although different expectations of the role of the health care social worker often exist, social workers still feel a need to be part of the system or the team in which they work. Resnick and Dziegielewski (1996), in a study of 144 health care social workers and other professionals who completed discharge planning, found that overall 86% of these professionals reported satisfaction with their jobs. It is important to note, however, that overall job satisfaction was linked to (a) finding purpose in what they do; (b) being able to see the outcome of one's work; (c) having contributed something to some patient's life; and (d) believing that what was done has benefited the patient served, Overall, Resnick, and Dziegielewski (1996) found that if health care social workers knew they were providing a service that benefited their patient, they were more pleased with their jobs and their own performance.

The role of the health care social worker can be a difficult and misunderstood one. Concrete suggestions to be considered in making the working environment more conducive to health care social work include:

First, developing creative and challenging ways for social workers to get feedback is important. Feedback after service discharge is sorely lacking in the health care arena. Some studies have shown that increased feedback can result in increased job satisfaction. This can be accomplished through introducing mail-back surveys, computer-based evaluations, scheduled telephone interviews, and utilizing other types of Rapid Assessment Instruments (REIs) to assist with identifying concepts and measuring concrete evaluation measures. For more detail on this idea, see the chapters on evidence–based practice strategy.

A second way to create a more conducive environment for health care social work is to facilitate and increase communication between referral sources and the health care service. This can be accomplished by implementing reply-transfer summaries that need to be returned to the original provider. In these situations, the receiving service would do a brief arrival note and return it to the sending service. For facility-based health care social workers, this can be further accomplished electronically by sending an update or the more traditional way by introducing patient follow-up issues into medical rounds that are generally a part of most inpatient units. This way the service providers can see the "environmental" benefit of their labor, and may be more open to helping establish these gains for future patients. For health care social workers not part of an inpatient unit or collaborative professional team, updates on referrals and patient activities from the referee are important for continuity of care.

The last suggestion, when some type of collaborative team is delivering the care (multidisciplinary, interdisciplinary, intradisciplinary, and pandisciplinary—see Chapter 2 for definitions), it is essential to facilitate increased communication with and between team members. For example, when a social worker addresses biopsychosocial concerns with the patient, this information should be related to the team. This type of sharing allows the team to see the benefit of this interaction on the overall treatment process. The logic is simple: by understanding the role of the social worker more completely, other professionals will be more likely to support and encourage its inclusion in service delivery problems.

RECOGNIZING AND HANDLING STRESS

In conclusion, regardless of the responsibility areas of the social work director or social work provider, handling excessive stress in the work environment is an important component that needs to be addressed. When social workers feel stressed, they are more likely to avoid the traditional patterns of expected behavior and indulge in more conservative and self-protective behaviors in this high-pressure environment, there are many areas where health care social workers can manifest stress reactions. First, they may choose quick unrealistic strategies or engage in anxiety-releasing behaviors such as venting their frustrations to colleagues to avoid dealing with more complicated problem-solving behaviors. Throughout their busy days, health care social workers deal with numerous health issues that could result in life-or-death situations for their patients. The pressure of an immediate or a quick discharge can result in numerous problems, as documented in several case studies throughout this book. This pressure must be addressed, and any means of professional stress reduction to avoid this scenario is encouraged (i.e., exercise, recreation that is nonwork related, and time for self). Taking care of the self is paramount for any helping professional to recognize. As selfish as it may seem on the surface, if you neglect self-care all the best laid plans for intervention will most likely be thwarted. One situation that rings so true with this author was when she was talking to a social worker about a recent flood that left her community devastated. The social worker stated that she was working in a make shift shelter trying to help a victim who had lost her home and could not find her children. At the same time, she was checking the recovery board every few minutes as she was not sure of what had happened to her own husband. As a social worker, however, she saw the devastation around her and put her own needs aside and stepped up to the plate to help others. This social worker said the greatest gift she ever received was the social worker who came from out of state to help with the situation. The other social worker asked her where she was from and when she heard she lived in the same area of devastation as the patient she was serving, she told her she was here to take over and that the local social worker should take care of her own affairs first and she would handle this. The social worker said she just sat down and cried she was so thankful and started checking the lists that were being posted without guilt. The lesson here related to self-care is clear. Take care of your own needs first as you may be too conflicted to help anyone else. The most successful interventions start with self-care and this relates to all professionals and emergency responders that too have experienced the emergency within their own family. Recognition of potential problems and some type of plan to assist those close to the situation always needs to be in place.

Second, strategies that involve risk-taking to improve patient services may be left unconsidered. This may lead to decreased advocacy for the patient and his or her family. Choosing conservative programs may decrease risk taking rather than picking less conservative ones that could create increased agency or public attention. In the behavioral care environment, the importance of advocacy for our patients needs to involve all related disciplines at all levels of health care practice (Lustig, 2012).

Third, communication patterns can be decreased, de-emphasized, or devalued in an attempt to quickly get a group consensus. Simply reducing the numbers of participants in decision making, or just letting the team decide without the social worker's input can accomplish this. For example, oftentimes in "patient care" conferences, there can be a delayed initiative to involve the patient or family members in the planning and discussion of treatment. Unfortunately, because of the time-consuming nature of their input, it may be discouraged, although it is mandated as part of the care reimbursement. In the case of a stressed health care social work director, a style of authoritarian management might be assumed that would allow him or her to gain greater control over the other social workers and the subsequent events resulting from the decision process.

A fourth result of stress in the social work health care director or provider can be more rigid patterns of rule concentration or importance. Here, the "rules" are identified and held responsible for decisions being made—not the decision maker (e.g., "I must go along with this because it is the rule"). This directly removes the responsibility from the director or provider and places the "rule" into a position where it cannot be easily addressed, changed, or reasoned with.

Lastly, the director or provider may be more likely to perceive routine tasks or decisions as more complicated and difficult to make than they actually are. This can result in procrastination or an increased emphasis on groupthink to solve quickly what seems overwhelming to the director or provider. Stress is a normal part of life. In excess, it can make decision makers uncomfortable and inflexible in their decision-making role. In the health care field in particular, stress is a psychological hazard that can cause distress and decision difficulty.

CHAPTER SUMMARY AND FUTURE DIRECTIONS

In closing, it is important to note that many health care social workers in practice today are witnessing unprecedented changes. For example, from an administrative perspective in the hospital setting, many private hospitals and veterans' health centers over the last 10 years drastically changed the structure and responsibility for the provision of social work services. The traditional departments of social work that were located in each of these facilities have changed. Social workers are often being reassigned to units, wards, or directly into service provision areas (such as discharge planning). Oftentimes, their supervisors are no longer social workers; rather, they are nurses or other health care administrative personnel. This has started to revert back but the process is slow.

The problems and limitations of this "splitting" are obvious. As a social work consultant, the most common complaint I have heard from social workers in this type of setting is that this splitting makes health care social workers feel that they are losing their identity and the strength that comes with having a solid departmental structure. Also, this lack of connection and delayed response from the professionals on the medical team can lead to case referrals where the problems are significant in terms of discharge planning or adjustment. This makes these types of referrals more time and labor intensive and much less cost-effective. Therefore, in the utilization review process where the emphasis is on service provision outcomes, being referred only the most complicated cases can make it appear that social workers have lower productivity rates. Others report that they are losing the camaraderie and support of having other trained social work professionals to cover for them, reassign work, and so on. In addition, the lack of direct supervision can present a significant problem for some social workers, particularly those who need regular visits and documented supervision by a licensed social worker to secure their own licensing.

Unfortunately for many, structural changes such as these will dictate practice reality. Although this change may at first appear threatening, it can prove to be positive. This structural change can be used to the advantage of the health care social worker to help open yet another door and gain recognition and increased importance as a part of the health care delivery team.

Coordinated Care: Domains of Change

Cost Effectiveness and Payment	Services and Timing
Outcomes for Ensuring Quality	Roles and Structure

The fact is simple, whether health care social workers like it or not: interdisciplinary teamwork is as much a part of the present as it is the future (Abramson, 2002). By being physically located on the unit, social workers can be recognized as part of the team and not just outsiders providing a service. These social workers will gain easy, quick, and convenient access to the patient and his or her family members. During the discharge process, in particular, this could be helpful. In addition to assisting the patient, if the health care social worker adapts quickly to this change, she or he will be able to capitalize on the newness of the situation and assist all team members in building group spirit and cohesion. This, in turn, will lead to greater unification and support for direct service provision and referral.

As stated earlier, the changes that have occurred in health care service provision and delivery, through the inception of behavioral managed health care, are unprecedented. This shift toward separation of social workers from other professionals in health care, and the movement back embraced by coordinated care, opens opportunities for recognition and expansion. In preparing for changes health care social workers will be expected to face in the future, the phrase "we have only just begun" seems most appropriate.

Glossary

Assimilation   When used regarding hiring and evaluation of employees, it refers to acknowledging that in the evaluation process differences based on diversity can exist and therefore can affect job performance, yet the director may either avoid or deny the existence of such factors when implementing decision making regarding the employee.

Budget   A record of funds, credits, and debts that is kept by an agency.

Bureaucracy   A formal organization with specific tasks, goals, and a clearly established hierarchy of decision making. Administrative and organizational procedures, rules, and regulations are clearly defined.

Bureaucratization   The recent pull for social organizations to become more rigid (centralized) in terms of policies and procedures.

Case mix system provides a standardized method or venue   For improving service quality that is to be used across numerous agencies and service providers in regard to service provision.

Continuous quality improvement (CQI)   In this method, data on clinical outcomes are gathered and integrated in a problem-solving format.

Employment contracts   These contracts can vary, but basically they provide either verbal or written communication of expectation of the job requirements and basic employer and employee rights. Requests for this type of contract are becoming more common in the health care field.

Equal Employment Opportunity Commission   Established by Title VII of the 1964 Civil Rights Act. Enforces equal employment opportunities.

Essential health care providers   This distinction generally refers to physicians and nurses as they are viewed as a necessary professional in the health care arena.

Halo effect   Where the director allows personal influences of one or more notable traits to influence the overall rating given.

Hawthorne effect   The prospect of change will produce some type of an effect without the change actually occurring.

Idealization   When a director allows an overestimation of individual attributes to influence employee decision making.

Incrementalism   Used in social planning, involves compromising and reaching agreements based on the needs and wishes of various political forces.

Quality assurance   Organizational procedures to assess whether services or products meet required standards.

Quality indicators   Concrete and measurable criteria that allow for the comparing of outcomes and best practice efforts.

Line item budgeting   Financial planning technique in which each proposed expense for a given year is identified and compared with the year before.

Title VII   Provision of the 1964 Civil Rights Act that prohibits discrimination in hiring, placement, and so forth on the basis of race, color, religion, sex, or national origin.

Use review A variety of mechanisms for monitoring and evaluation of the provision of "quality care" provided. See definition of *quality assurance.*

Utilization review A review process that is conducted in health care facilities, designed to ensure quality of care.

Questions for Further Study

1. What changes can social work professionals expect regarding the provision of core clinical skills?

2. What changes do you believe will be made in the standards for social work provision when they are revised?

3. What are some specific ways social workers can prepare for and address ethical decision making in the health care field?

4. What are appropriate ways to document disclosure of patient intent to harm self or others?

5. What are the different guidelines for ethical decision making offered by the various mental health associations?

Websites

Health Resources and Services Administration [HRSA]
Federal agency that is responsible for improving access to health care services for people who are uninsured, isolated, or medically vulnerable.
www.hrsa.gov/index.html

National Institutes of Health [NIH]
The NIH conducts research and communicates biomedical information.
www.nih.gov

National Institute of Mental Health [NIMH]
NIMH is the foremost mental health research organization in the world.
www.nimh.nih.gov/

American Medical Association [AMA]
The AMA promotes the art and science of medicine and the betterment of public health.
www.ama-assn.org

International Federation of Social Workers [IFSW]
An international organization of professional social workers.
www.ifsw.org/

National Council for Community Behavioral Healthcare
Advocates in Washington to advance the interests of members and consumers.
www.thenationalcouncil.org/

Society for Social Work Leadership in Health Care [SSWLHC]
Individuals seeking to promote effective social work health care administration
www.sswlhc.org/

PART **II**

Foundation Skills Necessary in Today's Health Care Environment

CHAPTER 5

Concepts Essential to Clinical Practice

Although the practice of health care social work has evolved through the years, the core concept in coordinated care and health service provision has remained constant. This core concept serves as the foundation on which all health care services are provided, and for social workers, it emphasizes the implementation of a *biopsychosocial and spiritual* approach to practice. This approach, particularly the focus on the biopsychosocial in its many varied forms, has traditionally been viewed as the basis for social work practice often utilized in the health care area to facilitate transdisciplinary practice and continuity of care (Egan, Combs-Orme, & Neely-Barnes, 2011). This approach to understanding the human condition helps the worker to view the patient and to understand that the patient's experiences result from the interactions among biological, psychological, and societal and cultural processes (Gilbert, 2002; Newman & Newman, 2003; Straub, 2012).

The purpose of this chapter is to present the concepts that are essential to clinical practice in the health care setting where the biopsychosocial–spiritual approach remains the cornerstone for which all intervention strategy rests. For the social worker in this setting, working as part of a collaborative team is expected while providing support for ensuring quality care services to the patients served. The view of the patient/client/consumer (hereafter referred to as the patient) in relation to his or her environment provides fertile ground for the delivery of comprehensive care.

UNDERSTANDING THE BIOPSYCHOSOCIAL– SPIRITUAL APPROACH

The biopsychosocial approach considers three overlapping aspects of the patient's functioning. The "bio" refers to the biological and medical aspects of a patient's health and well-being. The "psycho" involves the psychological aspects of the patient, such as individual feelings of self-worth and self-esteem. The "social" considers the social environment that surrounds and influences the patient. This mind–body approach to understanding the patient allows for the view of the medical situation through multiple contexts (Straub, 2012). When all three of these domains are assessed and addressed, the biopsychosocial model of practice intervention is being applied (Rock, 2002). For example, identifying all three aspects of the biopsychosocial model to the problem of "stress" is thought to be necessary to treat the problem comprehensively (Lawrence & Zittel-Palamara, 2002). In today's behavioral health care environment, this traditional perspective continues to be used with an emphasis on competency acquisition measured through behavioral outcomes.

In 1978, Regensburg referred to the biopsychosocial approach as the "wholeness, oneness and indivisibility of every human being" (p. 9). Engel (1977) further conceptualized the biopsychosocial model as a system-based approach clearly embedded in system's thinking; and Sperry (1988) applied it to treatment issues, calling it biopsychosocial therapy. Rock (2002) noted that the biopsychosocial model tries to integrate a view of the patient as a person-in-situation and indicated that this model recognizes that understanding biological factors is necessary but insufficient for "understanding a human person in a social world" (p. 11). When this approach is further examined through a life course perspective, age-related factors are all considered (Straub, 2012).

From this perspective, social workers need to remain mindful that the application of this type of model includes all three domains. Van Dijk-de Vries et al. (2012) note the importance of the biopsychosocial approach particularly in the area of chronic care and highlight the importance of not only recognizing its importance but also getting a commitment from all parties involved. It is important for the "bio" in biopsychosocial not to be ignored by social workers. The remaining elements of "psycho" and "social or cultural" were always highlighted and placed on a continuum, with the psychological aspects at one end and the social elements at the other. This artificial separation serves to fragment the fundamental perspective of viewing the individual from the wholeness perspective. Concepts fundamental to social work, such as "person-in-situation" and "person-in-environment," foster this sense of wholeness, making this artificial separation inconsistent with traditional clinical practice.

Gilbert (2002) has pointed out that although many practitioners may recognize the importance of a biopsychosocial approach, few may really adopt this approach in either their clinical practice or their research because adopting this approach requires a paradigm shift that can affect all aspects of practice. In fact, Egan et al., (2011) point out that utilizing this approach without taking into account neuroscience remains poorly formulated and poorly taught and can disrupt efforts for improved continuity of care. However, having an understanding of these three factors is essential in understanding the human condition within the health care setting. Each part should be weighed equally; and separation into its subsequent components is not as important as ensuring that each element gets the attention that it deserves. This is particularly true when that attention is needed for continued growth in the other areas.

Treatment may focus on one domain during the initial stage of the intervention and shift to the other domains during subsequent stages as the therapeutic process evolves. For example, if someone is suffering from an acute medical condition that must be addressed or stabilized for continued survival, certainly the medical (or biological) aspect must be addressed first. However, the social and psychological aspects of this condition cannot be ignored; and once the medical needs of the patient have been met, these aspects need to be addressed. Some examples of psychological difficulties include feelings of depression, the realization of being forced to face one's own mortality, and the struggle with life-and-death issues. These feelings and pre-existing beliefs can clearly affect the judgment of the patient and how their interpretation of the health services offered (Chang et al., 2012). Examples of social problems that may need to be addressed include occupational, recreational, or significant-other difficulties with family members. It is the balanced perception of these elements that makes the health care social worker's skills so necessary and unique in the provision of health care services.

Although most supporters of the biopsychosocial perspective propose the importance of these three primary areas, authors such as Rankin (1996) advocated for the inclusion of a fourth area. This fourth area targets the spiritual needs of the patient being served. The modified term considers a biopsychosocial–spiritual perspective. In this perspective, the spiritual component "focuses attention on the essential being of the individual, the role of the transcendent in the person's life, and the spiritual qualities of the belief system that person holds" (Rankin, 1996, p. 516). Rankin believes that by considering the addition of this factor, the health care professional is able to consider a much broader concept of the patient and the factors that can contribute to his or her development. Taking into account a spiritual perspective allows for recognition of the beliefs of the patient and how these beliefs will affect the care he or she receives. Spiritual qualities can affect interpretation of the health system and the services offered (Straub, 2012). It can influence compliance and affect health care at its most basic level. If a recipient does not believe that a certain practice is necessary or views it as invasive, supporting and informing the patient of the potential outcomes allows for informed choices. Providing this information on informed choices can result is an essential task for the health care social worker.

Biomedical Approach to Practice

The dominant model for understanding disease is generally referred to as the *biomedical model* (Wise, 1997). It derives its roots from basic scientific facts and focuses on the derivation of empirical evidence (Engel, 1977). From a traditional perspective, this model often considers disease as an entity yet does not directly recognize social behavior. This biomedical model is basic to medicine and the other medical sciences (Gilbert, 2002; Rock, 2002). It focuses primarily on increasing understanding of medical condition including its origin, signs, and symptoms with the end result being the subsequent treatment procedures, protocol, and prognosis for any physical health condition. Many professionals in the medical field, particularly those in family medicine, have long argued that the biomedical approach is not enough. When the biomedical approach alone is used, emphasis is placed on curing or resolving the patient's physical complaints. However, focusing only on the reporting of the patient's physical symptoms (e.g., wasting of muscle, loss of weight, sweating) leaves out the systemic and interrelated nature of the problem. Therefore, a more comprehensive approach that takes into account the biopsychosocial and spiritual perspective provides a more inclusive treatment model. This more holistic account also takes into account and expands the social aspects to include cultural aspects such as person's values, feelings, and expectations and how this can affect continuation of care (Straub, 2012).

Regardless of the limited scope of the biomedical approach to practice, social workers need to understand it to converse accordingly with other health care professionals. Familiarities with the medical terminology will assist the social worker to communicate openly and effectively both independently and as a member of the team. For example, social workers unable to understand medical terms or the jargon used in the medical field are at a significant disadvantage. Being aware of terminology and remaining aware of the problems that this lack of knowledge can cause will help the worker to avoid legal pitfalls that may result in litigation by a dissatisfied patient (Woody, 2012). Therefore, for practical and legal issues, the inclusion of this content in schools of social work is essential. Although there are complete dictionaries devoted to medical terminology, Tables 5.1 and 5.2 provide a brief primer to assist social workers in becoming more familiar with some of the basic terms, terminology, and medical conditions often used in the medical setting that are reflective of the biomedical approach to practice.

One of the major problems confronting a biomedical approach today relates to the process of the *deprofessionalization* of medical care. The essence of the biomedical approach to practice rests in the assumption that the professional possesses some type of special esoteric knowledge and skill that can be applied to the patient. In the past, the physician–patient relationship was rarely questioned. There was a great deal of faith in the specialized knowledge that only he or she could access that would eliminate a patient's pain or suffering. With the advent of an increased education and alternative professional

Table 5.1 Medical Terminology

Medical term	Definition
Abdomen	The part of the trunk that lies between the thorax and the pelvis; can include the pelvic area
Acidosis	A state characterized by actual or relative decrease of alkali in body fluids in relation to acid content
Activities of daily living	The general performance of basic self-care and family care responsibilities needed for independent living
Amputation	The cutting off of a limb or other parts of the body
Amputee	A person with a amputated limb or part of a limb
Anatomical	Relating to anatomy
Anemia	Any condition in which the number of blood cells, the amount of hemoglobin, and the volume of packed red blood cells are less than normal
Anesthesia	The loss of sensation resulting from pharmacological depression of nerve function or from neurological dysfunction
Antigen	Any substance that, as a result of coming in contact with appropriate cells, induces a state of sensitivity or immune response
Apgar rating	A score given to an infant to indicate the relative health of an infant
Aphasia	The inability to use language skills that were present in the past
Artery	Carries blood away from the heart (red rich color)
Carcin	Cancer
Carcinoma	A malignant neoplasm (a cancerous tumor)
Cardio, cardiac	Pertaining to the heart
Caries	Decay of the teeth (cavity is the lay term)
Cephal, cephalo	Relating to the head
Chondro	Cartilage, granular, gritty
Cirrhosis	Progressive disease of the liver
Cyst	Refers to the bladder, or an abnormal sac containing gas, fluid, or semisolid material, with a membranous lining
Cyt, cyto, cyte	Cell

(continued)

Table 5.1 Medical Terminology (*continued*)

Medical term	Definition
Degeneration	A worsening of mental, physical, or moral qualities
Derma	Skin
Dermatitis	Inflammation of the skin
Ecto	Outside
Endo	Within, inner
Entero	The intestines
Gloss	The tongue
Gyn, gync	Woman
Graph	A recording instrument
Hormone	A chemical formed in one organ or a part of the body and moves to another part or organ (can alter functional activity)
Hema, hem, hemato	Blood
Hepato	Liver
Hist	Tissue
Hydro	Water, hydrogen
Hyper	Excessive, above
Hypo	Below, deficiency
Hystero	Uterus
Ia, iasis	A condition
Kin	Movement
Lipo	Fat, lipid
Leuk	White
Logy	Study of
Litho	A stone
Macro	Large
Micro	Small
Masto	Breast

Table 5.1 (*continued*)

Medical term	Definition
Node	A circumscribed mass of tissue
Neur	Nerve
Oculo	Eye
Odont	Tooth
Oophor	Ovary
Orchi	Testis
Oste, ost	Bone
Path	Disease
Phos, phot, photo	Light
Phren	Diaphragm
Psyche, psych, psycho	The mind
Rrhea	A flowing or a flux
Rhino	Nose
Salpingo	Tube
Sacro	A muscular substance
Scler	Hardness
Scope	An instrument for viewing
Scopy	The use of an instrument for viewing
Somato	Relating to the body
Toxi	A toxin or poison
Tricho	A hair-like structure
Stom, stoma	Mouth
Therm	Heat
Thromb	Blood clot
Vaso	A duct or blood vessel
Vein	Carries blood toward the heart
Virus	A group of infectious agents that are capable of passing through fine filters that retain most bacteria

Table 5.2 Medical Conditions

Medical condition	Brief definitions[a]
AIDS	Generally a fatal disease caused by infection of the HIV
AIDS dementia complex	Impairment of cognitive functioning because of infection related to the HIV
AIDS-related complex	An imprecise term that refers to the signs and symptoms
Diabetes mellitus	A deficiency in the body results in chronic inability to create insulin, which results in too much sugar in the blood and urine
Diarrhea	An abnormally frequent discharge of semisolid or fluid fecal matter from the bowel
Emphysema	A disease of the respiratory system that results in continued episodes of difficult breathing and breathlessness
Epilepsy	A chronic disorder characterized by paroxysmal neuronal brain dysfunction related to excessive activity and characterized by the development of seizures
Failure to thrive	A condition in which an infant's weight gain and growth is far below what is expected for that level of development and age
Hepatitis	Inflammation of the liver
Hypertension	High blood pressure
Migraine	A symptom complex occurring periodically and related to pain in the head
Mitral valve prolapse	A problem related to the mitral valve in the heart
Multiple sclerosis	A common demyelinating disorder of the central nervous system
Palsy	Paralysis or paresis

[a]These definitions have been simplified and in many cases presented within a brief nontechnical context.

opinions, a range of options may call this authority into question. Patients want to have choices and participate in their own health care decisions as the blind obedience by the patient in the patient–doctor relationship is a product of the past.

Generally, most professionals now agree that in health care, a biomedical approach to health care delivery alone is not enough. The dominant conceptions of this model whether openly embraced can linger and still make incorporating the psychosocial aspects difficult (Meikle, 2002).

Therefore, although recognition of the roots of the biomedical model and the terminology that results remain important, a coordinated approach provides greater depth and understanding for all supporting the continuum of care.

Psychosocial Approach to Practice

In this traditional approach to clinical health care practice, the professional seeks to establish a relationship with the patient for the specific purpose of helping the patient overcome specific social or emotional problems and achieve identified goals for problem resolution and well-being (Barker, 2003). The types of problems that patients often encounter (as recognized by this perspective) include interpersonal conflicts, psychological and behavior problems, dissatisfaction with social relations, difficulties in role performance, problems of social transition, inadequate resources, problems in decision making, problems with formal organizations, and cultural conflicts.

The tenets of psychosocial learning theory were postulated by Lewin in the late 1940s. Lewin (1947) described three phases that patients must successfully negotiate to learn and incorporate an event. These phases include (a) "unfreezing," where a patient recognizes that there is a need to learn and becomes willing to incorporate this learning into current behavior; (b) "moving," where the patient participates actively in the learning process; and (c) "refreezing," where the learned behaviors are incorporated and subsequently integrated into the behavior scheme of the patient. From this timeless perspective, the therapist focuses on interpersonal and social concerns.

In completing a *psychosocial assessment*, the social worker summarizes the various issues that he or she sees as problems that need to be addressed. Oftentimes this assessment can include diagnostic labels, results of psychological tests, a brief description of the problem that needs to be addressed, assets and resources the patient may have, the prediction or prognosis, and the plan designed to address the problem (Barker, 2003). The psychosocial assessment can never be treated as a static entity, and the social worker must constantly change and update his or her appraisal to reflect progress on the issues the assessment is designed to address (Dziegielewski, 2010a). It is clear the health cannot be determined by one factor, and it is this interaction that sets the tone for problem identification and treatment (Straub, 2012).

BEHAVIORAL HEALTH CARE AND THE BIOPSYCHOSOCIAL APPROACH

The biopsychosocial approach has traditionally been used to integrate the biomedical and the psychosocial approaches to practice. Beginning in the 1980s, however, the demand for concrete-based services was required. This meant that a type of behavioral health care that focused on "outcomes" and performance standards derived in service provision was needed (Franklin, 2002). These clinical outcomes had to be related to the expected change that a patient would experience based on services received. This new integrated type of "behavioral-based psychosocial approach" provides health care social workers a theory base that can be used to support the services and interventions they provide. In addition, the focus on behavioral outcomes further attracts funding agencies, providing a basis for measuring service effectiveness and accountability. Similar to any method of practice, it does not answer every question or concretely address each possible situation. It is an abstraction or guideline that can be used to guide practice—in what could otherwise be a complicated process (Dziegielewski, 2010a).

The use of the biopsychosocial approach based in behavioral outcomes continues to have merit in practice delivery. All other disciplines involved in health care delivery understand and recognize the importance of this approach. Because the biopsychosocial approach is valued by other professions, social workers are able to provide leadership in understanding the "psycho" and "social" factors impacting patients (Rock, 2002). In addition, the emphasis in today's health care environment on maintaining health and wellness provide avenues for social workers to assume leadership roles (Dziegielewski, 2010a, 2010b). Here, the input of the social worker can be viewed as essential in predicting, anticipating, and developing ways to address probable health issues that may arise. The value of this input is contingent on the value others place on the behavioral biopsychosocial perspective within the current chronic care model of treating illness.

Today, there are believed to be a multiplicity of factors that contribute to health and wellness that must be addressed. From this perspective, it is clear that some life circumstances and social processes have more relevance than others (Lee & Motzaku, 2012). Although service may be rushed the social worker needs to always take the time to establish rapport with the patient. Establishing rapport is time well spent as it can serve to speed up the therapeutic process (Shulman, 2002). From this perspective, service provision focusing on health and wellness will need to provide a continuum of service, making the role of the social workers role consistent and comprehensive.

A coordinated behavioral biopsychosocial approach provides a firm basis for health care social workers to practice in today's turbulent environment. In practice, this model is consistent with competent and ethical social work practice as it works within current treatment restraints while emphasizing patient empowerment and self-determination. On the basis of competition from other allied health professionals, health care social workers, now more than ever, need to emphasize and rely on the strength of our practice profession—remaining an active member in the planning process for the patient.

Unfortunately, in adhering to this model, there are negative factors that need to be discussed. One problem embedded in this method of service delivery is the hierarchy of power that the approach assumes. From a behavioral biopsychosocial approach housed in the medical model, the primary care physician remains the gatekeeper and typically has the discretion in planning and referral for the general welfare of the patient. He or she is generally given service-entry decision-making power, whether it is based on an individual, multidisciplinary, or interdisciplinary team approach. Although these decisions are influenced by the factors that surround the patient's situation (i.e., medical condition, service availability, reimbursement potential, and team members suggestion), the entry to service and in many cases ultimate responsibility rest with the primary care physician. This power to make final decisions regarding patient care can often allow him or her to determine the ultimate course of treatment. In this model, the health care social worker is bound by the physician's decision—even when these decisions involve psychological or social issues.

A second possible problem with the behavioral biopsychosocial model stems from the blurring and mixing of tasks that professionals who subscribe to this method of service delivery provide. Ambiguous role definition allows other professionals to see themselves as performing the same function as social workers (Holliman et al., 2001). In some instances, this has led to other professionals actually being ascribed the tasks that were initially considered the role of the social worker. The problem with the psychosocial area of delivery is that the tasks performed do overlap and can be varied in relation to the patient need. Therefore, social workers need to remain active in establishing their "turf" and the actual roles and services they perform.

COLLABORATION AMONG HEALTH CARE PROFESSIONALS

Social workers are only one part of a unified health care delivery team. Social workers are expected to work together with other professionals to ensure that the best possible care is provided. In the health care arena, every patient, whether an individual, a family, or a group, must have an individualized plan for service delivery. The established plan that is reflective of the biopsychosocial–spiritual approach to practice must address the needs of the patient regarding the current problem as well as prepare for continued health and wellness.

One important way that social workers differ from other professions providing health care is their training. Social workers are generally trained to provide a large range of professional services in diverse settings. Although training requirements vary, most health care professionals—regardless of specialty—are trained to work exclusively in the health care field. Many of the collaborative efforts that social workers make with other professionals may be colored by the fact that these professionals are trained in a narrower field of practice. The training the social worker receives and the varied job expectations of this professional help the social worker to provide the diverse forms of helping that is needed in the health care field. However, it can be confusing to other professionals who do not understand exactly what it is that social workers do—or to professionals who put less emphasis on accepting psychosocial interventions as an essential part of medical intervention.

Striving to obtain a clear definition of what the health care social worker does can help lay the groundwork for acceptance as part of the team by the other professionals. In case management, social workers may be trained in a broader area than health care alone; the roles and services they provide in the health care field are often similar to other helping professionals. The similarities in professional training and purpose among health care professionals make struggles and competition for a unique service delivery niche more difficult. For example, social work has generally been viewed as the discipline that spans all areas of the health care continuum. Today, nursing is active in advocating for an expanded role for nurses similar to that of what was once believed the domain of social work and continue to advocate for involvement in every aspect of patient care from primary, secondary, and tertiary services to mental health issues.

There are several forms of collaborative practice in which social workers in health care settings engage. The first is a type of *case-by-case collaboration*. Carlton (1984) describes this as practitioners from different disciplines coming together to share and participate in a mode of service delivery or an individualized intervention plan designed to assist the patient, family, or community in need. Generally, this form of collaboration is considered the oldest and most commonly occurring. It may be conducted on a formal or an informal basis.

A second form of collaboration between health care professionals is *consultation*. The National Association of Social Workers (NASW) defines consultation as the provision of expert advice that can either be accepted or rejected by the consultee (National Council on Practice of Clinical Social Work, 1994). Caplan (1970) defines consultation as a process of interaction between two professional persons; where one is viewed as an expert who is called on to help the other regarding current work problems. In social work, the NASW practice standard number 7 for the NASW *Practice Standards of Clinical Social Work* (currently soon to be revised in 2012) recommends that social workers with at least 5 or more years of clinical practice experience still consider using consultation on an as-needed or self-determined basis. Basically, the consultant is considered an expert in the area, and the consultee seeks the expert's advice. However, although the consultee seeks the clinical advice of the consultant, he or she is not obligated to follow it or incorporate any of the ideas shared into the treatment context (National Council on Practice of Clinical Social Work, 1994). This identifies one of the major differences between professional supervision and consultation. Consequently, a supervisor could be sued for the mistakes a supervisee makes, but it would be difficult to sue a consultant for this because it is up to the professional consultee whether the consultant's input is adopted or not.

A third form of collaborative effort is the provision of strengths-based patient *education*. In this form of collaboration, the social worker offers his or her expertise to train other health care providers. When engaging in education to nonsocial work professionals, three fundamental kinds of knowledge need to be possessed by the social work practitioner/educator. All education efforts start with empowerment, and this means knowing the discipline of social work itself; being able to understand and incorporate the values and apply the skills inherent in the area of health care social work practice. Second, when educating consumers, social workers need to be aware of the professional standards to which those being educated must subscribe. Understanding the ethics and values of the profession will help the social worker to better address and anticipate service-delivery needs. Finally, social workers need to know how to educate and how to impart information to others effectively. They need to be skilled in different methods of teaching and aware of different learning styles. They also need to understand the patient's individual and family systems building on his/her self-help and identifying helping networks already part of the patient's system.

The last type of collaborative effort is the *team approach*, which includes the multidisciplinary, interdisciplinary, and transdisciplinary team concepts as they all can play an important role. In these collaborative team efforts, it appears evident that other disciplines are now moving into new areas and performing many of the tasks that used to be considered the domain of the health care social worker. Social workers can still maintain viable players in this arena, however. In today's practice environment, the collaborative team efforts among health care professionals to serve the patient better are expected. Collaboration of services is a product of our current health care system that does not appear to be wanting.

One important factor that helps in the marketability and service utility of the social worker is that they are cost-effective. In reality, even though many of the other health care professionals can do a similar job to the health care social worker, the social worker can be important in the cost-savings to the agency or the patient. This makes social workers viable and attractive team members regarding efficiency and cost-effectiveness of service provision.

Multidisciplinary Teams

The term *multidisciplinary* can best be explained by dividing it into its two roots, "multi" and "discipline." Simply stated, "multi" means many or multiple professionals. "Discipline" means the field of study in which a professional engages. When these two terms are put together, it, therefore, refers to "representatives of more than one discipline directing their efforts toward a common problem" (Carlton, 1984, p. 126).

The multidisciplinary team (MT) is composed of a mix of health and social welfare professionals, with each discipline in most part working on an independent or a referral basis (Siple, 1994, p. 50).

Generally, the multidisciplinary team is composed of several different health and social welfare professionals. These professionals can include physicians, nurses, social workers, physical therapists, and so on. Each of these professionals generally works independently to solve the problems of the individual. Afterward, these opinions and separate approaches are brought together to provide a comprehensive method of service delivery for the patient. The role of each professional on the team is usually clearly defined, and each team member knows the role and duties that they are expected to contribute. Many times, communication between the professionals is stressed, and goals are expected to be consistent across the disciplines, with each contributing to the overall welfare of the patient. The multidisciplinary team approach seems to be losing its appeal in today's health care environment, and inclusion of a more collaborative and integrative approach is being highlighted.

Interdisciplinary Teams

In today's health care environment, a transition appears to have occurred, de-emphasizing the multidisciplinary team concept of the past, while encouraging the continued development of interdisciplinary teams.

The interdisciplinary team (IT) also consists of a variety of health care professionals, but in this model different skills and expertise are brought together to provide more effective, better coordinated, and improved quality of services for patients (Siple, 1994, p. 50). In health care service, "when patients are different, services are similar, and the size of the service delivery organization is inadequate to justify a great deal of specialization, the primary need is for expertise in dealing with patient differences" (Duncan, Ginter, & Swayne, 1992, p. 341). This makes the role of the interdisciplinary team both convenient and cost-effective to health care administrators.

Anticipating the continued emphasis that will be placed on this team approach, Carlton (1984) used the term interdisciplinary interchangeably with collaboration. Carlton believed that collaboration in the true sense of its definition meant "two or more practitioners from two or more fields of learning and activity, who fill distinct roles, perform specialized tasks, and work in an interdependent relationship toward the achievement of a common purpose" (p. 129). This, in turn, is the same definition that can be applied to the interdisciplinary team.

The interdisciplinary team, similar to the multidisciplinary team, consists of a variety of health care professionals. The major difference between the multidisciplinary approach and the interdisciplinary approach is that the latter takes on a much more holistic approach to health care practice. Interdisciplinary professionals work together throughout the process of service provision (Abramson, 2002). Generally, all members of the team develop a plan of action collectively. In service provision, the skills and techniques that each professional provide can and often do overlap. A combining of effort similar to the multidisciplinary team is achieved; however, inter-dependence throughout the referral, assessment, treatment, and planning process is stressed. This is different from the multidisciplinary team, where assessments and evaluations are often completed in isolation and later shared. In the interdisciplinary team process, each professional team member is encouraged to contribute, design, and implement the group goals for the health care service to be provided.

For successful interdisciplinary practice, the following factors should always be considered: (1) recognize the values and ethics of the profession; (2) take into account the individual and the environment; and (3) recognize and understand the interdependency of practice and the contributions and expertise of colleagues that support the helping process. These elements are relevant to multidisciplinary or interdisciplinary teams, regardless of the model employed.

Transdisciplinary Teams and Pandisciplinary Teams

Two newer forms of teams identified in the health care literature are transdisciplinary and pandisciplinary teams. In its most simple definition, the *transdisciplinary team* is a group of health care professionals and nonprofessionals that freely share ideas and work together as a synergistic whole where ideas and sharing of responsibilities is a common place in routine care. Bruder (1994) defined it as an approach where team members share roles and work systematically across discipline boundaries. Very similar to the interdisciplinary team, this method of collaboration highlights the sharing of information and skills across team members and should always include the person and the family in the intervention efforts. The team meetings are planned and held on a regularly scheduled basis, and the input of all professionals and nonprofessionals are all considered part of the team approach. Somewhat different from the interdisciplinary team in that the individual and those that make up the family system are always considered a part of the educational and treatment team.

The *pandisciplinary team* is a more specialized team where a group of health care professionals work together in a specialized area. This is a very specialized team of professionals where each member of the team is seen as equal in the delivery of care with similar skills for assisting the patient. There are no distinctions, and the professional is considered an expert in the area in which he or she works and generally not linked to a professional field. For example, if working in geriatrics, all individuals would be considered a skilled professional listed by subject area rather profession.

Quality Improvement Teams

In today's health care environment, health care organizations are faced with conflicting demands. The public demands quality service provision, that organizations and the health care professionals who serve them be innovative, that they deliver high-quality care, and that they do this while containing costs. Often quality of care and containing costs can be conflictive, if not mutually exclusive (Gibelman, 2002). This challenges health care organizations and the professionals who serve them to develop new and innovative ways of balancing these two factors. With the problems in the current models of the delivery of care, new methods of delivery are emerging. Behavioral health providers are working together to create a better fit between the patient creating a model of care that is most comprehensive to his or her needs while taking into account the financial restraints indicative of the times (Fox, Hodgson, & Lamson, 2012).

Although we typically think of hospitals as the setting where measuring quality of care and establishing quality assessment teams are most important, they are not the only health care delivery organizations that are affected by these processes. The need for quality assurance, sometimes referred to as quality improvement (QI), transcends all health service delivery organizations and includes coordinated care agencies, clinics in medically underserved areas, rural locations, administrative and headquarter operations, nursing homes, hospices, and group homes. Social workers and other health care professionals will most assuredly serve in this capacity in some way as the programs and services they deliver are evaluated. All medical, health, mental health, rehabilitation, disease prevention, and health promotion programs need to be monitored.

QI processes and *continuous quality improvement* (CQI) were originally most popular in the manufacturing world rather than health care (Statit Quality Software, 2007). With rising costs and the fact that the underlying foundation of medicine is similar in terms of isolating variables, changing the process, and measuring the outcome, it is no surprise that CQI has gained a prominent role in health care delivery. Because almost all programs and services offered in the area of health care delivery are evaluated, positive results for measuring success are expected.

To assist programs to meet these societal and economic demands, many health care organizations are now implementing *continuous improvement* (CI) teams. These teams are formed to solve specific problems. They take knowledge and insight from several different areas, including statistics, operation management, organizational theory, strategic planning, information management, and service delivery (Batalden, Mohr, Strosberg, & Baker, 1995). Team membership and actual function may vary based on the health care service delivered; however, those chosen to participate in the team must have some *stakehold* in the service that is being delivered. This means that the participants can benefit from timely and cost-effective solutions to the problem with service delivery under investigation. In the past, one reason for failure in attributing CI teams was related to trying to implement it at the upper level of health care management rather than with the workers who are the most involved (Schalowitz, 1995). To address this weakness, organizations are encouraged to create teams that consist of both management and practice professionals.

Hart, Coady, and Halvorson (1995) continued to emphasize the importance of implementation of a team concept and described the professionals that should participate on the teams. The first member of the team, and surely the most important, is the *team leader*. Traditionally, social workers have not been overtly active in this process, although their involvement has been inevitable. Although not referred to by Hart et al. (1995), it is as the team leader that the health care social worker can be best used—assuming this role will allow the health care social worker to become an active and leading member in the workings of the QI health care delivery team.

In general, it is expected that the team leader be active in leadership and involvement in all areas of service delivery. The team leader must also be skilled in the political, social, and cultural environment to anticipate and initiate changes that need to be made. "The call for universal health care coverage with dramatic expansion of resource use becomes a significant challenge to health care leadership. Their ability [the leader] to proactively lead this effort and to simultaneously engage the delivery system in change is a significant challenge" (Hart et al., 1995, p. 61), and a challenge that social workers have always embraced. The diversity of the activities of the health care social worker makes him or her an excellent candidate for this leadership role.

To prepare for assuming this role, health care social workers need to be educated in the concepts of CQI methods. The skills they possess, with the general knowledge base from which they operate, make them excellent choices for leadership in this area. Although it is beyond the scope of this book to explain the entire QI process, its importance in the teaching and preparing of social workers who choose to practice in the health care arena should not be underestimated. To facilitate preparation for health care professionals as team leaders, professional training in this area is needed. Recognition of this knowledge and skill needs to be offered in all training programs for professionals. Schools of social work need to adapt this as part of training, particularly for those who choose to specialize in the area of health. Whether social workers serve as team leaders or merely as team members, they will undoubtedly be expected to participate in these teams. To participate actively and productively, professional education in this area will be essential. In addition, Guild (2012) reminds us of the importance of the roots of the profession and with the environment and our economy in such a state of depression advocacy on a social and political level is also needed.

Once the team leader has been selected, the members of the team must all work together for the common good of the patients served. It is here that the role of the physician is considered essential as a member of this team. The first major task of the health care team is to develop health care guidelines. It is these guidelines that often provide the basis for the CQI team to address. The guidelines must address issues of appropriateness, effectiveness, efficiency, and efficacy of the service delivery. In the development of these guidelines, input from the physician is essential. This input requires that physicians be encouraged to think beyond their own role and embrace the total system of service delivery (Hart et al., 1995).

The formulation of guidelines may create the greatest challenge that the physician will face, as he or she must learn to recognize the dominance of system influences that interact and permeate the health care arena. Physicians generally receive limited training on the influence of the environment. Many times they are not encouraged to supplement this training in practice, as patient care rewards are generally linked to the concrete service(s) they provide. Because of constant time restraints, it is not uncommon for physicians to depend on other members of the health care delivery team to address adequately the issues that go beyond direct patient care. Although this acceptance seems to be easier when relating to primary care physicians, it can be problematic for all physicians as members of the health care delivery team. In working with the physician, the social work team leader needs to prepare for this, by sharing with the physician his or her knowledge of environmental and practice systems that can influence guidelines for quality practice.

Another essential member of the QI health care delivery team is the nurse. Nurses are important members for inclusion on the team because they can be excellent resources as leaders or facilitators in the process. Nurses can assist in making suggestions for improving the process of patient care. It is also important to note that in our changing health care environment, there may also be some medical services that are now delivered solely by the nurse. This can make them a solo or entirely responsible medical practitioner regarding some of the patient care services provided. As independent practitioners, their input in establishing guidelines as part of the quality control team is essential.

A third member for inclusion of the QI health care delivery team is the administrator or middle-level manager. This person can provide valuable input because he or she is knowledgeable about the daily processes and administrative concerns involved in service delivery. Managers can help to predict problems that will occur within a system and suggest practical solutions for dealing with service changes from an administrative perspective. Traditionally, on QI teams, it has been the administrator or the middle-level manager who has often assumed the primary leadership role. The advantage of using the social worker as a team leader in addition or as replacement for the middle manager is the sensitivity that the social worker brings through knowledge of practice issues. The health care social worker can blend practice insight with administrative considerations, while integrating the needs of patients and their families.

Optional team members for inclusion in the QI team can include board members or consumers of the service as well as administrative support personnel, such as receptionists or other front line contact workers. If a health planning board exists, including one of more of these individuals as participants can be helpful. Members of these boards often consist of patients who use or live in the area where the service is being provided. This participation will allow board members to become empowered through education and understanding while participating in the basics of implementation. If board members are not available or no board exists, inviting individual patients to serve can be invaluable. Meeting the needs of the patient is the ultimate objective, and patient participation gives input into service delivery designed to address his or her needs. Including the receptionist and other front-line workers can also be helpful. Given their often daily contact with patients, these individuals are in opportune positions to evaluate front-line needs and desires (Hart et al., 1995).

In summary, the QI process, no matter what form it takes in the future, is here to stay. In the future, continued education and training in this area will probably be the responsibility of the coordinated care organizations or the service providers themselves. If social workers are taught how to implement, educate, and lead the movement in this form of quality assurance, they will be able to increase employment desirability as well as ensure and improve the measures that lead to continued patient health and wellness.

Social workers have a real advantage as team leaders because they are not limited, unlike so many health care executives that cannot engage in direct practice. Social workers can not only understand and anticipate trends in the turbulent environment disregard but they can also use their practice expertise to recognize and advocate for system changes that can lead to greater patient empowerment and advocacy.

CHAPTER SUMMARY AND FUTURE DIRECTIONS

In current social work health care practice, a combination approach that takes into account the behavioral, cognitive, and somatic aspects of health care delivery is recommended. This emphasis highlights the biopsychosocial–spiritual approach that integrates the biomedical, psychosocial, and cultural aspects and links it to behavioral outcomes in measuring service necessity, utility, and effectiveness (Straub, 2012). It has become clear that patients/clients/consumers are not an isolated system, and the beliefs they hold can indeed affect openness and response to health service delivery (Chang et al., 2012). Utilizing an integrated approach that takes into account not only the biological, psychological, sociological, cultural, and spiritual aspects provides health care social workers with a theory base that can be used to simplify what could otherwise be a complicated process.

Today the emphasis is strong to link these behavioral-based biopsychosocial and spiritual issues with medical outcomes data (Rock, 2002). Most of the other health-related disciplines also subscribe to this approach, making the social worker a leader in understanding and interpreting the "psycho," "social" and cultural factors while remaining aware and respectful of the spiritual needs in a patient's condition. On the basis of competition from other allied health professionals, health care social workers, now more than ever, need to emphasize and rely on the strengths of the practice profession, which include remaining active in the planning process for the patient.

Teamwork and collaborative efforts to assist patients are the present as well as the future of health care social work. Because many professionals truly do not understand the differences between the multidisciplinary, interdisciplinary, transdisciplinary, and pandisciplinary approaches, some time discussing these distinctions is central. The interdisciplinary and transdisciplinary approaches encourage overlap of roles and integration of services, and the transdisciplinary also recognizes the patient and the identified family system at each stage of the intervention. Social workers need to embrace these changes and allow themselves, as the other professionals are doing, to become more active in areas of service that are not considered traditional. In provision of health care service, there is overlap, blurred definitions, and diffuse boundary distinctions that are being made. This is not happening by accident—the interdisciplinary team concept is requiring it. Social workers by their nature can be flexible and should not fear assisting in all areas of the patient continuum of care. It is only by being assertive and reaching for more, as the other professions, that social workers can help the profession and the patients served. By increasing the marketability of the profession, social workers can also ensure that the services that they have traditionally provided to patients will not go unpracticed.

To expand the role of social work, the quality review process should be considered. The quality review process is part of health care delivery that will not go away. Health care social workers can make excellent team leaders and can guide this process, while ensuring quality care services to the patients served. Now is the time for social workers to reach out for new uncharted areas of practice and service delivery. After all, it is clearly efforts such as this that are needed to help secure and maintain the place for social workers at the health care delivery table.

Glossary

Biopsychosocial   In this approach to health care practice, the "bio" refers to the biological and medical aspects of an individual's health and well-being; the "psycho" involves the individual aspects of the patient, such as individual feelings of self-worth and self-esteem; and the "social" considers the larger picture and relates to the social environment that surrounds and influences the patient.

Biopsychosocial model of practice   When all three areas (the bio, psycho, and social) are identified, assessed, and addressed, a biopsychosocial model of practice intervention is implemented. This approach to practice is viewed primarily as the basis for social work practice in the health care area.

Biopsychosocial–spiritual perspective   This perspective is a modification of the biopsychosocial perspective that includes recognition and influences of patient spiritual needs.

Case-by-case collaboration   This is when practitioners from different disciplines come together to share and participate in a mode of service delivery or an individualized intervention plan designed to assist the patient, family, or community in need.

Collaboration   This term is often used interchangeably with the term interdisciplinary. In its most general sense, it means different yet related disciplines working together for the ultimate benefit of the patients served.

Consultation   In this form of collaboration, expert advice that can either be accepted or rejected by the consultee is given.

Continuous quality improvement   A specific method and plan for ensuring that quality care is obtained. The foundation of this method originally comes from a managerial perspective other than health care.

Depersonalization   The essence of the biomedical approach to practice rests in the fact that the professional possesses some type of special esoteric knowledge and skill that can be given to the patient. With the advent of increased education, consumers are becoming more knowledgeable and questioning the special knowledge that professionals have traditionally been considered to possess.

Education   In collaborative education, the social worker offers his or her expertise to train other health care providers.

Empowerment   The process of helping patients and their families or significant others to increase their interpersonal, social, socioeconomic, and political goals.

Interdisciplinary teams   Consist of a variety of health care professionals who are brought together to provide effective, better coordinated, and improved quality of services for patients.

Multidisciplinary teams   Are composed of a mix of health and social welfare professionals, with each discipline primarily working on an independent or a referral basis.

Pandisciplinary team   A specialized team where each member of the team is considered an expert in a specific area (e.g., gerontology) and in the delivery of health care all team members are considered equal for assisting the patient. These types of teams are linked to a skill rather than a professional discipline.

Quality assurance   The process or guidelines that a service delivery organization sets to ensure that services measure up to the standards set.

Quality improvement   This term is generally used interchangeably with quality assurance. See definition for *quality assurance*.

Stakehold To have some vested interest in serving as part of the quality assurance team.

Team approach This type of collaborative effort links professionals from different health care disciplines together to achieve enhanced patient outcomes.

Team leader This generally refers to the individual who is responsible for the coordination, education, and enhanced functioning of the quality assessment team.

Transdisciplinary team This is a group of health care professionals and nonprofessionals that freely share ideas and work together and meet together regularly as a synergistic team including the patient/client/consumer and identified support system members.

Questions for Further Study

1. What are the major weaknesses of using a biopsychosocial approach to practice?

2. What are some of the strengths of using the biopsychosocial approach to practice?

3. What forms of collaborative efforts should health care social workers participate in, and how could these roles be expanded?

4. Interdisciplinary teamwork seems to be the current trend in health care practice. Do you believe it will continue and why?

5. What new roles would you recommend that health care social workers assume as part of the health care delivery team, and how would these roles benefit the profession and the patient/client/consumer served?

Websites

American Public Health Association (APHA)
www.apha.org/membergroups/sections/aphasections/socialwork/

4 Interdisciplinary Teamwork in Health Care
www.med.unc.edu/epic/module4/m4to.htm

Society for Social Work Leadership in Health Care
www.sswlhc.org/

Today's Health Care Social Worker

Name: Lea Patterson-Lust, LMSW
List State of Practice: Alabama
Professional Job Title: Director of Social Work Services

Duties in a Typical Day
I am employed at a regional medical center as the Director of Social Work Services.

Although I am the director, this title is somewhat of a misnomer since I am the only person in my department. However, as department director I do oversee and act as a direct service provider, providing 100% of all the social work service needs for this 115-bed inpatient facility, with its full complement of outpatient services as well. It is my responsibility to make sure all of The Joint Commission's (TJC's) standards are met for social services. I wear a beeper 24 hours a day, seven days a week and I am often on call over the weekends for all social service emergencies.

My duties are varied as a health care social worker, but primarily I am responsible for: Adoption Assistance, Discharge Planning, Advance Directives, Court Ordered Placements (i.e., involuntary commitments, nursing home placement), Domestic Violence, Child Abuse and Neglect, Elder Abuse and Neglect, and Inpatient Services (working with uninsured or underinsured).

What do you like most about your position?
Providing direct services to patients and working with other professionals as part of a team.

What do you like least about your position?
What I like the least is the hospital bureaucracy. Also, the unrealistic expectations held by other medical professionals in regard to what the service system can provide.

What "words of wisdom" do you have for the new health care social worker considering work in a similar position?
It is important to remember that when working in an acute care setting that social work is generally perceived as a nonrevenue producing service. With all the decreases in health care reimbursement, social work services often feel the brunt end of such cuts. Social workers often are expected to meet the psychosocial needs of patients in crisis, including very complex problems. Although this is a critical service, because it is often not directly linked to reimbursement, it is often not valued.

CHAPTER 6

Practice Strategy: Considerations and Methods for Health Care Social Workers

A revolution in health care delivery is underway. Time-limited therapeutic approaches help social workers to be viewed as more competent, effective, and efficient. These approaches remain an integral part of our past, our present, and lastly, can create the basis for our future survival in health care.

—Dziegielewski

INFLUENCE OF BEHAVIORAL HEALTH CARE

In the field of social work, there is much diversity in what is considered the best theoretical or methodological basis for current practice (Dziegielewski, 2010a). This fluctuating trend also remains problematic in the field of health care social work practice. Furthermore, in this area of social work practice, the pressure is even greater because so many health care social workers simply do not do traditional social work counseling. Therefore, so many of the services provided include clinical case management that has two essential features—improving quality care to vulnerable populations and cost containment when providing this care (Frankel & Gelman, 2012). This means that psychosocial interventions with patients/clients/consumers (hereafter referred to as patients) who suffer from chronic disease will be more comprehensive and take into account both the biological and social aspects of the condition (Deter, 2012).

To complicate methodological intervention strategy further, health care social workers are often forced to go beyond the traditional bounds of their practice wisdom. For these social workers, selecting the best practice strategy must also be firmly based within the reality of the environment. For the health care social worker who must select a method of intervention, it is not uncommon to feel influenced and subsequently trapped within a system that is driven by social, political, cultural, and economic factors. With the widespread movement of behavioral health care, there are many factors in the environment that not only influence current health care practice—they dictate it.

Health care social workers generally work for and are obligated to behavioral health care agencies. The entire health care system is being reorganized by this concept and the bottom line is to reduce health care costs (Franklin, 2002; Rosenthal, 2011). *Fee for service* is decreasing, and insurance systems are requiring more partial or full risk *capitation* (Rock, 2002). Similar to its inception in the 1990s, managed behavioral care, often abbreviated to behavioral care, remains an alternative within the fee-for-service environment. This means that managed care organizations must compete with one another to secure contracts to provide service. Given that the United States has the highest health care expenses per capita of any industrialized nation, this cost of care impacts everyone (Boughtin & Orndoff, 2011). In the attempt to secure contracts for service, budget restrictions are implemented. Financial incentives are created that encourage the provision of limited service, thereby limiting the number of inpatient or outpatient days (Chambliss, 2000).

What this means for health care professionals who accept these contracts is that they will receive a probable decrease in earnings. This trend of declining income potential for physicians can have direct implications for social work professionals. Therefore, although the implication for health care social work practice is not found directly in the failing of physician incomes, it is found in the reasons for the decline. Two primary reasons for this decline are (a) less money available for health care and (b) the continued push toward further health care cost reduction. For most managed care organizations, the key strategy for reducing costs is limiting unnecessary health service use. This is generally accomplished by altering the treatment process and services offered in various ways. These cost-reduction and cost-shifting policies have caused the process of providing health care service to change dramatically over the years. To complicate the selection of a service method further, the provisions of counseling, treatment, and discharge planning need to be set within reimbursement parameters, and this will need to take into account the type and amount of insurance a recipient has.

In conjunction with cost-saving strategy, the guidelines and practices developed through quality improvement programs can also be used as pre-established criteria for service delivery (Heeschen, 2000). These pre-established criteria for practice delivery can cause health care social workers to be limited in the treatment plans they are able to create or the types of case management strategy they are allowed to employ (Dziegielewski, 2010a).

It is believed that the biggest test for health care social workers engaged in practice of any type today (therapeutic or concrete service delivery) will be to link the service to reimbursement patterns. Once this link is made, social workers can only stand to benefit. This will help the health care social worker to be able to justify time spent in the provision of time-limited therapy for increasing patient overall health and wellness.

ESTABLISHING THE TIME-LIMITED SERVICE STRUCTURE

Selecting the most appropriate intervention method in today's health care environment requires that a multitude of factors be considered in the selection process. In addition to these numerous factors, general support for "traditional methods of time-limited intervention," "lack of a formal space for counseling," and the "time constraints" health care social workers must face in trying to offer services cannot be overemphasized. Many times members of the health care delivery team do not recognize the importance of the role played by the social worker as part of the nurse/social worker team (Bristo & Herrick, 2002).

Unfortunately, other professionals on the team often believe that the social worker should concentrate on the provision of more concrete services (Holliman et al., 2001). However, this view remains debatable as the other professionals continue to recognize the importance and assist in providing for the psychosocial needs of the patients served. Unfortunately, in the health area, there is one issue that must be considered in selecting a practice structure—the concentration on balancing quality of care and cost effectiveness that cannot be avoided when selecting a mode for practice. As reinforced throughout the book, when there is a battle between them, it is generally cost effectiveness that wins. Therefore, health care social workers are expected to provide what they believe is the most beneficial and ethical practice possible, while being pressured to have completed it as quickly and efficiently as possible. There is no simple answer. The healthcare setting, as well as managed care contracts, capitation policies, and direct insurance reimbursement, can clearly affect the choice of health care counseling strategy to be used.

A further complication when selecting a structure for practice intervention for health care social workers is that defending a type of intervention "as in the best interest of the patient" may not truly reflect the patient's wishes. Traditionally, Americans have been resistant to allowing any interference by political and social factors in service provision relating to the provider–patient relationship. Today, however, based on the promise of lower premiums and lower health care expenditures, this remains an important area of exploration. It is not uncommon for patients to be more interested in receiving a service that is time limited or reimbursable, regardless of the expected benefit that they may gain from an alternative, possibly longer-term treatment strategy.

Time-Limited Service and Behavioral Care Principles

Today, time-limited brief practice methods remain in a state of transition, which simply reflects the turbulence found in today's general health care environment (Dziegielewski, 2010b). Evidence-based medicine and the importance of randomized controlled trials are expected to support all selected interventions (Deter, 2012). In choosing a method of practice, health care social workers, similar to other professionals, are being forced to deal with numerous issues (e.g., limited reimbursement patterns, declining health care admissions, capitation). Struggling to resolve these issues, as discussed previously, has become necessary based on the inception of prospective payment systems, managed care plans, and other changes in the provision and funding of health care.

The turbulence in the current health care environment requires health care social workers to struggle with not only picking a practice structure that is efficacious and efficient but also one that can enhance effectiveness in the briefest amount of time. In today's practice environment, practice strategy must encompass two things: maintaining quality of care and joining quality of care with an emphasis on cost containment (Dziegielewski, 2008b). It is no secret, however, that many social workers believe that whether openly stated or not, the emphasis is on ensuring cost containment. Stated simply, in selecting a form of time-limited intervention strategy, health care social workers must remember the importance of remaining viable "dollar generators" or they will feel the brunt of initial dollar line savings attempts.

Intermittent Therapy: Application of a Time-Limited Structure

In the health care setting, similar to other practice settings, it is not uncommon that patients expect that intervention will be brief. In addition to the limitations set by insurance reimbursement patterns, many patients simply do not have the time, desire, or money for longer-term interventions (especially the poor). It has become obvious that simply using clinical judgment not supported in evidence and claims that the patient simply feels better will no longer be allowed. In the medical setting, as in so many other areas of counseling practice, the days of insurance covered long-term therapy encounters have ended (Dziegielewski, 2010a).

In today's health care practice environment, reality dictates that the duration of most therapeutic sessions, regardless of the intervention used or the orientation of the therapist, remains relatively brief. In social work practice, most of these therapeutic encounters generally range from 1 to 12 sessions (Frankel & Gelman, 2012). Generally speaking, the least number of sessions is 1, and the greatest number is 20. There are some areas in the health care setting where this can apply, but generally patient contacts are generally much shorter with one- and two-meeting encounters being the norm rather than the exception. Actually, if polled, many health care social workers would agree that short-term treatment interventions in the traditional sense have become a product of the past. What is used today in this high-pressure environment is more adequately termed *intermittent therapy* where every session is considered complete and treated as if it is the only session that may occur.

Realization of limited availability and brief encounters rather than planned sessions makes social workers aware that quality therapeutic time is often limited. This makes well-utilized sessions essential. Without this framework for practice, encounters can result in numerous unexpected and unplanned terminations for the patient as well as feelings of failure and decreased job satisfaction for the social worker.

In time-limited intervention strategies, there are generally two types of practice delivery formats that have emerged: traditional brief intervention and intermittent brief intervention. To capitalize on professional time and the need for "face-to-face" contact, a combination of both formats may also be used. In the traditional format, patients begin and terminate intervention in a close-ended therapeutic environment. When using intermittent formats, which were rarely used in the past, the social worker captures the opportunity to work with the patient and planned encounters are not necessary. Intermittent approaches work well when responding to the limitations instituted by managed care policies. In health care, an intervention plan carried out in one session and monitored periodically over time can provide attraction for funding sources. An intermittent format for therapy usually employs fewer sessions; however, sessions can be spread out over a longer period. This attraction stems from the fact that when an intervention is engaged from an "as-needed basis," less time, resources, and funds are required. For health care social workers, use of an intermittent format can provide a new twist on intervention within the time-limited constraints of the behavioral health care setting.

In summary, for a model to be considered a viable, time-limited approach, it must include mutually negotiated concrete and realistic goals, a plan for measuring effectiveness, and a specific time frame for conducting and completing the service.

Development of Time-Limited Goals and Objectives

No matter what method of time-limited service provision a health care social worker selects, accurate assessment that includes establishing clear goals and objectives is at the heart of social work intervention (Engstrom, 2012). To establish a plan of intervention that is generally of an interdisciplinary nature, establishing behavioral goals and behavioral objectives are required as part of the intervention strategy. Simply stated, a goal constitutes what you and the patient want to accomplish; the behavioral objectives state exactly what the patient plans to do to address the identified goal(s) (Dziegielewski & Powers, 2000). However, it is important to note that many social work professionals do not make the fine distinction between goals and objectives and use the terms interchangeably.

Goals need to be clearly defined and provide direction and structure for the professional practice intervention. This is particularly important when dealing with an individual in the medical setting where clear goals and objectives are part of the patient's overall treatment plan. Many times it is this treatment plan that influences accreditation, certification, or reimbursement levels. When social workers take an active role in treatment planning, they can help enhance the plans effectiveness by making sure the patient maintains an active role in this process and goals and objectives are not overlooked or disregarded (Auslander & Freedenthal, 2012).

Clearly defined goals not only help the patient but also help the practitioner allowing for decisions related to whether she or he has the skills or desire to work with the patient. In time-limited service, provision to be sure that the individual will be able to secure the services that are needed and, in turn, to ensure that the practitioner is able to help the patient focus in on change efforts that will allow a healthier homeostatic balance to emerge. The goals and behavioral objectives chosen also help to outline the needed intervention and the particular practice strategies and techniques that will be needed. Finally, goal setting is a crucial element in measuring the effectiveness of service provision as it can provide the standards against which progress is measured.

To start the therapeutic process, the social worker and the patient need to work together to define problems into workable and solvable units. To start this process, goals that are reflective of the problem need to be identified. These goals and subsequent objectives need to be specific, clear, verifiable, and measurable. This remains consistent with the patient's overall plan, where the established goals need to be as concrete and behavior specific as possible. Therefore, the objectives should be designed to further quantify the goals. For example, if an individual was suffering from a grief reaction regarding the sudden illness of a loved one, the social worker would want the goals and objectives to be specifically related to the restoration of equilibrium.

In social work, goals and objectives need to be mutually negotiated between the helping professional and the patient. This may seem difficult in time-limited service provision where the health care social worker is pressed for time. However, the role of the practitioner regardless of the method of intervention should be always one of facilitations helping the patient to maintain an active role in all helping efforts. The patient must also help determine whether the goals and objectives sought are consistent with his or her own culture and values. It is up to the therapist to help the patient structure and establish the intervention strategy; however, emphasis on mutuality is central to the development of goals and objectives.

In implementing the method of intervention, the role of the social worker is essential in ensuring that the problem that needs to be dealt with is addressed. Goals and objectives should always be stated positively and realistically so that motivation for completion will be increased. It is also essential, in establishing the effectiveness of what is being done, that the goals (particularly the objectives) be stated in as concrete and functional terms as possible. Also, remember to take into account the health care setting as when important face-to-face meetings are expected to discuss the designated goals and objectives and the subsequent treatment plans, the simpler the goal and the more involved the patient the quicker the approval. Attendance of care plan meetings by patients and family members is often mandated as part of the care plan, but such meetings can be time consuming, so the more clear, concise, and relevant the plan the better (Beaulieu, 2012).

FACTORS IN TIME-LIMITED SERVICE PROVISION

Establishing a model for the phases of service provision for the health care social worker can be an arduous task. These phases of intervention are generally related to traditional forms of time-limited intervention where there is a predetermined beginning and end. Unfortunately, this is not usually the case for the health care social worker, where intermittent and single-session formats have become a practice reality. Although the traditional forms of brief intervention (with clear plans that are monitored periodically) are attractive to funding sources, they may be impractical to implement. This is particularly problematic when concrete indicators, such as discharge planning, education, and after-care provision, are the primary objectives expected at the completion of service.

In the health care setting, there is a great deal of intervention that is done on an "as-needed basis," so it is important to be flexible in anticipating and experiencing the intervention phases. In time-limited service provision, the phases of intervention may cross several encounters, where at others time, they may be condensed into one. Regardless, objectives that lead to the desired outcome must be addressed at each phase of the service provided (Frankel & Gelman, 2012). Generally, in the *initial phase* of service provision, a hopeful environment is created where the patient begins to feel confident that his or her problem can and will be addressed. It is important that the social worker communicates and starts to build rapport. Many times health care social workers may actually initiate service provision in a hallway or at a patient's bedside. No matter where the process starts, it is important that the patient feels safe, comfortable, and free to talk about his situation. In the hurried rush of the health care social worker's day, it is all too easy to neglect this essential ingredient, which is basic to the start of a successful interventive encounter.

The social worker must further help the patient to break down problems into concrete terms, which, once identified, establish the groundwork for the development of concrete goals and objectives (Dziegielewski, 2008b). Generally, an initial contract is formulated. It does not matter if this is written or verbal, but a clear understanding of what will transpire is essential. It is important that early in the intervention process, the social worker start to think about assessment and assistance to obtain patient behavior change. Diagnosis and assessment measures will be covered in greater depth in a following chapter; however, initiation of a well-rounded and comprehensive assessment at this initial phase is considered essential (Dziegielewski, 2008b). Measurement of initial individual, group, or social functioning needs to be established. If measurement scales are not implemented to serve as a baseline, an initial ranking to compare patient functioning at the beginning and end of intervention is suggested. Measures for assessment should include physical and functional performance (including sexual performance), community integration, and other types of social and recreational activities that will allow for readjustment in the environment (Mpofu & Oakland, 2009).

Finally, an agreed-on time frame for service provision needs to be established (Walter & Peller, 2000). The patient needs to know what he or she can expect from the health care social worker and how much time will actually be devoted to addressing his or her problem(s). The social worker needs to identify what can be done to address the situation and what effect the potential solution may have in the long term (Frankel & Gelman, 2012). In the initial phase, the measurement of effectiveness will be finalized. It is here that the health care social worker must decide and plan for implementation of how she or he will measure the effectiveness of the intervention strategy employed.

The *main phase of intervention* is generally based on the model and format chosen in the initial phase. This is the most active of the stages because this is when concrete problem solving actually occurs. Guidelines that can assist in this stage regardless of the model chosen include planning each session in advance, summarization of each session, and maintaining flexibility if renegotiation needs to occur in regard to the problem-solving process.

For the health care social worker, planning each session in advance requires the need for commitment of time outside of the formal session. Most times this planning is not reimbursable to the social worker or the health care agency. Therefore, both the patient and the social worker must be willing to commit this time to planning outside of the traditional session. For the health care social worker, this is particularly important when preparing health and wellness counseling. Generally, there is limited time to do this and not only must the social worker be prepared to discuss the topic but he or she also must have written materials that will assist him or her to make the most of the service time available.

Another area where advanced planning is beneficial concerns the medical aspects of the patient's condition. Many times patients suffer from medical problems that complicate the psychosocial–spiritual aspects the patient is experiencing. Social workers need to know enough about the "bio" in the behaviorally based biopsychosocial aspects of practice to assist the patient in addressing these needs. Also, the issue of medication influence within the counseling environment should not be ignored (Dziegielewski, 2010b).

Many times patients are taking medications. The social worker needs to know how these medications can affect the patient. Medications can influence actions toward family members or significant others as well as impact other social relationships. With the increased use of medications for all types of health and mental health problems has a pronounced affects on the practice of health care social work (Dziegielewski, 2010b).

No matter how many sessions are being implemented, the technique of *summarization* should be incorporated into each session (Dziegielewski, 2010a). When incorporating this technique, initiation of each formal encounter is dedicated to the patient actually stating the agreed upon objectives that are to be addressed. This will allow both patient and social worker to quickly focus on the task at hand. Summarization should also be practiced at the end of each session. This will allow the patient to recapitulate what she or he believes has transpired in the session and how it relates to the stated objectives. Patients should use their own words to summarize what has transpired. In acknowledging and summarizing the content and objectives of the session, (a) the patient takes responsibility for his or her own actions; (b) repetition allows the session accomplishments to be highlighted and reinforced; (c) the patient and the social worker ascertain that they are working together on the same objectives; and (d) the therapeutic environment remains flexible and open for renegotiation of contracted objectives.

Finally, this phase will require arrangements be made for future follow-up. Social workers want feedback, and getting this information cannot only benefit the patient but also the social worker. Receiving feedback on how the therapeutic encounter is progressing can lead to overall levels of job satisfaction. At this stage, in the intervention process, it is important to ensure that proper attention is given to the measurement of feedback and follow-up, particularly if an unplanned termination results. This is important to prepare for, as frequently quick and unplanned terminations occur in the health care environment.

In the *final phase* of intervention, a follow-up contact is established. Here, the social worker meets with the patient utilizing intermittent in-person sessions or can arrange for telephone communication to review and evaluate current patient progress and status changes. When completing follow-up, a recommended time lapse of no more than 1 to 4 months is recommended. The social worker should prepare in advance for this meeting to continue and reaffirm previous measurement strategies. Because long-term therapy is generally not possible, when indicated a referral would be expected (Frankel & Gelman, 2012).

Time-Limited Service Provision Has Replaced Traditional Psychotherapy

Alperin (1994) and other psychotherapists, particularly those who support psychoanalytic therapy, believe that managed care policies are biased against them. They believe that making changes in a person takes time and that rushing into changes could lead to further heightening of complications in future health and wellness. They urge social workers to realize this danger and advocate strongly for its continuance before it becomes an extinct mode of practice delivery in today's "big business" practice environment.

The problems of conducting traditional forms of psychotherapy are not unique to the health care environment. For years, the emphasis on the applicability and effectiveness of time-limited methods of practice has been well established (Dziegielewski & Powers, 2000; Ligon, 2002). Even with the rich history of the psychodynamic approaches, it is easy to see how time-limited interventions have gained in popularity, particularly in the health care setting. This approach when combined with the overall objective of bringing about positive changes in a patient's current lifestyle that often accompanies little face-to-face contact makes this method conducive for change. It is this emphasis on effectiveness and applicability leading to increased positive change that has helped to make time-limited brief interventions popular. In the health care area, time-limited approaches are the most requested forms of practice in use today.

The major difference between traditional psychotherapy and time-limited approaches is that the foundation for each is different. This difference requires social workers to re-examine some basic premises that have been taught regarding long-term therapeutic models used in a more traditional format. There are seven factors that can be identified that highlight the difference between these two methods.

First is the primary difference in the way the patient is viewed. Traditional psychotherapy approaches linked individual problems to personal pathology. This is not the case from a time-limited perspective where the patient is seen as basically healthy with an interest in increasing personal or social changes.

Second, time-limited approaches may be most helpful when administered during critical periods in a person's life (Roberts & Dziegielewski, 1995). This provides a basic difference from the use of traditional psychotherapies that are seen as necessary and ongoing over a much longer period. Third, in time-limited interventions, the goals and objectives of the formal encounter are always mutually defined by both the patient and the social worker. This can be different from the traditional psychotherapies where goals were first recognized and defined by a therapist and later shared with the patient.

The time-limited environment requires that goals and objectives be concretely defined and extend beyond the walls of the actual formal encounter. Oftentimes, homework or *bibliotherapeutic* (outside reading) interventions are included as a standard part of the practice strategy. In the medical setting, it is also not uncommon for medicines to be considered a part of the treatment regime that must be incorporated. The term "bibliotherapy" refers to the use of a medical intervention, such as medicine, outside reading materials, and brief intervention techniques. This is different from traditional psychotherapy in which memories of what happened outside of the session are actually the focus of intervention. In the traditional psychotherapy approaches, issues are generally addressed during the sessions only—not generally outside of them (Budman & Gurman, 1988). This is because the presence of a therapist is seen as a powerful catalyst necessary for change. The patient needs this direction to make the therapeutic changes required.

The fifth difference between the time-limited approaches and the traditional psychotherapeutic methods is one of the hardest for social workers that were educated in traditional psychotherapeutic methodology to accept. Simply stated, in time-limited service provision, regardless of the model or method, little emphasis is placed on insight. Neither recognition nor addressing "insight-oriented change" is considered essential. This is different from traditional psychotherapy where development of problem-oriented insight is considered necessary before any type of meaningful change can occur.

Sixth, in time-limited approaches, the therapist is seen as active and directive. Here, the social worker goes beyond just active listening and assumes a consultative role with the patient. Social workers are now expected to be active and directive within the change process, which results in the development of concrete goals and problem-solving techniques. This is different from traditional psychotherapeutic approaches where emphasis was placed on a more nebulous "inner representation of satisfaction."

Finally is the issue of termination where ending the therapeutic environment is discussed early in the process, generally in the first session. Many times discussion for setting a specific time frame for intervention can happen in the first session; termination issues are discussed continually throughout the intervention process. Many times in traditional psychotherapy, termination is not determined in advance; therefore, it is not considered an essential part of the process of therapy.

WHEN THERE SIMPLY IS "NO TIME" FOR THERAPEUTIC INTERVENTION

Social work professionals complain that in the health care setting, there is often no time for time-limited brief interventions as discussed previously. However, it is important to note that this practice reality should not discontinue attempts at conducting it. This lack of time does not mean that if it were available the patient would not benefit.

When it is impossible, however, concentration still needs to remain on setting appropriate objectives in the health care setting (Rock, 2002). Also, it is essential to remember that the focus on any service offered today in the health care area is not generally process driven, but rather it is outcomes based. For social workers, the focus needs to be placed on the *outcome* that is desired. One easy way to remember where to put the emphasis in measuring outcome (no matter how little time is available) is to be sure to measure *what comes out at the end*, which is the actual outcome that needs to be identified.

No matter what method of intervention used, you must be prepared to collect outcomes data. Regardless of the clinical health care setting, if you routinely collect and identify the outcomes related to your service provision, you will be able to clearly justify the service that was provided. Always remember that the best place to begin in setting and determining outcomes is "to start where the patient is." What does the patient say about the problem? The easiest way to develop specific outcome measures is to use and focus on "behavioral" identifiers. First, the behavior pattern can be established regarding problem gathering, subsequent frequency, and intensity and duration information about it. Questions to ask include the following:

* **Identify the problem:** Can you briefly define the problem that needs to be addressed?
* **Circumstances surrounding the problem:** What events in your life make this problem happen? What specific things help the problem to reoccur? How do others react when the problem occurs? How do others directly contribute to the problem?
* **Effect of the problem:** Can you tell me how the problem affects your life?
* **Starting the problem-solving strategy:** If you could solve the problem what would you do?

Once this has been completed, you can help the patient to redefine and re-examine the problem behavior. In this way, the patient is encouraged to focus on specific problem-related talk and strategy. All service provision needs to incorporate this "attention focus limitation," as the health care social worker is generally limited by service restrictions and time constraints to go beyond this dimension. Once the problem has been defined, the social worker needs to urge the patient to explore and identify solutions to solve the problem. In general, does the patient believe he or she can control the problem, and if so, what types of things have been tried in the past? What new or modified strategies could be tried in the future?

PRACTICE METHODS USED IN TIME-LIMITED SERVICE PROVISION

In this section, several methods usually linked to the provision of clinical health care social work services will be briefly summarized: cognitive-behavioral approaches, interpersonal psychotherapeutic/psychodynamic approaches, strategic or solution-oriented methods, crisis intervention, and an introduction to health, education, and wellness counseling. Regardless of what model is being discussed, concentration on the measurement of behavior change will always be emphasized. In today's health care environment—for reimbursement and marketability purposes—this emphasis is considered essential. It is not uncommon to hear the new terms "managed behavioral health care" or the methods of "behavioral health care management." These are terms social workers in health care need to cement into their practice vocabulary as they introduce and later define the methods of intervention that they will select for service provision (Franklin, 2002).

Cognitive–Behavioral Intervention Approaches

In the early 1970s, the importance of applied behavioral analysis and the power of reinforcement on the influence of human behavior were explored (Skinner, 1953). However, many theorists believed that behavior alone was not enough and that human beings acted or reacted based on an analysis of the situation and the thought patterns that motivated them. Here, the thought process, and how cognitive processes and structures influence individual emotions, was highlighted (Roberts & Dziegielewski, 1995). In cognitive–behavioral approaches (cognitive–behavioral therapy [CBT]), it is recognized that measuring the behavior alone is not enough. Attention needs to be given to the thought as it relates to the behavior. Therefore, CBT is considered a number of related theories that focus on recognizing the importance of cognitions in the psychological process (Vonk & Early, 2002).

Therefore, CBT is associated with demonstrable behavioral results—cost effectiveness—but with the emphasis of expanding the patient's sense of self-efficacy, independence, participation, self-monitoring, and control in their treatment. It can be utilized with various treatment groups (e.g., individual, groups, couples, families) and modalities (e.g., in person, electronic, Internet). However, this therapeutic intervention can suffer from service restrictions such as insurance plan billing and reimbursements, and it is unclear how these limitations can affect the effectiveness in treatment (Dziegielewski, 2010a).

Similar to other settings when employing this method of practice, the health concern and the way the person views the problem are identified. In the application, especially when depression exists, the development of a *schema* occurs (Beck & Weishaar, 2000). This schema is referred to as the cognitive structure that organizes experience and behavior (Beck & Freeman, 1990). Schemas involve the way individuals view certain aspects of their lives, including relationship aspects such as adequacy and the ability to depend on their own physical limitations. Once a schema is identified concretely, the critical incidents that define it can be interpreted and thus reacted to by the individual. When physical limitations are identified as a result of a medical situation, the individual can feel betrayed by his or her own body. The identification of the problem situation can be clouded with negative and self-defeating feelings. The first step in the process involves identification of these feelings and how they affect the resulting behavioral response. Identifying the cognitive distortions can be difficult as in the start of the problem-solving process, it can seem overwhelming to the patient. Cognitive–behavioral approaches to identifying the problem focus on the present and seek to replace distorted thoughts or unwanted behaviors with developing clearly established goals (McMullin, 2000).

In the health care area, similarly to other areas of practice, goals should always be stated positively and realistically so that motivation for completion will be increased (Dziegielewski & Powers, 2000). Also, to facilitate the measurement of effectiveness, objectives must be stated in concrete and

functional terms. In setting the appropriate objectives, the focus is not necessarily on process but rather on the outcome that is desired. The adaption of
cognitive and behavioral principles in the time-limited framework creates a
viable climate for change. In health care, this means helping the patient to
clearly identify the problem, thoughts, and feelings that influence the behavioral reactions to it.

In the health care setting, the application of CBT interventions is most
helpful when coupled with other medical treatment modalities in an integrated approach. From this perspective, the medical aspects are joined with
the psychosocial/cognitive ones. The techniques utilized in CBT are ideal for
working with depression or other anxiety problems that can accompany a
medical condition. This approach allows social worker to be relatively confrontive, yet respectful of the patient being served. The health care social
worker can identify difficulties and concerns and the negative schemas that
surround them related to safety, trust, power and control, self-esteem, and
intimacy (Keane, Marshall, & Taft, 2006). Identifying these concerns is essential for identifying problematic thoughts and how this may interfere with the
problem-solving process increasing the ability for patient independence and
positive self-regard.

Anxiety related to medical concerns can impact an individual's ability
to self-regulate the emotion resulting in reactions where information is incorrectly attributed and impaired. (Fruzzetti, Crook, Erikson, Lee, & Worrall,
2008). The application of the cognitive model allows for the identification
of these concerns, bringing them into conscious consideration and allowing the patient to intentionally evaluate and compare the cognitive reaction
experienced to what has actually happened. This allows for the identification of the precipitation of physiological and cognitive reactions, which
when left unrecognized can create a self-perpetuating cycle that intensifies
anxiety and depressive feelings (McEvoy & Perini, 2009; Siev & Chambless,
2007/2008).

Another useful component of CBT is that it addresses the misperception of threat and danger assessments (real or imagined) and the activation
of fear, terror, rage, and worry which are common when faced with a health
concern. The CBT model of practice can be helpful in addressing anxiety,
allowing for self-monitoring, cognitive restructuring (including evaluating
and reconsidering interpretive and predictive cognitions), relaxation training, and rehearsal and coping skills (Siev & Chambless, 2007/2008). It is a
present-based therapy that reinforces the patient's focus on the now and reality test to sustain functioning, while addressing and increasing coping capabilities and restructuring thoughts and behaviors.

One cognitive–behavior based intervention is Albert Ellis' *rational emo-
tive behavior therapy* (REBT) (Ellis, 2008; Ellis & Grieger, 1977). In the health
care setting, this can be particularly helpful for patients "catastrophizing,"
personalizing, or imagining the worst case events where the individual is
responsible for the catastrophic outcome or the behavior cannot be completed. When used in the health care setting, REBT can help to identify the

patient's irrational and unrealistic thoughts. Once identified these cognitions can be replaced with more functional and adaptive alternatives.

The "ABCDE" format provides structure for the analysis of cognitions. The A is defined as the activating event (real or imagined); B is the belief that the person has about A (rational or irrational belief; functional or dysfunctional); C is the consequence (emotional, behavioral, or both); D is the disputation of the distorted beliefs (provide evidence for belief); and E is the new effect or philosophy that evolves out of the rational belief replacing the faulty belief (Ellis, 2008). The patient is taught that an irrational or faulty belief he or she has about A causes C. From this perspective, it becomes clear to the patient that everyone, including the patient, is a fallible and imperfect human being. It teaches the individual to develop unconditional self-acceptance and unconditional acceptance of others. REBT employs active-directive techniques, such as role playing, assertiveness training and conditioning, and counter-conditioning procedures (Ellis, 1971).

In the health care setting where time is often limited, self-help interventions can provide both practical and cost-effective interventions. These types of interventions allow for the extension of therapeutic session while promoting individual health and well-being. Inclusion of web-based self-help groups, books, and other computer-based materials can benefit and maximize treatment time. These supplemental interventions are also a hallmark of the philosophy of cognitive–behavior therapy as they can be applied utilizing Internet-based services, especially where automatic decision making is generated (Andersson, 2009). When used from a CBT perspective, this supporting information can assess individuals' decision making and provide educational protocols and support to increase awareness and motivation. The Internet can make intervention accessible through self-help materials, computer-based live group exposure sessions, and direct therapist support and encouragement online, through online chats or via email (Andersson, 2009).

In summary, it is clear that medical problems often happen quickly, and individuals may be frustrated with their inability to perform in areas in which they previously were proficient. When faced with a medical situation, consumers may develop negative schemas or ways of dealing with the situation that can clearly cause conflicts in their physical, interpersonal, and social relationships. Specific techniques, such as identifying irrational beliefs, and using cognitive restructuring, behavioral role rehearsal, and systematic desensitization, can assist the patient to adjust and accommodate to the new life status that will result. In the health care setting, CBT can help the patient to not only recognize the need for change but also assist with a plan to provide the behavior change needed for continued health and functioning. In the managed care setting, the basic ideas from this method of health care service delivery remain essential. Oftentimes, whether or not this method is used directly, the ideas and principles that it explicates are incorporated into service delivery. This focus on cognitive-behavioral relationships fits ideally into the behavioral health care delivery services of today, and using web-based technology is one way to enhance the time-limited services provided.

Interpersonal Psychotherapy

Interpersonal psychotherapy therapy (IPT) is an approach that highlights the psychodynamic aspects of therapeutic practice. IPT is an approach rich in tradition that remains one of the most popular forms of short-term psychotherapeutic therapy used in medical setting today for reducing symptoms and dealing with interpersonal problems. Originally, IPT was formulated as a time-limited outpatient treatment for depressed patients (Rounsaville, Malley, Foley, & Weissman, 1988). Recent studies to support its effectiveness have been reviewed throughout the years (Borge, Hoffart, Sexton, Markowitz, & McManus, 2008; Krupnick et al., 2008; Lipsitz, Gur, Forand, Vermes, & Fyer, 2006; Lipsitz et al., 2008). Using this framework, many conditions such as depression, anxiety disorders, and substance problems have been treated. Although the results of some of these studies are mixed, it appears IPT clearly appears more effective than no treatment.

From a "biopsychosocial" perspective, this form of therapy has gained credibility and recognition among several of the related health care disciplines—particularly, medical settings that employ physicians and nurses as core members of the patient care team. In this time-limited model, therapists are seen as active, supportive, and a contributing factor in therapeutic gain (Lipsitz et al., 2006). IPT is recommended for professionals such as MDs, PhDs, MSWs, or RNs and has been used with individuals, couples, and families. Efficacy has also been stressed for the treatment of anxiety and depression (Lipsitz et al., 2008).

Currently, IPT is highlighted as a viable short-term acute treatment to directly address symptom removal and prevention of relapse. In addition, it is also viewed as helpful for patients having difficulty relating to significant others, careers, social roles, or life transitions. IPT treatment generally addresses a patient's present situation, and focus on the "here and now" is generally assumed. The focus on recent interpersonal events is stressed, with a clear effort to link the stressful event to the patient's current mood.

In treatment, assessment that includes a diagnostic evaluation and psychiatric history is gathered. Particular attention is paid to changes in relationships proximal to the onset of symptoms. The patient's interpersonal situation is highlighted. The focus of intervention is directed toward interpersonal problem areas, such as grief, role disputes, role transitions, or deficits. Focusing on one of these interpersonal areas will allow the health care social worker to identify problems in the interpersonal and social context that need to be addressed.

Once the goals and objectives have been established, a treatment strategy is applied. Treatment strategy is directly related to the identified interpersonal problem. For example, if there was a role conflict between a patient and his or her family member regarding limitations of a particular medical condition, treatment would begin with clarifying the nature of the dispute. Discussion of the medical condition would result, with an explanation of usual limitations that may be beyond the control of the patient.

Limitations that are causing the greatest problem would be identified, and options to resolve the dispute are considered. If resolution does not appear possible, strategies or alternatives to replace it are contemplated. In some cases, application manuals can be acquired and followed that give specific treatment approaches regarding certain interpersonal problem areas (Rounsaville et al., 1988).

In using IPT as a treatment model, attention needs to be provided regarding the varied and diverse types of training that each member of the interdisciplinary team has received. When using different health care professionals with differing backgrounds and education levels, the use of treatment manuals may be of benefit to highlight psychosocial areas of intervention. The use of manuals continues to gain in popularity based on the current pressure to use specific goals and objectives.

Finally, when using IPT, the social worker seeks to incorporate change strategy into the therapeutic environment. Generalization of what was learned in the clinical appointments is related to situations or symptoms that may arise in the future. However, it is important to note that the therapist cannot expect to solve all the issues involved in an interpersonal conflict. Therefore, at the end of treatment, it is possible that some concerns might not be completed. These issues will be left up to the patient to continue to address.

In summary, when using this method of intervention, the role of the health care social worker is essential in helping the patient to identify treatment issues of concern and provide the groundwork for how they can be addressed. Many times, this includes helping the patient to learn how to recognize the need for continued intervention. This is especially important when problems seem greater than what the patient is capable of handling at the time. The social worker is influential in helping the patient to feel comfortable about seeking additional treatment when needed. This help-seeking behavior is an important step in establishing and maintaining a basis for continued health and wellness.

The application of this method of practice in the different health care social work settings is variable. Based on the "medical model" and the fact that "therapeutic treatment" is planned and coordinated throughout the sessions, it may be best suited for an inpatient or a therapeutic case management setting. Today, this method continues to be used primarily in the inpatient setting or structured rehabilitative setting, which generally involves the work of a coordinated interdisciplinary team. The use of manuals and specifically outlined steps to structure the intervention process has made it a viable practice methodology for managed care and other service reimbursement considerations.

Solution-Focused Intervention Strategy

In solution-focused intervention strategy, sometimes referred to as "solution-focused brief therapy," it is assumed that patients are basically healthy individuals. All patients possess the skills they need to address their problems and remain capable of change (De Shazer, 1985). In this approach to health care practice, specific problem solving is not the focus; rather, it is an exploration that is designed to find, identify, and consider "alternative solutions" for implementation. There does not need to be a causal link between the antecedent and the actual problem; this connection is not needed to establish a link between the problem and the solution (O'Hanlon & Weiner-Davis, 2003).

In this model of intervention, the social worker is active in helping the patient to find and identify strengths in his or her current functional patterns of behavior. A dialogue of "change talk" is created rather than "problem talk" (Walter & Peller, 1992). In "change talk," the problem is viewed positively with patterns of change highlighted that appear successful for the patient. Positive aspects and exceptions to the problem are explored, allowing for alternative views of the problem to develop. Once the small changes have been highlighted, the patient becomes empowered to elicit larger ones (Green, Oades, & Grant, 2006). The key ingredients in a solution-based approach to time-limited health care practice appears to be (a) focusing on what the patient sees as the problem; (b) letting the patient establish what is the desired outcome; (c) beginning to analyze and develop solutions focusing on the individual strengths the patient can contribute; (d) developing and implementing a plan of action; and (e) assisting with termination and follow-up issues if needed. Murphy (2008) outlines four key assumptions.

1. If it works do more of it.
2. Every patient is unique, resourceful, and capable of change.
3. Cooperative relationships enhance solutions.
4. Patient feedback improves outcomes.

For more specifics on how to apply this model, see De Jong (2002) and or De Jong and Berg (2012). One reason for this attention and favor rests in the method of measurement that is highlighted as part of the intervention. Often, "scaling questions" that involve specific aspects of a patient's life, which can be translated into numbers and reflect progress, are used. For example, if a patient is depressed about his or her medical condition, a self-reported level of scaling this depression is used. A scale can be devised that reflects the way the patient perceives the depression. Current mood could be rated from 0 as feeling "free" from depression, 3 or 4 as in the middle, and 7 as feeling "completely" depressed. Once completed, the identified solutions are tied to the ratings and can be tracked over time.

Simply stated, in "solution-focused" interventions, the emphasis in practice is placed on constructing probable solutions to a problem. The idea that it is easier to construct solutions than it is to attempt to change problem behaviors prevails. By not spending a great deal of time on the cause of the problem, the emphasis on the intervention is switched away from the past toward present or future survival. A meta-analysis of recent studies in the area shows promise for continuing to use this approach (Kim, 2010). There is often more than one solution, and it becomes the role of the health care social worker and the patient together to help construct alternative and possible scenarios of assistance. Basically, the role of the practitioner with this type of intervention strategy is to create an interactive process that formulates solution-focused questions from the language or meaning reflected in the patient's answers (De Jong, 2002).

SOLUTION-FOCUSED QUESTIONS

- What would have to occur to make the problem more tolerable for you?
- What specific changes would you need to achieve to make you feel more comfortable with the problem?
- What can you do to make these changes occur?
- If you woke up tomorrow and the problem was solved, what would be different?
- In what ways is it different?

Crisis Intervention

Because of a growing awareness of the need for principles and techniques of time-limited clinical intervention that deal with survivors of crisis, crisis intervention has come to be accepted as a viable modality for health care social work practice. Crisis intervention addresses acute problem situations and can help the individual discover an adaptive means of coping with a particular life stage, tragic occurrence, or problem that generates a crisis situation (Laube, 2002). Today, crisis intervention is used in a wide range of primary and secondary settings and with many different individuals, families, communities, and groups. Health care settings where crisis intervention techniques are often employed include hospitals (especially hospital emergency department), public health agencies, hospice services, home health care agencies, and almost all other agencies that employ health care social workers. In addition, crisis intervention has been found to be successful in the health area with survivors of rape, domestic violence, mental illness, and numerous other medical or life-threatening illnesses.

A major characteristic of the implementation of crisis intervention that is inherent in all time-limited intervention approaches is the short duration of the therapeutic experience. Brief time-limited intervention is important because the state of crisis is self-limiting by its nature (Roberts, 2000). Time-limited intervention is intended to accomplish a set of therapeutic objectives with a sharply limited time frame, and its effectiveness appears to be indistinguishable from that of long-term treatment (Reid & Fortune, 2002). Using minimum therapeutic intervention during the brief crisis period can often produce a maximum therapeutic effect. Empowering patients by identifying supportive social resources coupled with focused intervention techniques can be used to facilitate therapeutic effectiveness. Crisis intervention is a dynamic form of intervention that focuses on a wide range of phenomena that affects individual, family, or group equilibrium.

Generally, the term "crisis" is defined as a temporary state of upset and disequilibrium, characterized chiefly by an individual's inability to cope with a particular situation. During this crisis period, customary methods of coping and problem solving do not work. According to James and Gilliland (2012), crisis is a perception of an event or situation as an intolerable difficulty that exceeds the resources and the coping mechanisms of the individual. This is further supported by Roberts (2000), who stated that a person in a crisis state has experienced a hazardous or threatening event; is in a vulnerable state; has failed to cope and lessen the stress through customary coping methods; and, therefore, enters into a state of disequilibrium. However, it is important to note that any definition of a crisis must remain somewhat subjective because what precipitates a crisis state in one individual might not generate such a response in another (Roberts, 2000).

With the techniques used in crisis intervention, the crisis situation can eventually be reformulated within the context of growth. Ultimately, the patient is expected to reach a healthy resolution where he or she can emerge with greater strength, self-trust, and a greater sense of freedom than before the crisis event occurred (Roberts, 2000). In crisis intervention, the social worker practices with the assumption that acute crisis events can be identified, controlled, and lessened. Therefore, successful resolution is achieved when social workers apply crisis intervention techniques to help patients successfully resolve the emotional crisis. The health care social worker is essential in helping the patient reach a healthier resolution of the problem. Most health care practitioners agree that assisting an individual in a state of crisis can provide an important opportunity for achieving patient-oriented health–behavior change.

Stages of Crisis Intervention

Generally, in the application of crisis intervention, a psychosocial assessment is implemented to identify the triggering or precipitating event, or particular problem that started the chain of events leading to an acute crisis state. In behavioral health, emergency medicine, and surgical recovery, the application of Roberts's seven-stage crisis intervention model is imperative (Roberts, 2000). The first stage refers to assessing the nature and extent of the life-threatening illness or psychiatric emergency that is overwhelming the patient at the time. The second stage involves helping the person in crisis to prioritize his or her concerns. The first and second stages of intervention often lead to what is referred to as the middle phase. In this middle phase, the crisis intervention approach should focus on encouraging the person in crisis to talk to the counselor about the event; understand and conceptualize the meaning of the event; and integrate the cognitive, affective, and behavioral components of the crisis. The third stage of intervention consists of helping the person in crisis to solve problem and find effective coping methods.

In the middle phase of intervention, social workers are encouraged to view a psychological crisis as both danger and opportunity. Generally, when an individual is in this crisis phase, he or she is open to the future and has heightened motivation to try new coping methods. The outcome of a crisis is either a change for the better or a change for the worse. Although uncomfortable, this active crisis state provides an important turning point and energy for the change effort. The patient's individual personal resources, problem-solving skills, adaptability to withstand sudden intensely stressful life events, and social support networks need to be assessed. It is here that the worker can start the process to assist with the flow of the intervention (Vonk & Early, 2002).

In the final phase of intervention, whether the patient is seen in person or counseled on the telephone (as a hotline caller), the patient needs to be prepared to deal with recurring problems stemming from the original crisis event. For example, violent crime victims in the aftermath of gunshot wounds may experience flashbacks or intrusive thoughts about the victimization. The patient will need to be prepared for common reactions that may occur. Another example is the person who has recently been diagnosed as HIV positive who may receive mixed messages from those she or he encounters. In the final session, it would be useful to help the patient decide on the best person to turn to for support in dealing with delayed or posttraumatic reactions if they should develop, even if at the present time they are not being experienced. The working through of the actual traumatic event and integrating the self is considered the primary goal in the middle phase. In the final phase of intervention, emphasis is placed on the ability of an individual to adapt or restore himself or herself to a balanced state—preferably one that exhibits restored or enhanced levels of confidence and coping.

In the application of crisis intervention, it is important to note that psychological trauma can be understood as an "affliction of the powerless" (Herman, 1992, p. 33). Threats to life and bodily integrity overwhelm normal adaptive capabilities, producing extensive symptomatology. Adopting a pathological view of symptomatology is not helpful; it is more beneficial when patients can comprehend their symptoms as signs of strength. Symptoms that are understood as coping techniques developed by the survivor to adapt to a toxic environment can enhance self-esteem (Roberts & Dziegielewski, 1995).

In the health care setting, crisis intervention can be severely limited by resources and agency role and function. Oftentimes, the health care social worker simply does not have the time to follow through with the formal intervention described here. In these cases, recognition of the problem, assessment of immediate danger, and referral with subsequent follow-up cannot be overstated. Because many individuals present in hospital emergency department as well as before surgery in acute crisis, it is important when feasible for

Applications: Roberts's Seven-Stage Crisis Intervention Model in the Health Care Setting

Effective intervention with survivors of trauma precipitated by a crisis requires a careful assessment of individual, family, and environmental factors. A crisis by definition is short term and overwhelming. According to Roberts (2000), a crisis is described as an emotionally distressing change. The crisis can cause a disruption of an individual's normal and stable state where the usual methods of coping and problem solving do not work.

Roberts (1991, 1995, 2000) describes seven stages of working through a crisis that involve (a) assessing lethality and safety needs; (b) establishing rapport and communication; (c) identifying the major problems; (d) dealing with feelings and providing support; (e) exploring possible alternatives; (f) formulating an action plan; and (g) providing follow-up. Roberts's seven-stage model applies to a broad range of crises addressed by health care providers and has been recommended as the framework for time-limited cognitive treatment throughout the book.

To enhance the application of this crisis intervention, the following assumptions are made: (a) all strategy will follow a "here-and-now" orientation; (b) the intervention period will be time limited (typically 6–12 sessions); (c) the adult survivor's behavior is viewed as an understandable (rather than a pathological) reaction to stress; (d) the assumption by the mental health worker of an active and directive role; and (e) the intervention strategy will strive to increase the survivor's remobilization and return to the previous level of functioning.

STAGE I

Psychosocial and Lethality Assessment

There are many hazardous events that can initiate a traumatic response. Listed below are some of the hazardous events or circumstances that can be linked to the recognition or reliving of traumatic events. These events can have the likelihood of triggering anxious responses from patients so that they seek help, even if the traumatic event is not immediately identified as the crisis issue: (a) growing public awareness of the prevalence of the traumatic event or similar traumatic events; (b) the acknowledgment by a loved one or someone that the patient respects that he or she has also been a victim; (c) a seemingly unrelated act of violence such as rape or sexual assault being committed to the patient or someone they love; (d) the changing of family or relationship support issues; and (e) the sights, sounds, or smells that trigger events from the patient's past (these can be highly specific to individuals and the trauma experienced).

Immediate Danger

With the number of suicides on the rise, intervention requires careful assessment of suicidal ideation, and the potential for initial and subsequent hospitalization or medication may be required. Questions to

(continued)

(*continued*)

elicit pervasive symptomatology should be asked (e.g., depression, suicidal ideation, anxiety, eating disorders, somatic complaints, sleep disorders, sexual dysfunction, instances of promiscuity, substance abuse, psychological numbing, self-mutilation, flashbacks, and panic attacks). On the basis of the age and the circumstances of the trauma experienced, the patient's living situation should be assessed to assure that the patient is still not in danger and that an adequate support system does exist. Several structured and goal-oriented sessions may be needed to help the patient move past the traumatic event, generating an understanding that what happened in regard to the traumatic event may have been beyond his or her control.

In these initial sessions of therapy (session 1–3), the goals of the therapeutic intervention are recognizing the hazardous event and acknowledging what has actually happened. For some reason (based on the triggering catalyst), the survivor of trauma is currently being subjected to periods of stress that disturb his or her sense of equilibrium. (It is assumed that the individual wants to maintain homeostatic balance and that physically and emotionally the body will seek to regain equilibrium.) As stated earlier, the survivor may not present with the actual crisis event, and the mental health counselor may have to help the survivor get to the root of the problem (i.e., the real reason for the visit). During these initial sessions, the survivor becomes aware and acknowledges the fact that the trauma has occurred; and once this happens, the survivor enters into a vulnerable state. The impact of this event disturbs the survivor, and traditional problem-solving and coping methods are attempted. When these do not work, tension and anxiety continue to rise, and the individual becomes unable to function effectively. In the initial sessions, the assessment of both past and present coping behaviors of the survivor is important; however, the focus of intervention clearly must remain in the "here and now." The mental health worker must attempt to stay away from past issues or unresolved issues unless they relate directly to the handling of the traumatic event.

STAGE II

Rapidly Establish Rapport

Many times, the survivor of trauma may feel as though family and friends have abandoned them or that they are being punished for something they did or did not do. These unrealistic interpretations may result in feelings of overwhelming guilt. It is possible that the capacity for trust has been damaged, and this may be reflected in negative self-image and poor self-esteem. A low self-image and poor self-esteem may increase the individual's fear of further victimization. Many times, survivors of trauma question their own vulnerability and know that re-victimization remains a possibility. This makes the role of the counselor in establishing rapport with the patient essential.

(*continued*)

Applications:Roberts's Seven-Stage Crisis Intervention Model in the Health Care Setting (*continued*)

Whenever possible, the mental health professional should progress slowly and try to let the survivor set the pace of treatment. Let the patient lead, because he or she may have a history of being coerced; and forcing confrontation on issues may not be helpful. Allowing the patient to set the pace creates a trusting atmosphere, which gives the message "the event has ended, you have survived and you will not be hurt here." Survivors often need to be reminded that their symptoms are a healthy response to an unhealthy environment. They need to recognize that they have survived heinous circumstances and continue to live and cope. The trauma victim may require a positive future orientation, with an understanding that they can overcome current problems and arrive at a happy, satisfactory tomorrow. Hope that change can occur is crucial to the survivor's well-being.

Perhaps more than anything else, throughout each of the sessions, these patients need unconditional support, positive regard, and concern. These factors are especially crucial to the working relationship because a history of lack of support, "blaming," and breach of loyalty are common. The therapeutic relationship is seen as a vehicle for continued growth, development of coping skills, and the ability to move beyond the abuse.

STAGE III

Identify the Major Problems or Crisis Precipitants

Once the major problems relevant to the particular event are identified and addressed; the concept of support remains essential. Group participation has been effective, as well as the use of journal writing, relaxation techniques, physical exercise, and development of an understanding that the victim needs to be good to him or her.

In these next few sessions (session 3–6), the mental health worker needs to assume an active role. First, the major problems to be dealt with and addressed must be identified. These problems must be viewed in how they have affected the survivor's behavior. Education in regard to the effects and consequences of this type of trauma will be discussed. Here, the precipitating factor, especially if the event was in the past, must be clearly identified. Complete acknowledgment of the event can push the person into a state of active crisis marked by disequilibrium, disorganization, and immobility (e.g., the last straw). Once the survivor enters full acknowledgment, new energy for problem solving will be generated. This challenge stimulates a moderate degree of anxiety, plus a kindling of hope and expectation. This actual state of disequilibrium can last 4 to 8 weekly sessions or until some type of adaptive or maladaptive solution is found.

(*continued*)

(continued)

STAGE IV

Dealing With Feelings and Emotions

The energy generated from the survivor's personal feelings, experiences, and perceptions steer the therapeutic process. It is critical that the social workers demonstrate empathy and an anchored understanding of the survivor's world. These symptoms are seen as functional and as a means of avoiding abuse and pain. Even severe symptoms such as dissociative reactions should be viewed as a constructive method of removing one's self from a harmful situation and exploring alternative coping mechanisms. Survivors' experiences should be normalized so that they can recognize being a victim is not their fault. Reframing symptoms is a coping technique that can be helpful. In this stage (session 6–8), the survivor begins to reintegrate. The survivor gradually begins to become ready to reach a new state of equilibrium. Each particular crisis situation (i.e., type and duration of incest, rape) may follow a sequence of stages, which can generally be predicted and mapped out. One positive result from generating the crisis state in stage 3 is that in treatment, after reaching active crisis, survivors seem particularly amenable to help.

Once the crisis situation has been obtained, distorted ideas and perceptions regarding what has happened need to be corrected and information updated so that the patient can better understand what he or she has experienced. Victims eventually need to confront their pain and anger so that they can develop better strategies for coping. Increased awareness helps the survivor to face and experience contradicting emotions (anger/love, fear/rage, dampening emotion/intensifying emotion) without the conditioned response of escape. Throughout this process, there must be recognition of the patient's continued courage in facing and dealing with these issues.

STAGE V

Generate and Explore Alternatives

Moving forward requires traveling through a mourning process (generally in sessions 8–10). Sadness and grief at the loss need to be experienced. Grief expressions surrounding betrayal and lack of protection permit the victim to open to an entire spectrum of feelings that have been numbed. Now accepting, letting go, and making peace with the past begins.

STAGE VI

Implement an Action Plan

Here, the mental health worker must be active in helping the survivor to establish how the goals of the therapeutic intervention will be completed. Practice, modeling, and other techniques, such as behavioral rehearsal, role play, the process of writing down of one's feelings, and

(continued)

Applications:Roberts's Seven-Stage Crisis Intervention Model in the Health Care Setting (*continued*)

an action plan, become essential in addressing intervention planning. The survivor has come to the realization that he or she is not at fault or to blame. The doubt and shame of what his or her role was and what part he or she played becomes clearer and self-fault less pronounced. The survivor begins to acknowledge that he or she did not have the power to help him or herself or to change things. Oftentimes, however, these realizations are coupled with anger at the helplessness a patient feels to control what has happened to him or her. The role of the mental health professional becomes essential here in helping the patient to look at the long-range consequences of acting on his or her anger and in planning an appropriate course of action. The main goal of these last few sessions (session 10–12) is to help the individual reintegrate the information learned and process it into a homeostatic balance that allows him or her to function adequately once again. Referrals for additional therapy should be considered and discussed at this time (i.e., additional individual therapy, group therapy, couples therapy, family therapy).

STAGE VII

Follow-Up

This area is important for intervention in general, but one that is almost always forgotten. In the successful therapeutic exchange, significant changes have been made for the survivor in regard to his or her previous level of functioning and coping. Measures to determine whether these results have remained consistent are essential. Oftentimes, follow-up can be as simple as a telephone call to discuss how things are going. Follow-up within one month of termination of the sessions is important.

Other measures of follow-up are available but require more advanced planning. A pretest/posttest design can be added to the design by simply using a standardized scale at the beginning of treatment and at the end. Scales to measure depression, trauma, and so on are readily available. See Corcoran and Fischer (2007) as a source for potential measurement scales that can be used in the behavioral sciences.

Finally, it is important to realize that at follow-up many survivors may realize that they want additional therapeutic help. After they have adapted to the crisis and have learned to function and cope, they may find that they want more. After all, returning the survivor to a previous state of equilibrium is the primary purpose for the application of this brief crisis intervention therapy. If this happens, the health worker should be prepared to help the patient become aware of the options for continued therapy and emotional growth by giving the appropriate referrals. Referrals for group therapy with other survivors of similar trauma, individual growth-directed therapy, couples therapy that is to include a significant other, or family therapy should be considered.

social workers to apply Roberts's seven-stage sequential practice model of crisis intervention. Practice models can serve as a guideline to help the health care social worker act quickly and confidently. Health care social workers may be the first helping professional these individuals meet that is willing to spend time with them. Many times, simply normalizing or giving permission to feel as they do is critical to starting the return to healthy homeostatic balance (Feigelman, Jordan, McIntosh, & Feigelman, 2012).

The importance of assessing patient danger to self or others is also essential. Individuals in crisis are experiencing feelings and emotions that they are not able to resolve by the usual methods of coping. This means that "unusual" or "permanent" solutions may be selected to handle what could be viewed as a temporary setback. The role of the health care social worker is essential in assessment of the situation and helping to provide service to combat the stress, whether that is done directly through intervention or indirectly through planned and actively assisted referral.

INTRODUCTION TO PROMOTION AND WELLNESS EDUCATION AND COUNSELING

For the most part, health literacy is defined as the currency that enables patients to obtain the benefits of the health care delivery system (Smith, 2011). As presented by the Centers for Disease Control and Prevention in *Healthy People 2020*, health promotion remains an important part of the nation's health delivery agenda (Centers for Disease Control and Prevention, 2012a). However, despite the growth and emphasis placed in this area, health promotion and recognition of the importance of health literacy remains fragmented. Poor communication between the disciplines involved can contribute to this lack of interaction between the research and the practice communities.

Many times in the medical field, health care social workers are called on to participate in a type of counseling that is not considered traditional. This type of counseling can include many different techniques; however, at a minimum, it must be time limited, and goal and objective focused, and assist patients to address present and future health and wellness issues. More and more health care social workers are being called on to provide this type of "health counseling" or "health education," yet rarely is it openly discussed and accepted as a method of providing social work practice.

In today's current health care environment, many believe that counseling to maintain health and wellness is essential (U.S. Department of Health and Human Services, 2009). Openly acknowledging this method as part of health care social work practice can assist social workers in identifying with this commonly provided service. There is also a need to include marriage and family therapy techniques especially in ensuring that the needs of historically underserved populations are addressed (Davey & Watson, 2008). Recognition of the patient and his or her family as part of the support system will make substantial contributions for reducing racial and ethnic disparities, increasing wellness in both health and mental health treatment. Social workers are in a unique position to participate in health counseling and prevention services. The overall practice of social work is health oriented, both conceptually and philosophically. The social worker can serve as a link between the person and a system of support and assist in maintaining health, detecting illness early or preventing deterioration of existing problems.

CHAPTER SUMMARY AND FUTURE DIRECTIONS

Health care provision continues to change rapidly and so are the health and behavioral health agencies that provide these services. Public demand is clear, and the expectations for health care similar to mental health call for practice strategy that goes beyond the traditional bounds of service provision. The public being served expects to be treated with state-of-the art technology, but they also want to be supported in a system of delivery where hope is fostered and wellness is stressed. This has required the development of innovative initiatives with practice strategy that seeks novel approaches to addressing the whole person where each method selected is responsible for demonstrating measurable outcomes that remain cost effective. Health promotion is so important to our future that the Centers for Disease Control budget for FY 2012 requested $705.378 million for new chronic disease prevention and health promotion programs with the expectation of improved coordination and health outcomes.

The need for supportive counseling with measurable outcomes has never been more important. The resistance to use only cognitive–behavioral approaches may be softened by utilizing a method with a rich history such as IPT where problem-solving efforts take into account some measure of the past, and in this newer model of psychodynamic practice, the unconscious is considered immediately accessible and changeable.

When IPT is used in the medical area, learning to identify personal problems and the concrete means to address them are considered essential. In the solution-focused therapies, a solution (or course of action) is identified, and specific attempts are made to attain it. In the cognitive–behavioral approaches, focus on understanding the complex relationship between socialization and reinforcement as it affects thoughts and behaviors in the current environment is stressed. This results in a clear emphasis on specific goals and objectives that can measure practice effectiveness. Crisis intervention highlights the use of crisis to enhance therapeutic effect. Interpretation of this traditional framework into a single-session intervention can assist the health care social worker to deal with the time-limited immediacy of a situation. In the last model outlined, social workers focus on providing health counseling and education based on the principle of creating and maintaining wellness. In general, health care social workers have not traditionally viewed health counseling as a viable method of therapeutic social work practice. Refuting this assumption, and recognizing the need for its inclusion, a model for empirically incorporating it into practice is described later in this book.

Regardless of what type of time-limited intervention is selected, it is clear that health and behavioral health care agencies need approaches that demonstrate measurable outcomes supported by services that provide alternatives to costly attempts at service provision that do not show direct measurable benefit to the patient/client/consumer served. This has caused an increased interest in time-limited home-based care and community programs and services that are recovery focused and often peer-run to help the individual return to the environment. It has also caused some to request the consideration of family therapy approaches sensitive to the needs of the nontraditional family and successful return to the community (Hodgson, Lamson, Mendenhall, & Crane, 2012).

Many health benefit plans do not recognize the importance of supportive and strategic counseling strategy. To complicate this situation further, too many social workers in this field are quick to say that we do not do counseling anymore. With the desperate need for this type of intervention in the health care setting, commentaries such as this should be avoided. Health care social workers should not allow administrative pressure to provide only reimbursable concrete services in their practice strategy. The bottom line is patients need and continue to want supportive counseling that takes into account the behavioral as well as the social and environmental circumstances in the health care setting that surround the identified medical concern. It is true that the number of people suffering from anxiety and depressive disorders, self-destructive acts, and life-threatening illnesses has steadily risen, making the need for these comprehensive supportive services paramount. To receive and continue to qualify for reimbursement for such services, social workers need to remain aware and active in the social and political climate that surrounds the health care practice arena.

Generally, social and political changes do not happen quickly. In the meantime, health care social workers are encouraged to engage in time-limited methods. These time-limited methods of practice offer promise for meeting urgent biopsychosocial and spiritual needs as well as identifying any crisis-related needs of patients identified as in distress. Regardless of what intervention method is selected, an emphasis on strength building and helping the patient to identify his or her own resources allows for empowerment. All methods of practice used in the health care area need to help patients/clients/consumers reframe their thinking patterns and use patient strengths.

Based on the turbulence and insecurity in our current health care environment, patients need the help and assistance that can be given only by competent professional social workers. Consequently, social workers experienced and trained in the area of health care need to be knowledgeable of the methods, tools, and techniques that are currently being used to provide this service.

For health care social workers, the importance of clearly stated behavioral objectives and the outcome result (not the practice method that is used) remain the "bread and butter" of the billing process. Stated simply, the goal becomes the overall task that the health care social worker wants to establish; however, it is the clearly stated behavioral outcome-based concrete objective that will help to ensure reimbursement and facilitate the measurement of service effectiveness. Never forget that the resultant objective must be clearly related to the outcome measure. This means that regardless of what time-limited method is used in the helping strategy, it will only be considered important to funding sources when it brings about changes in outcome (i.e., the end result).

Glossary

Bibliotherapeutic intervention   The assignment of reading materials to the patient generally completed as therapeutic "homework" to expand the formal limits of the counseling session.

Capitation   Under this provision, providers are paid a certain amount to provide a fixed amount of care for a certain period.

Cognitive–behavior therapy   This method of practice uses the combination of selected techniques incorporating the theories of behaviorism, social learning theory, and cognition theories to understand and address a patient's behavior.

Crisis   Generally, the term "crisis" is defined as a temporary state of upset and disequilibrium that is characterized by an individual's inability to cope with a particular situation.

Crisis intervention   A therapeutic practice used to help patients in crisis regain a sense of healthy equilibrium.

Fee-for-service   Defined simply, it is the amount of money paid for the service that is delivered.

Goals   A statement of the overall process a patient wants to achieve.

Intermittent therapy   A type of intervention strategy, used in the health care setting, in which every session is considered complete and treated as if it is the only session that may occur. Acknowledgment of this format allows for planned intervention and closure with each therapeutic encounter.

Interpersonal therapy   A form of time-limited treatment used in the medical setting. Generally, an assessment that includes a diagnostic evaluation and psychiatric history is gathered. The focus of treatment is directed toward interpersonal problem areas, such as grief, role disputes, role transitions, or deficits.

Managed behavioral health care   In this type of health care, coverage services are based, determined, and/or assessed by clear and specific outcome criteria.

Objectives   Specific statements that tell specifically how the goal will be accomplished.

Outcomes   These are the consequences of a situation, or, simply stated, attention is focused on what comes out at the end of the intervention process.

Psychotherapy   A form of therapy that involves understanding the "inner processes" of the individual regarding his or her personal situation.

Schema   This is considered a pattern of thinking that is referred to as the cognitive structure that organizes an individual's experience and behavior.

Summarization   The process of describing what has occurred in a situation, highlighting the addressing of goals and objectives that have been accomplished in the session. This technique should always be completed at the beginning and end of every time-limited session.

Questions for Further Study

1. What can health care social workers do to stress the value of the counseling services they provide?

2. What can social workers do to increase reimbursement potential on the counseling services they provide?

3. Which form of time-limited service provision seems most appropriate to use in the hospital setting and why?

4. Which form(s) of counseling seem to be most beneficial in the public health setting and why?

5. What things can social workers do to support the inclusion of counseling as part of the services provided in the managed care system?

Websites

Psychotherapy Finances
News related to financing for psychotherapy and behavioral health care
www.psyfin.com/

Yahoo Social Science/Social Work
A website for social workers with links, articles, and forums
dir.yahoo.com/social_science/social_work/

The Centers for Disease Control and Prevention (CDC)
Provides health news, publications, software, data, and statistics
www.cdc.gov/

Today's Health Care Social Worker

Name: L. Daisy Skinner, MSW, LCSW
List State of Practice:
Professional Job Title: Nephrology Social Worker

Duties in a typical day
The typical day of a nephrology social worker begins with the
pressing problems with patients on the first shift (treatments
between 5:00 a.m. and 9:00 a.m.). These issues include having no
transportation that morning, utilities being shut off due to non-
payment of bill, the need for medical equipment (walker, wheelchair, etc.), and/or personal issues. The information is given to the
nurse or patient care technicians, and they refer it to me to address.

1. **What do you like most about your current position?**
   People who have end stage renal disease have a myriad of
   medical problems that range from diabetes to hypertension
   (both the leading causes of kidney failure) to cancer and ampu-
   tations. That said, what I enjoy most about this job is the ability to work with physicians, nurses, and patients to join the
   psychological with the physical pieces in a way that benefits
   the patients to their maximum potential. It is critical to guide
   and provide supportive counseling to the patient through the
   complicated transplantation process. Working with families to
   help patients through the medical maze as well as helping to
   address end-of-life issues with them are the most rewarding
   aspects to this multifaceted job.

(continued)

(continued)

---

2. **What do you like least about your position?**
   Arranging for and fielding problems with daily transportation through the countywide transportation system for the disabled and older adults.

3. **What "words of wisdom" do you have for the new health care social worker who is considering working in a similar position?**
   Breathe! And, use humor. Breathe because the problems are numerous and varied, and you must be able to "switch gears" instantly. Humor because even though life is difficult for these patients, a laugh goes a long way. You must be a self-starter and have life's experiences to draw upon. Ask for or arrange a help-network with other nephrology social workers (they are your biggest supporters). Read past case notes, which provide a plethora of information. Above all, when the going gets rough, remember your reason for being there in the first place: you're making a difference in the patients' lives.

CHAPTER 7

Documentation and Record Keeping in the Health Care Setting

With the rapid growth of behavioral care social workers in health care settings are forced to become more skilled in identifying and responding to the needs of patients/clients/consumers (hereafter referred to as patients) and the changing practice environment. Practice strategy reflective of intermittent and time-limited therapeutic encounters must clearly reflect assessment and treatment progress while demonstrating worker efficiency, effectiveness, and accountability. In the health care setting, preplanned intervention and support services rarely occur. This requires versatility in all areas, especially the documentation that clearly outlines the services provided. Without organized and complete patient records, helping professionals cannot accurately document the services that they provide (Kagle & Kopels, 2008).

Social workers who work in health care settings realize the importance of accurate documentation and record keeping because they have been forced to become skilled in identifying and responding to the needs of patients. Whether a social worker is involved in indirect health care practice (focusing on health care policy and advocacy or health care administration) or direct practice (involving health-related assessment, intervention, prevention, and alleviation of negative situations), accurate and comprehensive documentation skills remain essential for quality intervention. Limited resources, specific program guidelines, and expectations inherent for insurance reimbursement make it increasingly imperative that social workers be responsive to growing expectations of accountability and improved program effectiveness.

The pressure for evidence-based interventions is so extensive that providing individualized care strategies must carefully examine the needs of the patient, ensuring continuity of care. Because each patient's situation is unique, service often requires individualized treatment strategy, and when offered in a time-limited or intermittent setting, individual change efforts can become more difficult to measure as opposed to being conducted in a planned, more formalized setting (Dziegielewski, 2010a, 2010b). Because service provided is not always conducted in a clearly defined environment and may include unplanned and brief encounters, measuring intervention success can be problematic. Rushed and high-pressured encounters do not always allow for clear plans depicting assessment and intervention. Yet, despite the complications inherent in rushed and brief service encounters, there is a need for well-organized and complete patient records. Service delivery records that reflect accurate assessment and individualized treatment approaches are needed to clearly outline progress within the services provided (Kagle & Kopels, 2008; Sidell, 2011).

The emphasis on accountability also requires that documentation show evidence-based changes, and when this is not clear, the result can be the loss of insurance coverage from third-party payers (Dziegielewski, 2010a, 2010b). Therefore, each individualized plan needs to outline efficacy, necessity, and effectiveness of the health care services provided with a clear link to outcome success and patient/client/consumer change (Dziegielewski, 2008a; Rubin, 2008). Comprehensive documentation is needed that clearly outlines the problem, describes the efforts to address the problem, and explains what makes this type of service provision necessary (Monette, Sullivan, & DeJong, 2005).

Service records must clearly reflect assessment and treatment progress while demonstrating worker efficiency, effectiveness, and accountability. The record will also need to include behavior-based measures that support patient engagement and participation that is reflective of physical and functional performance as well as community engagement on discharge (Mpofu & Oakland, 2009). Without organized and comprehensive patient records, helping professionals cannot accurately document the services that they provide. Documentation, when related directly to supervision, is important as it verifies that the service actually occurred (NASW 2003b).

EDUCATION AND TRAINING IN RECORD KEEPING

Dziegielewski (2008b) stressed the importance of training for all health care social workers in the area of documentation. In addition, training in this area cannot be static as record-keeping formats can change constantly based on agency preference and insurance requirements through third-party billing. A trial-and-error approach can have devastating consequences and may lead to uncertainty related to the nature, duration, and outcomes of the therapeutic encounter. For many social workers, particularly those in long-term care, it is considered time consuming, repetitive, and burdensome (Beaulieu, 2012). Therefore, social workers need to avoid supporting the notion that this type of activity is fruitless and that the time required for ensuring complete and accurate records only results in less quality time to spend with patients.

In fact, it can lead to more quality time when the information gathered adds to the therapeutic encounter and clearly documents exactly what happened. This can be easily added to therapeutic techniques such as active listening that provide more than a supportive ear. When looked at as something that one must do, it can result in a strong desire to postpone or defer documentation to a later time. It is understandable that the pressure to document exactly what has happened in measurable terms can raise anxiety.

Yet, all information that is not documented clearly is considered not to have happened, so accurate and comprehensive documentation is essential to all treatment efforts.

Documentation Rule Number One

If you did not document it … it did not happen.

To achieve comprehensive documentation, there is an expectation in most human service agencies that new social work employees know how to document patient progress and how to identify what information should be included in the files. Therefore, be sure to always address the potential consequences of brief and unplanned interventions and, regardless of the setting, know how to apply evidence-based procedures with an individualized plan that reflects the continuity of care. Education and training in documentation should include at a minimum an evidence-based treatment approach; a plan to assess the feasibility and manage the quality of the intervention; a plan to ensure that all helping efforts are grounded in culturally sensitive practices efforts; and finally, a plan for more sustainable empowering strategies that utilize the patient's own strengths and helping networks (Levkoff, Chen, Fisher, & McIntyre, 2006). Health care social workers need to be knowledgeable of the importance of documentation and the different types of professional record keeping that can lead to effective, efficient, and comprehensive documentation.

CONFIDENTIALITY, RELEASING INFORMATION, AND HIPAA

In the United States, a high value is placed on a person's right to self-determination and privacy. In health care, respecting and maintaining confidentiality sits at the forefront of almost all courses of action. To maintain a patient's privacy or confidentiality requires that information learned regarding the patient only be released in certain circumstances, and when it is released, the least amount of information needed is to be selectively disclosed (NASW, 2011). Overall, how to address confidentiality can be a complicated process, because there are certain circumstances in which breaching is sanctioned by both state laws and professional standards.

In social work, it is clear that confidentiality may be breached with or without the patient's consent to report instances of neglect and abuse. Other circumstances include times when a patient may be a danger to self or others, or when other compelling reasons exist, such as imminent harm to a patient or if the law requires disclosure. There are situations in which breach of confidentiality is certainly justifiable and expected, although the principles that surround maintaining confidentiality are central to gaining a patient's trust to disclose problem-related information. For health care social workers, similar to others in the field, this can create a complex issue that must rest firmly in ethical decision making.

The 1996 NASW *Code of Ethics* (revised by the Delegate Assembly in 2008) provides lengthy standards with regard to privacy and confidentiality, clearly stating that social workers should "respect patients' right to privacy ... and ... should protect the confidentiality of all information obtained in the course of professional service, except for compelling professional reasons" (NASW, 1996, Standard 1–1.07, p. 10). In practice and in maintaining documentation of such, all social workers should make every attempt possible to adhere to the rules of confidentiality and remain keenly aware of what to do if it may need to be broken. In health care, the same standards apply.

In addition, on August 21, 1996, Congress enacted the Health Insurance Portability and Accountability Act (HIPAA), which was instituted to protect the consumer and combat health care fraud while simplifying health care administration and insurance. HIPAA requires that entities limit disclosures of patient information to the minimum necessary related to a specific purpose, with a few exceptions.

In addition, the Health Information Technology for Economic and Clinical Health (HITECH) Act has specified that the entity that is disclosing the information is the one responsible for determining the minimum amount of information necessary for the purpose requested. Also, when information is disclosed, entities should limit the information as much as possible and use a limited data set that has been stripped of identified information. If this is not possible and identifiers are needed, only the minimum amount of information requested is to be revealed. This latest change became effective in 2009; however, additional regulations to redefine what is meant by "minimum necessary" are forthcoming.

HIPAA has been important for providing oversight for protected health information and set clear ground rules for what information related to a patient could or could not be revealed. These regulations continue to shape how medical information is transmitted between facilities and how records are stored (Beaulieu, 2012). Outlined within the HIPAA regulations are what constitutes a covered agency and what information can be shared with and without patient permission. To facilitate the process, a list of 18 HIPAA identifiers was prepared that outline the patient information protected under this Act. See Table 7.1 for an abbreviated list of the HIPPA identifiers.

When it comes to HIPAA or simply ensuring confidentiality, in general, each social worker should be aware of the legal rules in his or her state

Table 7.1 HIPAA: List of 18 Identifiers

1. Names

2. All geographical subdivisions smaller than a state, including street address, city, county, precinct, zip code, and their equivalent geocodes, except for the initial three digits of a zip code, if according to the current publicly available data from the Bureau of the Census: (1) The geographic unit formed by combining all zip codes with the same three initial digits contains more than 20,000 people; and (2) the initial three digits of a zip code for all such geographic units containing 20,000 or fewer people is changed to 000

3. All elements of dates (except year) for dates directly related to an individual, including birth date, admission date, discharge date, and date of death; and all ages over 89 and all elements of dates (including year) indicative of such age, except that such ages and elements may be aggregated into a single category of age 90 or older

4. Phone numbers

5. Fax numbers

6. Electronic mail addresses

7. Social Security numbers

8. Medical record numbers

9. Health plan beneficiary numbers

10. Account numbers

11. Certificate/license numbers

12. Vehicle identifiers and serial numbers, including license plate numbers

13. Device identifiers and serial numbers

14. Web Universal Resource Locators

15. Internet Protocol address numbers

16. Biometric identifiers, including finger and voice prints

17. Full face photographic images and any comparable images

18. Any other unique identifying number, characteristic, or code (note this does not mean the unique code assigned by the investigator to code the data)

of practice and how to respond if situations arise. Because severe penalties could result, all social workers need to remain mindful that staying informed is the responsibility of the health care professional. Always keep in mind that in cases of willful neglect of the HIPAA requirements, serious monetary penalties can result. These penalties will come in addition to the harm that revealing this information does to the patient.

As the use of electronic records continues to grow, encrypted records with clear assurances for HIPAA compliance should be in place. All information stored in electronic records and shared with other contractual obligations or business associates who utilize this information should also be aware of the procedures for protection. If a breach occurs, the social worker will need to have a plan to mitigate any harm that might result. Most social workers are sensitive to the privacy concerns of patients seeking mental health treatment.

One practice standard reflective of the seasoned practitioner that those new to the field may find particularly helpful is that if the legal and moral code standards for ethical conduct do not match, simply follow the one that is most comprehensive. When following this practice principal, the social worker will find the document that is almost always the most comprehensive is the one held by the social work profession.

HIPAA requires that all health care workers be trained in the rules and requirements to help eliminate any confusion about what can and cannot be revealed. For a review of HIPPA requirements related specifically to social work, the reader is referred to NASW *Law Notes: Patient Confidentiality and Privileged Communications* (2011). This pamphlet is particularly helpful in breaking this down into a simple, concise, easy-to-read format and provides discussion of this topic and other topics related specifically to ensuring confidentiality.

As with other decisions made in social work practice, ethical decisions and maintaining confidentiality are not usually simple, right or wrong choices that can be made without a great deal of thought. Often they involve choosing between two undesirable actions with neither choice being the correct one, yet some considerations will outweigh others (Saxon et al., 2006). In social work practice, ethical decisions often must be made quickly but always ensure that time is allowed to process the situation assuring the best legal and ethical decision is made (Loewenberg et al., 2000). Furthermore, although helpful as a guideline, the NASW *Code of Ethics* does not provide specific direction when professional values clash, so examining each situation on an individual basis is always recommended. When needed, discuss decisions with a "jury of your peers" and do not hesitate to seek consultation when needed. However, NASW does provide a rich database of helpful information on confidentiality and how to handle privileged communications.

HIPAA Resource

U.S. Department of Health and Human Services

http://www.hhs.gov/ocr/privacy/

RECORD KEEPING AND JUSTIFICATION OF SERVICE

Professional record keeping can serve many purposes. First, record keeping can help health care social workers maintain the basic written information that is needed in the practice environment. To qualify for reimbursement, most third-party payers require that health care practitioners record specific assessment, goals, objectives, and the actual treatment process that will be employed in the helping environment (Kagle & Kopels, 2008). When feeling rushed, the temptation to jot down something quickly can be hard to overcome, especially when pressured to write it quickly and concisely. The key to remember when documenting in any record is that when a social worker is brief and concise in his or her documentation, she or he also needs to be relevant and comprehensive (Dziegielewski, 2010a).

Furthermore, in this society, litigation is common, increasing the pressure for adequate documentation that reflects the legal and ethical concerns employed in the helping relationship (Dziegielewski, 2010b; Woody, 2012). All social workers need to document carefully to avoid mistakes in assessment and treatment that could result in legally actionable mistakes (Woody, 2012). To stress the importance of accurate and concise record keeping, the following three catchy statements of expectation may be of assistance.

1. If the social worker did not record it, it did not happen.
2. The life expectancy of a document could be forever, so document carefully. Someday a social worker may leave an agency, but the document she or he has written could stay indefinitely.
3. If a social worker was summoned to court, could he or she defend what was written in the patient/client/consumer case record?

What is summarized in these three phrases constitutes simple common sense rules for documenting. In the first statement, the social worker is reminded that if information was not recorded in a record, it cannot be added after the fact. So many times in a hurried environment intervention, case management or discharge planning strategies could be addressed, but in the hurried time frame simply did not get recorded. If called to question, however, the documentation rule is clear: if it was not documented—it cannot be established as having happened. When a situation results, the only information that can be shared as reality is what was written in the case record. With this in mind, social workers should always be sure to take the extra time to document all that is relevant to the case, permissions obtained, and any safety plan information gathered and formulated. Documenting this information will protect the patient and the agency (Woody, 2012).

The second statement refers to the "life expectancy" of a record. In some states, records may be closed after 3 to 5 years, but there can always be exceptions to any rule. If a patient's record is ever ordered by a court, regardless of whether it happened years ago, could the social worker read his or her own notes and summarize clearly what happened? In addition, related to the third statement, if the record was subpoenaed to court, could the social worker defend what was written? In documentation, it is central to always write each record as if it stands alone so that if the note was separated from the rest of the record, it could outline the complete picture.

Social workers also need to be careful not to show personal feelings or bias in a record especially when feeling frustrated with a situation. This is not considered professional and should never be documented. Just stick to the facts. One rule that may help with this is to never document something when you are angry or upset. Give it some time whenever possible to be sure your professional dictations are not clouded with your personal interpretations. Because the life expectancy of a record could be stored electronically indefinitely or placed in the "cloud," it is quite possible it could be retrieved many years later.

Documentation Rule Number Two

Never make it personal; this is not about the social worker's feelings.

The written synopsis that describes assessment, intervention, and treatment strategy will always provide essential information that could be shared if subpoenaed to court. A clearly documented record protects the patient, the professionals involved in the care, and the health care facility. This documentation can provide essential information related to admission circumstances, the care given, and the follow-up received.

EVIDENCE-BASED PRACTICE: RECORDING GOALS AND OBJECTIVES

Accurate record keeping in the health care environment is central to the concept identifying treatment goals and measuring objectives as part of evidence-based practice. In evidence-based practice, maintaining objective and impartial records can assist in understanding, establishing, and justifying the intervention process that has been initiated. Accurate, clear, and concise record keeping can help to establish continuity of care. For example, was the information documented to show the rate of patient progress or nonprogress and retrogression? Were changes needed in the current program highlighted and was a specific plan to address them identified? Was the patient able to complete the tasks and behavioral requirements assigned, and if not, was there a plan documented that allowed for goal changes or returning to an earlier stage of intervention? Were factors that could impede progress identified? What problems have been stabilized and resolved? Finally, was the identified care plan and services provided delivered in the most cost-effective way possible (Dziegielewski, 2010b)?

The record needs to be accurate, stressing service accountability and addressing the needs for reimbursement. Continuous care organizations and other external reviewing bodies tasked with monitoring service can hold health care social work providers responsible for quality of care issues, length of service provision, level of care provided, use of ancillary and other therapeutic services, referral patterns and use, cost-restraining interventions, appropriateness or suitability of service, compliance to a standard set of provision criteria, the use of outcome criteria, and so on. Therefore, be prepared as often the health care service record is audited to determine whether professionals have applied the most affordable services prudently dedicated to quality service provision.

TYPES OF RECORD KEEPING

Throughout the history of health care social work, some type of medical record or recording process has been required. In the beginning, most records were in the form of *ledgers* and *narrative records*. This early form of record keeping merely provided the facts regarding the patient's situation (Timms, 1972). When public health services were delivered, they were documented, but little clinical interpretation generally occurred. This did change, and in the second half of the 19th century, a more sophisticated approach resulted. This new approach went beyond simply listing the problems to "making a case" for a patient's needs and resources (Sheffield, 1920).

In 1920, Ada Eliot Sheffield wrote a book titled, *The Social Case History: Its Construction and Content*. In this method of recording, she highlighted what the facts meant and how they could be applied to relieve suffering. Sheffield, similar to Mary Richmond, believed that accountability meant improving social conditions (public health) and delivering effective services and enhancing practitioner skills.

Process Recording

Historically, *process recording* is an early type of record keeping that clearly influenced health care social work. This form of recording became popular in the 1920s, and its introduction was influenced heavily by the field of sociology. It was expected to facilitate research and practice by allowing a patient to reveal the self by using his or her own dialogue (Burgess, 1928). Oftentimes, this type of recording format was used to (a) gather information for the development of social work practice theory and (b) monitor service evaluation. However, it did not take long, and this method of recording soon lost its favor. Many social workers thought it was too long, detailed, and cumbersome to use in the practice setting.

Today, process recording is generally not used in the health care practice setting. However, it is used in hospital training programs, cases involving the courts and legal issues, and other educational settings. For the most part, process recording is primarily used to assist beginning-level social workers and other health care providers to learn counseling and practice strategy. In training, it is not uncommon for students to be asked to create a detailed chronological format that includes a factual face sheet, goals, contracts, patient interpretations, and telephone and in-person contacts, all involved in the service that was provided. It can also be very helpful in preparing for testimony to be delivered in the legal setting, where in court every word shared is recorded. This makes choosing the words we use to describe an event a very careful and important process. It also requires that when we describe what has been documented, communication should be clear on both content and the resulting outcome.

Diagnostic Recording

A second type of early case recording that had its roots in a health and mental health setting was *diagnostic recording*. Hamilton (1936, 1946) grounded the development and use of this type of case recording in psychosocial theory. Diagnostic recording added to the basis of process recording in that the exploration of social causes was expanded to include those issues of a psychosocial nature. A trained diagnostician completed this assessment and interpretation. It was the use of diagnostic recording that is said to have cemented the relationship between practice, the practitioner, supervision, and the record (Kagle, 1995). The format for this type of recording often varied in length and content with little unifying structure. This form of record keeping quickly lost favor in the medical setting as it became too hard to find important information; and oftentimes, the information simply was not there to find at all, because what was to be recorded was at the discretion of the recorder.

In today's health care environment, this type of recording is rarely if ever used. Taking into account the current practice environment and stress on clear documented outcomes, the lack of style and format of this method clearly has caused it to lack in favor.

Audio and Video Recordings

Audio and *video recording* are methods of case recording, which are used in some medical settings today, particularly when research studies and other types of quality control measures are implemented. In the practice setting, this type of recording is almost always limited to training programs and is primarily used for educational purposes only. For example, oftentimes, this method is used to train primary care physicians, nurses, and so on, particularly in the area of family dynamics. Oftentimes, the interdisciplinary team reviews sessions, and suggestions for improving service delivery are made. This type of recording is consistent with family therapy, as often they view the practitioner as an "objective observer" where watching actions and behaviors become essential for refining current skills and exploring better ways of addressing a problematic situation.

However, audio and video recording are generally not used as the sole method of recording service delivery. In health care practice today, this method of recording alone is considered deficient and is never used without supplementation. Also, whether used in the practice or the research setting, any type of recordings that are made need to ensure that permission from the patient and, in the case of a minor, permission from his or her parent has been obtained. On the permission form, it is recommended that the form clearly state the purpose of the taping, how long it will be kept, and what will be done with the recording. This means outlining clearly the purpose of the recording as well as who will see the recordings, how it will be shared, and plans for disposal when the purpose is completed. Permission and clarity of purpose is particularly important if the patient is going to be participating in any type of taping that will be used in either the research or the practice setting.

Time Series Recording

In evidence-based practice, *time series recording* offers an efficient and effective way to establish whether an intervention is successful and to display this result graphically. Generally, this form of recording is most commonly associated with behavioral interventions and single-subject designs. This method of recording encourages the use of this type of design to document and measure specific patient problem behaviors. It can be helpful in providing information toward the movement of goals and objectives.

In this method, individual patient data are collected and displayed visually on a graph. The information gathered is later analyzed statistically or visually. One major weakness of this form of record keeping is that it requires expertise in the design and setup of the recording. One of the major limitations for the use of this type of design and other time series recording formats in the health care setting appears to be the lack of knowledge and support of the documentation format. Many health care supervisors and other medical professionals are not familiar with single-subject designs and the methods of recording generally practiced in this context. Therefore, they do not encourage its use.

A second reason for the lack of popularity of time series recording as a method of documentation is the charting procedure. This form of record keeping is limited to documenting only certain aspects of the patient's problem or situation. This makes it essential for health care social workers to know the basics of this approach to recording and stressing that others on the team follow the format and chart similarly. Time series recording is most helpful for showing patient progress to the individual or the team but not necessarily for recording in the record.

In time series recording, the *single-subject research design* is used. In this design, the individual is studied throughout the treatment process. Use of this type of design can help the health care social worker answer the question: "Is what I am doing working?" The attractiveness of this design in the health care setting is that it can be used with individual patients, a couple, a family, or a group.

It is beyond the scope of this chapter to go into depth in this area, but for further information on tips and techniques to improve documentation strategy, the social worker is referred to Sidell (2011) on *Social Work Documentation: A Guide to Strengthening Your Case Recording.*

Computerized and Standardized Records

Computerized or *standardized records* constitute the most common forms of record keeping utilized in most health care facilities. In the 1980s, agencies, hospitals, and other health care facilities began to recognize the benefits of computer technology in record keeping. Today, almost all health care agencies keep standardized and computerized administrative files. The most common use of computers involves word processing, making computers invaluable tools for writing assessments, progress notes, correspondence, and reports (Gingerich, 2002). There are some agencies that continue to use handwritten recordings, and more personal and problem-oriented notes that are maintained outside of a computer system are becoming rare. One concern that continues to grow is the problem of protecting patient confidentiality within the computerized record. The news is almost always filled with someone who has successfully accessed computer data files, leaving the sensitive information recorded inside open to misuse through unintended access.

To protect the confidentiality of the patient, information and computer access must be guarded. Guarded access is important to restrict information to only select professionals with a need to know. The use of computerized records is expanding so much that increasingly it has become the only type of record keeping used. In addition, computerized tools, often referred to as rapid assessment instruments (RAIs), are often used to supplement the record keeping. The use of these measures is most relevant for incorporating outcome measures such as symptom checklists, to be used as a diagnostic tool and for graphing or analysis of data (Gingerich, 2002). In terms of the future, evidence is strong that paper-based records will almost completely disappear, and checklists and computer-based files will constitute patient record keeping within a totally automated system.

Person- or Family-Oriented Recording

The *person-* or *family-oriented* record is a new type of record keeping found in the health care setting. Generally, this form of record keeping is seen most in a community-oriented practice model for health care delivery. In this record, a database, treatment plan, assessment, progress notes, and a progress review are included; however, special attention is given to the uniqueness of the patient and his or her family. Particularly, in the family-oriented record, a concentration on wellness is highlighted as information for everyone in the household may be viewed at the same time. The entire family is kept in one file. Similarly, in the patient-oriented record, the responsibility for the record rests with the patient. All information from numerous providers is all kept in one record, and, at times, the record may be released directly to the patient to ensure that continuity in health care treatment is documented. The emphasis in the family- and person-oriented record is measuring individual family or patient progress over time and different providers.

Problem-Oriented Recording

Among the various types of record-keeping formats, many health care facilities use problem-oriented recording (POR) (Dziegielewski, 2010a). Traditionally used in health care or medical settings, this type of recording was originally formulated to encourage multidisciplinary, interdisciplinary, transdisciplinary, and pandisciplinary collaborations and to train medical professionals. As members of these types of treatment teams, helping professionals find that problem-oriented case documentation enables them to maintain documentation uniformity while remaining active within a team approach to care.

For the health care social worker, POR emphasizes accountability through brief and concise documentation of patient problems, services, or interventions as well as patient responses. Although there are numerous formats for problem-oriented case recording, always keep comments brief, concrete, measurable, and concise. Many professionals feel strongly that POR is compatible with the increase in patient caseloads, rapid assessments, and time-limited treatment. By maintaining brief but informative notes, health care professionals are able to provide significant summaries of intervention progress. Generally, the health care social worker cannot select the type of POR that will be utilized as this choice is based on agency, clinic, hospital or practice's function, need, and accountability. Clear and concise documentation reflects the pressure indicative of evidence-based practice. This makes it critical for the health care social worker to be familiar with the basic types of POR and how to utilize this format within the case record.

One thing that all POR formats share in common is that all formats start with a problem list that is clearly linked to the behaviorally based biopsychosocial intervention (Chamblis, 2000; Frager, 2000). This problem-focused documentation helps the health care social worker to focus directly on the presenting problems and coping styles that the patient is exhibiting, thereby helping to limit abstractions and vague clinical judgments. Therefore, this type of documentation should include an inventory reflective of current active problems that are periodically updated. When a problem is resolved, it is crossed off the list with the date of resolution clearly designated. Noting that the active problems a patient is experiencing is considered the basic building blocks for case recording within the problem-oriented record.

Although numerous formats for the actual progress note documentation can be selected, the SOAP (subjective, objective, assessment, and plan) is considered the most commonly used. See Table 7.2 for SOAP, SOAPIE (subjective, objective, assessment, plan, implementation, and evaluation), and SOAPIER (subjective, objective, assessment, plan, implementation, evaluation, and response) recording formats.

Table 7.2 SOAP, SOAPIE, and SOAPIER Recording Formats

Subjective, Objective, Assessment, and Plan (SOAP)
Subjective, Objective, Assessment, Plan, Implementation, and Evaluation (SOAPIE)
Subjective, Objective, Assessment, Plan, Implementation, Evaluation, and Response (SOAPIER)
S = Subjective data relevant to the patient's request for service; patient and practitioner impressions of the problem.
O = Objective data such as observable and measurable criteria related to the problem. If patient statements are used, put the statement in quotes.
A = Assessment information of the underlying problems; diagnostic impression.
P = Plan that outlines current intervention strategy and specific referrals for other needed services.
I = Implementation considerations of the service to be provided.
E = Evaluation of service provision.
R = Patient's response to the diagnostic process, treatment planning, and intervention efforts.

SOAP is the most common form of POR, and became popular in the 1970s. In this format, the health care social worker utilizes the "S" (subjective) to record the data relevant to the patient's request for service and the things the patient says and feels about the problem. In this section, the health care professional can use his or her clinical judgment in terms of documenting what appears to be happening with the patient. Some professionals prefer to document this information in terms of major themes or general topics addressed, rather than making specific statements about what the practitioner thinks is happening. Generally, in this section, intimate personal content or details of fantasies and process interactions should not be included. When charting in this section of the SOAP, note the health care social worker should always consider whether this statement could be open to misinterpretation. If it is vulnerable to misinterpretation or it resembles a personal rather than professional reaction to what is said, it should not be included.

The "O" (objective) includes observable and measurable criteria related to the problem. These are symptoms, behaviors, and patient-focused problems observed directly by the social worker during the assessment and intervention process. In addition, some agencies, clinics, and practices have started to include patient statements in this section as well. If a patient statement is to be utilized as objective data, however, exact quotes must be used. For example, if in the session patient states that he will not harm himself, the practitioner must document exactly what the patient has said. What is said must be placed in between the quotation marks. Under the objective section of the summary, note it is also possible to include the results from standardized assessment instruments designed to measure psychological or social functioning.

The "A" (assessment) includes the therapist's assessment of the underlying problems, which if in the mental health setting might include a *DSM-IV-TR* multi-axial system. Because application of this framework is beyond the scope of this chapter, please see Dziegielewski (2010a) for more specific applications. In "P" (plan), the practitioner records how treatment objectives will be carried out, areas for future interventions, and specific referrals to other services needed by the patient.

With today's increased emphasis on time-limited intervention efforts and accountability, two new areas have been added to the original SOAP format (Dziegielewski, 2010a). This extension referred to as SOAPIE identifies the first additional term as "I," which stands for the implementation considerations of the service to be provided. Here, the health care social worker explains exactly how, when, and who will implement the service. In the last section of the SOAPIE format, an "E" is designated to represent service provision evaluation (Dziegielewski, 2010a). It is here that all health care professionals are expected to identify specific actions related to direct evaluation of progress achieved after any interventions are provided. When treatment is considered successful, specific outcomes-based objectives established early in the treatment process are documented as progressing or checked off as attained. In some agencies, a modified version of the SOAPIE has been introduced and referred to as SOAPIER. In this latest version, the "R" outlines the patient's response to the intervention provided.

A second popular POR format used in many health and mental health care facilities today is the DAP (data, assessment, and plan) format. The DAP encourages the social worker to identify only the most salient elements of a practitioner's patient contact. Using the "D" (data), the social worker is expected to record objective patient data and statements related to the presenting problem and the focus of the therapeutic contact. The "A" is used to record the diagnostic assessment intervention from the multiaxial format, the patient's reactions to the service and intervention, and the social worker's assessment of the patient's overall progress toward the treatment goals and objectives. Specific information on all tasks, actions, or plans related to the presenting problem and to be carried out by either the patient or the helping professional is recorded under "P" (plan). Also recorded under "P" (plan) is information on future issues related to the presenting problem to be explored at the next session and the specific date and time of the next appointment (Dziegielewski, 2010a). Again, similar to the SOAP, the DAP format has also undergone some changes. For example, some counseling professionals who generally apply the use of the DAP are now being asked to modify this form of record keeping to add an additional section. This changes the DAP into the DAPE (data, assessment, plan, and education) and adds a section where documentation under the "E" reflects what type of educational and evaluative services have been conducted. See Table 7.3 for a summary of the recording format.

Two other forms of problem-based case recording formats often used in health and mental health setting are the PIRP (problem, intervention, response, and plan) and the APIE (assessed information, problems addressed,

Table 7.3 DAPE Recording Format

Data, Assessment, and Plan (DAP) Data, Assessment, Plan, and Education (DAPE)
D = Data that are gathered to provide information about the identified problem.
A = Assessment of the patient in regard to his or her current problem or situation.
P = Plan for intervention and what will be completed to assist the patient to achieve increased health status or functioning.
E = Professional education that is provided by the mental health practitioner to ensure that problem mediation has taken place or evaluation information to ensure practice accountability.

Table 7.4 PIRP and APIE

Problem, Intervention, Response, and Plan (PIRP)
P = Presenting problem(s) or the problem(s) to be addressed. **I** = Intervention to be conducted by the mental health practitioner. **R** = Response to the intervention by the patient. **P** = Plan to address the problems experienced by the patient.
Assessed Information, Problems Addressed, Interventions Provided, and Evaluation (APIE)
A = Documentation of assessed information in regard to the patient problem. **P** = Explanation of the problem that is being addressed. **I** = Intervention description and plan. **E** = Evaluation of the problem once the intervention is completed.

interventions provided, and evaluation). See Table 7.4, where a similar structure to SEAP and DAP is employed. All four of these popular formats of problem-oriented case recording have been praised for supporting increased problem identification, standardizing what and how patient behaviors, and coping styles that are reported, thus providing a greater understanding of health and mental health problems and the various methods of managing them. This type of problem-oriented record brings the focus of clinical attention to an often traditionally neglected aspect of recording. It allows for recognition of a patient's problems and for quick familiarization with the central problem.

For health care social workers, utilizing a problem-focused perspective must go beyond merely recording information that is limited to the patient's problems. When the focus is limited to gathering only this information, important strengths and resources that patients bring to the therapeutic interview may not be validated. Furthermore, partialization of patient problems presents the potential risk that other significant aspects of a patient's functioning will be overlooked in treatment planning and subsequent practice strategy. Therefore, problem-oriented forms of case recording need to extend beyond the immediate problem regardless of whether coordinated care companies require it (Dziegielewski, 2010a; Rudolph, 2000).

DOCUMENTATION, TREATMENT PLANNING, AND PRACTICE STRATEGY

Throughout history, health care social workers have relied on some form of record keeping for clearly documenting information on patient situations and problems. Although the formats used by professionals have changed, the value of documentation in maintaining case continuity has remained a professional priority (Dziegielewski, 2008b). In its most basic form, case recording provides the helping professional with a "map" that indicates where the patient and practitioner have traveled in their treatment journey (Dziegielewski, 2008a). Because the treatment experience is often a dynamic interchange that goes beyond what written words can describe the exact words used must be chosen carefully. Add to this the implosion of technology and computer-based correspondence and record keeping makes the primary goal of case documentation an evolving process. Case documentation must also be geared toward maintaining high-quality service and preserving continuity of service when different mental health professionals are involved. In addition, well-documented diagnostic assessments and interventions can also protect the health care social worker in high-risk cases, making him or her less likely to be judged negligent in the legal setting (Bernstein & Hartsell, 2004; Hartsell, Hartsell, & Berstein, 2008). Understanding the relationship between identifying patient problems, interventions used, and patient progress enables the social worker to assess the interventions provided and make necessary changes in the intervention process.

The purpose of documentation and accurate record keeping is multifaceted, and comprehensive record keeping must (1) provide an accurate and standardized account of the information gathered; (2) support this information with introspective and retrospective data collection; (3) provide the information needed for good practice standards that include relevant ethical, legal, billing, and agency requirements; and (4) provide clearly stated information that will withstand scrutiny by external reviewers such as accreditation bodies, ombudsmen, lawyers, insurance companies, and quality assurance/improvement and control personnel.

For health care social workers, accurate case documentation is critical or most third-party payers will not reimburse for the start or continuation of services. Therefore, the link between clinical indicators and best practice strategy will always emphasize accountability and reimbursement, as it is mandated by the external reviewing bodies that monitor patient services (Dziegielewski & Holliman, 2001). All social workers are expected to justify and document patient eligibility for service, appropriateness for continuation of services, length of treatment, level of care, interventions provided, and the use of outcome criteria (Holliman, Dziegielewski, & Datta, 2001).

Utilizing a holistic framework that stresses the patient's behavioral and biopsychosocial factors allows health care social workers to play an important role in the efficient delivery of interdisciplinary psychological and social services. As part of a collaborative team, practitioners can support all members to document effectively while collaborating with each other on assessing patient progress. The importance of providing accurate, up-to-date, and informative records is vital to the coordinated planning efforts of the entire team.

With the advent of behavior-based care, however, high caseloads and shorter lengths of stay have caused health care social workers to adapt a style of documentation that is brief yet informative (Holliman et al., 2001). The challenge then is to evaluate practice by summarizing important patient information into meaningful yet accountable notes and treatment plans (Bloom, Fischer, & Orme, 2009). Given the litigious nature of our society, informative records that demonstrate treatment interventions and reflect legal and ethical values and concerns become important documents in legal proceedings (Cumming et al., 2007). These documents can be recalled long after the therapeutic intervention has ended. The pressure for accurate documentation rests in the growing emphasis and pressure to utilize evidence-based professional practice and justification for the course of intervention that will follow.

When utilizing evidence-based practice, clear documentation as reflected in the case record can be used for numerous purposes. According to Chambliss (2000) regardless of the helping discipline or practice setting, generic rules for efficient and effective documentation must always be employed.

- Clearly document problem behaviors and coping styles.
- Clearly outline behavioral symptoms as this will provide the basis for subsequent goals and interventions.
- The intervention plan must clearly reflect progress indicators and time frames, reflective and supportive of the identified problem.
- Case notes and intervention plan must clearly document and show response to interventions.
- Case notes are used to assess goal accomplishment and to evaluate the efficiency, treatment, and cost effectiveness of the service delivered.

Measuring Goals and Objectives

In the health care setting, the time-limited and/or unstructured nature of the setting clearly presents challenges for the social worker trying to measure the effectiveness of his or her interventions. Basically, no matter what evaluative effort is employed, it must be initiated early and brought to closure fairly quickly. In addition, in establishing effectiveness, this experience should not be seen as being intrusive in the helping process. Consequently, the purposes of both the intervention and the evaluation should be compatible and mutually supportive for building a bridge to evidence-based practice (Schoenwald, Kelleher, & Weisz, 2008). Therefore, the first task for the health care social worker is to help the patient not only to participate in the development of the change efforts, but also to express these efforts in specific time-limited goals and objectives. A goal stated simply is defined as the desirable objective that is to be achieved. Identifying goals also helps the practitioner to become aware of what is needed and whether he or she has the interest and skill to assist the patient with the problem behavior.

Brower and Nurius (1993) suggest two key characteristics that need to be present when designing effective intervention goals. First, goals need to be specific, clearly verifiable, and measurable as well as concrete and behavior-specific as possible. Therefore, the objectives should be designed to further quantify the goals. Second, whenever possible, both the social worker and the patient should mutually agree on all goals and objectives. The patient must also contribute to determine whether the goals and objectives sought are consistent with their own culture and values. It is up to the social worker to help the patient structure and establish the intervention strategy; however, emphasis on mutuality is central to the development of goals and objectives.

In social work, we have long realized the importance of goal setting that facilitates the intervention process. With the advent of coordinated care strategies, however, an increased emphasis has been placed on the means of assuring that a specific goal and the subsequent objectives have been accomplished. Therefore, for evidence-based practice to be meaningful, social workers must establish a climate where goals, and the specific objectives to meet them, are viewed as realistic, obtainable, and measurable. This suggests that no one methodological approach is likely to be appropriate for all types of patient problems or health care settings. The evidence-based challenge is to fit the method to the problem and not vice versa. This requires a thoughtful selection of research strategies, the various threads of which can be creatively woven throughout the broader fabric of the overall intervention plan (Dziegielewski & Powers, 2000).

Using Measurement Instruments as Outcome Indicators

Once the goals and objectives have been established, the difficult task of evaluating the clinical intervention in standardized or evidence-based terms must be addressed. This task is simplified when problems are addressed directly by the goals and objectives rather than when characterized in somewhat vague and nebulous language. With the emphasis on treatment efficacy and accountability in today's practice environment, it is essential that mental health practitioners learn to include objective measures that help to evaluate the interventions used within the health care setting. Included in these measures are standardized scales, surveys, and RAIs. These tools provide evidence-based data that identify the changes occurring over the course of the intervention (Corcoran & Boyer-Quick, 2002).

It is extremely important that health care social workers become familiar with and integrate measurement instruments in their practice and in their documentation to determine whether treatment interventions have impacted baseline behaviors and problems (Dziegielewski, 2008b). Gathering predata and postdata on a patient's problem enables both the practitioner and the patient to examine whether progress has occurred and provides regulatory agencies with tangible objective evidence of patient progress. Using a holistic framework that stresses the patient's behaviorally based biopsychosocial factors plays an important role for health care social workers in the efficient delivery of interdisciplinary health services.

One evaluation model that has historically gained and continues to receive widespread attention and use is goal attainment scaling (GAS) (Lambert & Hill, 1994). This type of scaling appears to be adaptable to a wide range of situations and was originally introduced by Kiresuk and Sherman (1968) as a way of measuring programmatic outcomes for community mental health services. GAS employs a patient-specific technique designed to provide outcome information regarding the attainment of individualized clinical and social goals. This structured quality, organized around the attainment of limited goals with concretely specified objectives, articulates especially well with the methodological requisites of standardized measures such as the GAS. The GAS requires that a number of individually tailored intervention goals/objectives be specified in relation to a set of graded scale points ranging from the least to the most favorable outcomes considered likely (Turner-Stokes, 2009).

Although at first it may seem somewhat dated, the goal attainment guide remains consistent in today's behavioral outcome-focused practice environment as it is constructed with a specific time frame in mind. With this type of measure, any number of goals may be specified for a particular patient, and any subject area may be included as an appropriate goal. Even the same goal can be defined in more than one way. For example, the goal of alleviating depression could be scaled in relation to self-report or in relation to specific cutoff points on a standardized instrument such as the Beck Depression Inventory (Beck, 1967). However, it is essential that all goals be defined in terms of a graded series of verifiable expectations in ways that are relevant to the idiosyncrasies of the particular case. In this approach, goals can be weighted to denote the importance to the patient and the treatment team (Turner-Stokes, 2009).

In summary, the GAS is given as an example of how goal/objective attainment can be weighted and prioritized to monitor and organize identified problems assisting with evidence-based practice initiatives. Basically, use of systems such as the GAS can provide a systematic yet flexible practice evaluation model that can help bridge the methodological gap between clinical and administrative interests.

Understanding and concretely defining terms such as stress, anxiety, and depression, and how these conditions can relate to the medical condition a patient is experiencing requires a full assessment of their biopsychosocial functioning. Although commonplace in our professional jargon, such terms tend to carry rather subjective connotations and as a result can be difficult to measure. This requires that establishing and monitoring a method for measuring effectiveness of the intervention process become a practice necessity.

The first step in measuring practice effectiveness, as stated earlier, generally begins with being able to show how mutually negotiated goals and objectives have been met. Change must be documented through some type of concrete measurement with clear clinical indicators indicative of patient progress. Once goals and objectives have been clarified, the importance of establishing baselines through the use of concrete and/or standardized measurement instruments begins (Lewis & Roberts, 2002). Therefore, it is often the task of the health care social worker to select, implement, and evaluate the appropriate measurement instruments. Most professionals agree that standardized scales (that have been assessed for reliability and validity) are generally recommended.

In recent years, social workers have begun to rely more heavily on the use of these types of standardized instruments in an effort to achieve greater accuracy and objectivity in their attempts to measure some of the more commonly encountered clinical problems. The most notable development in this regard has been the emergence of numerous brief pencil-and-paper assessment devices known as rapid assessment instruments (RAIs). As standardized measures, RAIs share a number of characteristics in common. They are brief, relatively easy to administer, score, and interpret, and they require very little knowledge of testing procedures on the part of the clinician. For the most part, they are self-report measures that can be completed by the patient, usually within 15 minutes. They are independent of any particular theoretical orientation and as such can be used with a variety of interventive methods. Because they provide a systematic overview of the patient's problem, they often tend to stimulate discussion related to the information elicited by the instrument itself. The score that is generated provides an operational index of the frequency, duration, or intensity of the problem. Most RAIs can be used as repeated measures and thus are adaptable to the methodological requirements of both research design and goal assessment purposes. In addition to providing a standardized means by which change can be monitored over time with a single patient, RAIs can also be used to make equivalent comparisons across patients experiencing a common problem (e.g., marital conflict).

One of the major advantages of RAIs is the availability of information concerning reliability and validity. Reliability refers to the stability of a measure. In other words, do the questions that comprise the instrument mean the same thing to the individual answering them at different times, and would different individuals interpret those same questions in a similar manner? Unless an instrument yields consistent data, it is impossible for it to be valid. But even highly reliable instruments are of little value unless their validity can also be demonstrated. Validity speaks to the general question of whether an instrument does in fact measure what it purports to measure.

There are several different approaches to establishing validity (Chen, 1997; Cone, 1998; Schutte & Malouff, 1995) each of which is designed to provide information regarding how much confidence we can have in the instrument as an accurate indicator of the problem under consideration. Although levels of reliability and validity vary greatly among available instruments, it is very helpful to the social worker to know in advance the extent to which these issues have been addressed. Information concerning reliability and validity, as well as other factors related to the standardization process (e.g., the procedures for administering, scoring, and interpreting the instrument), can help the professional make informed judgments concerning the appropriateness of any given instrument (Dziegielewski, 2008b).

The key to selecting the best instrument for the intervention is knowing where and how to access the relevant information concerning potentially useful measures. Fortunately there are a number of excellent sources available to the clinician to help facilitate this process. One such compilation of standardized measures is *Measures for Clinical Practice and Research: A Source Book* by Corcoran and Fischer (2007). These measurement scales can serve as a valuable resource of rapid-assessment instruments specifically selected for review because they measure the kinds of problems most commonly encountered in clinical social work practice. Corcoran and Fischer have done an excellent job, not only in identifying and evaluation a viable cross-section of useful clinically grounded instruments but also in discussing a number of issues critical to their use. In addition to an introduction to the basic principles of measurement, this book discusses various types of measurement tools, including the advantages and disadvantages of RAIs. Corcoran and Fischer (2007) also provide some useful guidelines for locating, selecting, evaluation, and administering prospective measures. The instruments in this text are listed in two volumes relative to their use with four target populations: couples, families, and children (volume 1) and adults (volume 2). They are also cross-indexed by problem area, which makes the selection process very easy. The availability of these, as well as numerous other similar references related to special interest areas, greatly enhances the social work professional's options with respect to monitoring and evaluation practice.

In summary, to further enhance the measurement of practice effectiveness, many social workers are feeling pressured to incorporate additional forms of measurement in the treatment plan (Dziegielewski, 2008a). The pressure to incorporate individual, family, and social rankings is becoming more common. This requires that specific measurement scores that establish functioning levels for the patients served are clearly measured and documented. To provide this additional measurement, more and more professionals are turning to the *DSM-IV-TR* and providing Axis V (Generalized Assessment of Functioning) rating scores for each patient served. In this method, functioning ratings are assigned as patients enter therapy and again on discharge (Dziegielewski, 2010a). The scales allow for assigning of a number that represents a patient's behaviors. The scale ranks these behaviors from 0 to 100 with the higher numbers being considered more indicative of higher levels of functioning and coping. In rating the highest level of functioning, a patient has maintained over the past year, and comparing it to current level of functioning, helpful comparisons can be made that help the social worker to quantify the patient problems and changes resulting within the counseling relationship.

This allows for a comparison of scores that can be viewed as representative of achieving increased patient functioning. See the *DSM-IV-TR* published by the American Psychiatric Association (2000) for scale rankings for the above.

Also, in the *DSM-IV* "Criteria Sets and Axes Provided for Further Study," there are two scales that are not required for diagnosis yet can provide a format for ranking function that might be particularly helpful to social work professionals. The first of these optional scales is the relational functioning scale termed the Global Assessment of Relational Functioning (GARF). This index is used to address family or other ongoing relationship status on a hypothetical continuum from competent to dysfunctional (American Psychiatric Association, 2000). The second index is the Social and Occupational Functioning Assessment Scale (SOFAS). With this scale, an "...individual's level of social and occupational functioning that is not directly influenced by overall severity of the individual's psychological symptoms ..." can be addressed (American Psychiatric Association, 2000).

The complimentary nature of these scales in identifying and assessing patient problems is evident in the fact that all three scales, the GARF, GAF, and SOFAS, use the same rating system. The ranking scale for each scale is the same and goes from 0 to 100 with the lower numbers being more representative of the more severe problems. The use of all three of these tools is encouraged as it can help social workers to employ concrete measurements from a more multifaceted perspective involving the clinical documentation of increased levels of functioning from the individual (GAF), family (GARF), and social (SOFAS) perspective.

Best Practices Start with an Individualized Treatment Plan

Developing best practice strategy always starts with the completion of a patient-centered individualized treatment plan. One reason for this popularity is that most programs require reimbursement, and this makes it important to follow the requirements and standards by organizations such as The Joint Commission (Maruish, 2002). This means that the plans must reflect the general and the unique symptoms and needs the patient is experiencing. Creation of an individualized treatment plan for the patient in the health care setting provides structure and helps to quantify the types of intervention services needed. Furthermore, a clearly established treatment plan can assist to deter any litigation by either the patient or a concerned family member (Bernstein & Hartsell, 2004). When the treatment plan clearly delineates the intervention plan, families and friends of the patient may feel more at ease and may actually agree to participate and assist in any behavioral interventions that will be applied.

Once the problem behaviors have been identified, this information can be utilized to start a treatment or intervention plan that will lead to best practice strategy. Each treatment plan will need to be individualized to the specific concerns or problems identified by the patient. In the health care setting, treatment plans have gained in importance. In developing the intervention plan, Maruish (2002) identifies several assumptions that are always considered in the health care environment.

* The patient is experiencing behavioral health problems.
* The patient is motivated to work on the problems.
* Treatment goals are tied to the problems identified.
* Treatment goals are achievable, collaboratively developed, and prioritized.
* Progress indicators are noted and tracked.

In formulating the plan, there are several critical steps that need to be identified (Jongsma, Peterson, & Bruce, 2006). First, problem behaviors, which are interfering with functioning, must be identified. In practice, it is considered essential that the patient and his or her family participate and assist in this process as much as possible in terms of identifying the issues, problem behaviors, and coping styles that are either causing or contributing to the patient's discomfort. Of the entire problem behaviors a patient may be experiencing, the ones that should receive the most attention are those behaviors that impair independent living skills or cause difficulties in completing tasks of daily living. Once identified these behaviors need to be linked to the intervention process. The identification of specific problem behaviors or coping styles can provide an opportunity to facilitate educational and communicative interventions that can further enhance communication between the patient and family members. Involving the family and support system in treatment plan formulation and application can be especially helpful and productive because at times individuals experiencing mental confusion and distortions of reality may exhibit bizarre and unpredictable symptoms. If support systems are not included in the intervention planning process, and the patient's symptoms worsen, the patient–family system environment may become characterized by increased tension, frustration, fear, blame, and helplessness. To avoid support systems from withdrawing from the patient. Thereby decreasing the support available to the patient, family members and key support system members need to either be involved or at a minimum be made aware of the treatment plan goals and objectives that will be utilized if the patient consents to their involvement.

Second, not only do family and friends need to be aware of the treatment plan initiatives, but they also need to be encouraged to share valuable input and support to ensure intervention progress and success. Family education and supportive interventions for family and significant others can be listed as part of the treatment plan for an individual patient. It is beyond the scope of this chapter to discuss the multiple interventions available to the family members of the mentally ill individual; however, interested readers are encouraged to refer to Dziegielewski (2010a) for sample treatment plans for working individuals who suffer from mental illness.

Next, to assist in treatment plan development, it is critical to state the identified problem behaviors in terms of behaviorally based outcomes (Dziegielewski, 2010a). In completing this process, the assessment data that lead to the diagnostic impression and the specific problems often experienced by the patient need to be outlined. Once identified the patients' problems are then prioritized so that goals, objectives, and action tasks may be developed. Third, the goals of intervention, which constitute the basis for the plan of intervention, must be clearly outlined and applied. These goals must be broken down into specific objective statements that reflect target behaviors to be changed and ways to measure the patient's progress on each objective. As subcomponents to the objectives, action tasks that clearly delineate the steps to be taken by the patient and the helping professional to ensure successful completion of each objective must be included.

Once the problem behaviors have been identified, the health care social worker must identify the goals and the behaviorally based objectives that can be used to measure whether the identified problems have indeed been addressed and resolved. If the problem behavior is ambivalent feelings that impair general task completion, the main goal may be to help the patient decrease feelings of ambivalence. Measurement of this goal will require documenting an objective that clearly articulates a behavioral definition of ambivalence. Once identified the ways that the ambivalence will be decreased are outlined along with the mechanisms used to determine whether the behavior has changed. The therapeutic intervention involves assisting the patient to develop specific and concrete tasks that are geared toward decreasing this behavior and consequently meeting the objective. The outcome measure simply becomes establishing whether the task was completed. No treatment plan can be all-inclusive, but each treatment plan must be individualized for the patient outlining the specific problem behaviors and how each of these behaviors can be addressed.

Measuring Change in the Health Care Setting

In health care, it remains obvious that the helping relationship is a complex one that cannot be measured completely through the use of standardized scales or assessment measures. To facilitate measurement of effectiveness, specific concrete goals and objectives must incorporate a number of direct behavioral observation techniques, self-anchored rating scales, patient logs, and a variety of mechanical devices for monitoring physiological functioning. Together these methods can provide a range of qualitative and quantitative measures for initiating evidence-based practice.

For the health care social worker, evidence-based practice interventions can lead to greater efficiency and effectiveness. For many social workers, this requirement to concretely identify all problem behaviors in clear terms or indicators has led to frustration as social workers are expected to operationalize the change behaviors as part of the assessment process.

For many health care social workers, the link between the actual practice components and the strategies needed to assess them can be elusive. For example, in the case plan, a problem statement along with behaviorally based goals and objectives must be clearly identified. The patient's capacity for self-determination must be recognized as well as the accountability issues that remain germane to the profession, the agency, and requirements and conditions relevant to service reimbursement.

MAINTAINING CLINICAL RECORDS

Because records can be maintained in more than one medium, such as written case files, audio or video recordings, and computer-generated notes, special attention needs to be given to ensuring confidentiality and the maintaining of ethical release of patient information. Probably the greatest protection a health care social worker has in terms of risk management for all types of records is maintaining accurate, clear, and concise clinical records (Reamer, 2002b). This means that an unbroken chain of custody between the social worker and/or the multidisciplinary/interdisciplinary team and the record must always be maintained. Because health care providers will ultimately be held responsible for producing a clinical record in case of litigation, this policy cannot be overemphasized. Furthermore, documentation in the health care record should always be clearly sequenced and easy to follow. If a mistake occurs, never change a summary note or intervention plan without acknowledging it. When changes need to be made to the clinical case record, the intervention plan, or any other types of case recording, clearly indicate that a change is being made by drawing one thin line through the mistake and dating and initialing it. Records that are legible and cogent limit open interpretation of the services provided. In addition, the mental health practitioner will always be required to keep clinical case records (including written records and computerized backup files) safeguarded in locked and fireproof cabinets (see Table 7.5). Most health care facilities, after service completion, are now using archiving types of storage systems such as microfiche or microfilm to preserve records and maximize space.

Table 7.5 Documentation Reminders

Because accurate and ethical documentation insures continuity of care, ethical, and legal aspects of practice, and provides direction for the focus of intervention, every record must have the following essential information:

---

* Date, time of entry, and duration
* Dates of all case-related telephone numbers and electronic contacts
* Interview notes that clearly describe the presenting problem and evidence-based format for recording of behaviors
* An intervention plan that clearly established overall goals, objectives, and intervention tasks
* Always use ink that does not run (ball point pens are best)
* Never using pencil or whiteout to erase mistakes
* Draw a line through an error, marking it "error" and initialing the error
* Print and sign social worker's name, title, and credentials with each entry
* Document all information in the case record as if you might some day have to defend it in a court of law

---

Criteria modified from Dziegielewski (2010a).

As the use of computer-generated notes continue to become more common, different forms of problem-oriented case recording will be linked directly into computerized databases (Gingerich, 2002). In terms of convenience, this can mean immediate access to fiscal and billing information as well as patient intervention strategy, documentation, and treatment planning. When working with computerized records, Bernstein & Hartsell (2004) suggest the following: (1) when recording patient information on a hard drive or disk, be sure to store in a safe and secure place; (2) be sure to secure any passwords from detection; (3) if you are treating a celebrity or a famous individual, use a fictitious name and be sure to keep the "key" to the actual name in a protected place; (4) always maintain a backup system and keep it secure; (5) be sure that everyone who will have access to the patient's case file reads and signs an established protocol concerning sanctity, privacy, and confidentiality of the records; and (6) take the potential of computer theft or crash seriously and establish a policy that will safeguard what will need to happen if this should occur. The convenience of records and information now being easily transmitted electronically produces one major concern. Because clinical case records are so easy to access and are portable, there is a genuine problem represented by the vulnerability of unauthorized access of the recorded information. This means that if a health care social worker is dealing with personal and confidential information about the patients who are served, every precaution should be taken to safeguard the information that is shared. In addition, because medical records are kept for the benefit of the patient, access to the record by the patient is generally allowed. When engaging in any type of disclosure or transfer issues to either the patient or third parties, however, a written consent from the patient is expected. Every effort to obtain consent from a legally competent adult, the legal guardian of an incompetent adult, or the executor/administrator of the estate of a deceased person, needs to be obtained (NASW, 2011).

ETHICS AND LEGAL CONSIDERATIONS IN RECORD KEEPING

Malpractice is negligence in the exercise of one's profession (Schroeder, 1995). Schroeder (1995) warns that one way to protect professionals against malpractice is to encourage them to keep careful records that clearly and accurately reflect the service that was rendered. Social workers in health care, similar to all social workers, have to be careful to protect the patient's right to privacy and confidentiality. Many times, these records involve personal information that can be damaging to the patient served, especially when records are subpoenaed into a court of law. For the most part, state and federal workers are exempt from responsibility as they carry qualified immunity against judgment (Schroeder, 1995). However, other professionals generally do not qualify for this exemption. This is particularly problematic for social workers that work in home health care agencies and so on.

To ensure protection, all social workers practicing in the health care field should contemplate maintaining their own malpractice insurance. The NASW sponsors a professional liability policy that should be considered. For clarification and more updated information on the malpractice insurance coverage available to health care social workers (e.g., rates, services, and policies), contact with the national office of NASW is recommended. Also, contacting NASW for updated information regarding ethics and legal implications is highly recommended. Sparks (2012) reminds us that social workers have the power to invoke change, but all change efforts must be grounded in the professions values and ethics.

CHAPTER SUMMARY AND FUTURE DIRECTIONS

Behavioral health care presents a type of service delivery where social workers are expected to show that the intermittent or time-limited brief services they provide are necessary and effective. This challenge has been a particularly vigorous one for the health care social worker because of the variation and lack of clarity in the types of interventions provided. Health care social workers must be aware and capable of using the different methods of record keeping often used in the health care setting. Regardless of the specific style or type of record keeping being used, all records need to include the following information (a) be able to identify, describe, and assess the patient's situation; (b) describe the reason or purpose for the service being provided; (c) describe the goals and objectives to be obtained listed as behavioral outcome measures; (d) establish the plan for intervention; and (e) evaluate the process and outcome of therapeutic process. Accurate record keeping is essential to quality social work practice.

It is the responsibility of the health care social worker to ensure that records are maintained that are both accountable and accurate. As a member of an interdisciplinary or multidisciplinary team, documentation is essential for effective and efficient communication with other team members. In health care delivery, the medical record is often considered central for treatment coordination; it generally reflects the patient care planning of the entire team. The social worker's written input as a professional part of the health care delivery team is indispensable in the documentation of services rendered.

Regardless of the type of record keeping employed, it is essential that the social worker be sure that patient information is accurate and complete. Comprehensive record keeping addresses both the ethical and legal aspects of practice. Every record must have basic information that includes the date and time of entry, interview notes that describe the patient and the problem or situation that requires treatment, an assessment and initial treatment plan, and therapeutic objectives and treatment responses. A time frame for intervention must be clearly established, and progress regarding that time frame must be documented. When family interventions are included, the time, date, and who was involved should always be inserted. Also, when discharge services are addressed, such as placement and so on, they need to be formally documented in the record.

The social worker practicing in today's coordinated care environment must be aware of the direct link between service delivery and good record keeping. The written connection to outcome measurement is essential. The process of assessing pretreatment, posttreatment, and follow-up measures of patient progress or change must be clearly demonstrated through this written exchange. When symptom description is made, it must be clearly stated in observable, demonstrable terms that can clearly relate to the measurable treatment intervention presented. The treatment plan should always include a detailed description of patient complaints with the specific interventions used to address them. Health care social workers need to always remember the importance and power that is ascribed to this written document—especially in this time of litigation, limited service delivery access, and the movement to control health care costs.

Glossary

Accountability   Coordinated care and other health care delivery reviewing bodies hold social workers and other health care professionals responsible for the services provided. Important elements for consideration include quality-of-care issues, level of care used, use of ancillary services and resources, appropriate referrals, and other activities that produce cost-effective and efficient service delivery.

APIE   A form of problem-oriented record keeping often used in the medical setting. *A* = assessment, *P* = problem identification, *I* = intervention, and *E* = evaluation.

Appropriateness   The degree of compatibility, suitability, and compliance with standardized sets of criteria for service provision and delivery.

ASAP   Affordable services applied by professionals.

Audio recording   This form of record keeping is often used for educational purposes in the medical setting. Generally, if this form of record keeping is used in establishing service provision, it is not used alone, and another form of recording, such as the problem-oriented format, is used to supplement its use.

Audit   A standard "criteria based" examination and review of written documentation and clinical practice provision.

Care management   Using the patient's allowed benefits; a program is established to determine eligibility and direct service provision to achieve maximum functioning.

Computer standardized records   This form of record keeping first became popular in the 1980s and has significantly grown as computer technology continues to grow. A particular concern in the use of this form of record keeping for social work professionals is ensuring the maintenance of patient confidentiality.

DAP or DAPE   A form of problem-oriented recording that is often used in health and mental health settings. D = data, A = assessment, and P = plan (DAP); or D = data, A = assessment, P = plan, and E = education (DAPE).

Diagnostic recording   This form of early social work record keeping was completed by a trained diagnostician. The notes were generally long and not uniform. It is rarely used as a form of record keeping in health care practice setting today.

Family-oriented records   This form of record keeping generally includes the entire household of a patient, and all information is generally recorded in the same file. This type of record is considered particularly good for prevention and wellness services as it relates to the entire family. For example, as one individual is in for treatment, the medical personnel can also screen for information relevant to other family members, which is all located in the same record.

Health Insurance Portability and Accountability Act (HIPAA)   This Act was implemented by U.S. Congress on August 21, 1996 to protect the consumer and combat health care fraud while simplifying health care administration and insurance. This Act and its subsequent revisions limit disclosures of patient information to the minimum necessary related to a specific purpose, with a few exceptions.

Ledgers   An early form of writing in the field of social work that recorded events after they occurred.

Malpractice   Is simply referred to as negligence in the practice of one's profession. Health care social workers must ensure accurate and effective record keeping has occurred that is reflective of the service that was rendered.

Narratives   A form of early social work documentation that simply documented what transpired with a patient seeking services.

Outcome criteria   Specific elements relative to evaluating end results in terms of the level of patient functioning.

Outcomes management Feedback related to the outcomes identified to improve service delivery continually.

Outcomes measurement The process of assessing pretreatment, posttreatment, and follow-up measures of patient change or progress.

Person-oriented record In this form of record keeping, an emphasis on wellness and prevention are stressed. In addition, the record is generally considered the property of the patient who ensures that different professional services are recorded in one central record. This type of record keeping seems to be most popular in community practice or rural health care delivery settings.

PIRP A form of problem-oriented recording that is often used in the health and mental health setting. P = problem(s), I = intervention, R = response, and P = plan.

Process recording An early form of social work recording that was used in the health care environment as a means of verbatim recording of the events that transpired in a session. This form of recording is still used in the medical setting; however, it is only used for educational purposes.

Problem-oriented records In this form of record keeping, emphasis is placed on limiting documentation to the problem being addressed. Today in the health care environment, this is the most popular form of recording with numerous variations in the formats used. Examples of such formats include the SOAP, SOAPIE, PIRP, DAP, DAPE, and so on.

Single-subject research designs These are designs that help a provider to establish whether the treatment provided to a patient works. Target behaviors are identified and tracked throughout the treatment process.

SOAP and SOAPIE This is one of the most popular formats for problem-oriented recording. This form is often used in medical and mental health settings. S = subjective, O = objective, A = assessment, and P = plan (SOAP); and S = subjective, O = objective, A = assessment, P = plan, I = intervention used, and E = evaluation (SOAPIE).

Time series recording This form of record keeping is continuing to evolve in the medical setting. Generally, target behavior(s) are clearly identified and followed over time.

Video recording This form of record keeping is often used in the medical setting for educational purposes. At times, recordings of surgery, procedures, and so on have been made to accompany the written record. This form of record keeping is usually supplemental.

Questions for Further Study

1. Do you believe there is a need for cost–benefit information to be included in the patient record?

2. How can empirical practice strategy best be reflected in the case-recording format chosen?

3. Why do you believe that problem-oriented records have gained in popularity over the years? With the advent of coordinated care, do you believe this popularity will decline?

4. When would you disclose confidential information from a patient's record? What would you do if you were not sure?

5. What is HIPAA and why is it important for social workers to be knowledgeable of what it involves?

Websites

American Recovery and Reinvestment Act of 2009, Title XIII, Health Information Technology, Subtitle D – Privacy (Pub. L. No. 111-5). thomas.loc.gov/cgi-bin/query/z?c111:H.R.1.enr

74 Fed Reg. 56123 (codified at 45 CFR 160). *HIPAA Information Privacy.* www.hhs.gov/ocr/privacy/hipaa/administrative/ enforcementrule/enfifr.pdf.

74 Fed Reg. 42739 (codified at 45 CFR 160-164). *Breach Notification for Unsecured Protected Health Information.* www.gpo.gov/2009/pdf/E9-20169.pdf

CHAPTER 8

Health and Mental Health Assessment

This chapter introduces the reader to the principles that outline the relationship between an individual's physical health and aspects of his or her mental health. This application is supported through the use of diagnosis and assessment skills, as too often artificial distinctions are made to separate physical health from mental health when often these two concepts cannot be separated. This artificial separation can lead the social worker to neglect important cultural health and mental health concepts that might otherwise be given minimal attention. The argument is made that the physical health and mental health of a person are always intertwined (Dziegielewski, 2010a). Health care practice strategy is highlighted, with an explanation and emphasis on the person-in-environment (PIE) assessment scheme, and later relating the scheme to the *Diagnostic and Statistical Manual of Mental Disorders, Fifth Edition (DSM-5)* multiaxial system. In addition, considerations for raising sensitivity for all members of the health care team are highlighted in each aspect of the chapter.

TERMINOLOGY CHANGES: ADAPTING TO THE BIOMEDICAL CULTURE

Over the years, the formulation of an *assessment* leading to a *diagnosis* has been a source of serious debate within the profession. Carlton (1984) believed that the debate essentially stems from the fact that the profession of social work has not always separated these two entities into distinct clinical aspects of practice. This means that the clinical features inherent in either one can and often do overlap. The terms are used interchangeably, and this shift can cause confusion and resistance by those that do not take into account the cultural surroundings that encourage the shift. This complicates explication and definition in many health care settings, which results in the completion of either service (diagnosis, assessment, or the diagnostic assessment) as being viewed as interchangeable (Dziegielewski, 2010a). It is this hesitancy and inability to differentiate between these concepts that can create obvious difficulties in practice reality.

Terminology needs to be reflective of the culture. This is why when elements between two similar yet conflicting terms are not considered to be distinct, the inherent concepts are allowed to blur and overlap. The process is further complicated by the multiplicity of meanings applied to the terms used to describe each aspect. In the assessment process, for example, the major reason for this difficulty is in differentiating clearly what each term means. This is explicated when examining the concept of "assessment," the concept of "diagnosis," and "the relationship between the mental diagnosis and the physical health condition" overlap. These overlapping concepts and the enmeshing between them can easily cause confusion. This lack of clarity within definitions and overlapping relationships causes social, personal, and professional interpretation to be varied and nonuniform in definition, practice, or approach.

To highlight the difficulty in differentiating between assessment and diagnosis further, it is important to note that the profession of social work did not develop in isolation. The roots of the social work profession, as well as of professional practice strategy, have been influenced greatly by such disciplines as general medicine, psychiatry, and psychology. There is a medical culture that develops among professionals in an area that causes all involved to adapt a certain mind-set or worldview. For social workers to remain competitive and viable as providers, the health care practice strategy provided needs to adhere to this culture. Remaining competitive therefore can mean being forced to adapt to the dominant culture. This can be seen in the simple terms that are used. For example, throughout this book those that have historically been called "patients" in the social work profession are referred to now interchangeably as "patients," "clients," and "consumers." The emphasis selected for continuity is using the word "patient," simply because that is what is primarily used in the literature. Using the dominant terminology allows for increased communication as it perpetuates shared meanings.

Another example is in the field of addictions where a patient who has previously used a substance and is able to overcome and stop using can fall back into a pattern of using again. The social worker has an active role in assessing the substance use as well as developing the treatment plans used to assist the consumer (Dziegielewski, 2005). To utilize shared terminology the term for someone who is again using the substance was historically referred to as "relapse." Today, however, it is not uncommon see this old term replaced by words such as "reinstatement" as opposed to "relapse." In the medical field, when a patient is not taking his/her medications as directed, it was previously referred to as "compliance" (Dziegielewski, 2010b). Today, however, if one examines the literature it is not uncommon to see it referred to as adherence and in some cases as a less medicalized term such as "ensuring consistency." The point is that terminology changes with the culture and so must the professional's interpretations and expressions. In this case, awareness is reflected in the terms used with other professionals and the explanations provided to the patient.

Adapting the dominant culture and the terminology used allows for increased communication and connection between the collaborating disciplines. Successful communication in health care is tied to science and although awareness is essential, use of the terminology requires awareness of not only the terms but also the implications of its use. As a social worker, the voice of the patients served needs to be clear and as the existing culture provides a broadening array of ambiguous choices, careful review is needed (Sparks, 2012).

This means that methodologies and theoretical foundations that support practice strategy must also be reflective and adaptive of these same expectations. These expectations generally deal with reimbursement for service, and conscious or not, guide the forces behind health care practice (Braun & Cox, 2005; Kielbasa et al., 2004).

Since most of the time health care social workers are part of the agency structure, they are forced to practice within the organizational budget. Social workers serve many roles such as assessment, case management, and discharge planning; advocacy for patients; and they serve on ethics committees, human review boards, and work with specialized populations offering direct assessment and treatment strategies. Estrine, Hettenbach, Authur, and Messina (2011) and their colleagues remind us clearly that recognition of culture is particularly important when providing service delivery to vulnerable populations. The power in social work is the ability of the worker to articulate a position clearly and affect change, taking into account their understanding of the ethical issues involved (Sparks, 2012). Furthermore, taking into account the "person-in-situation" and the "PIE," which remains the cornerstone of social work practice, allows for the realization that the quality of the medical care can also affect the course of the disease.

Masi (2012) reminds us neighborhoods differ in terms of ethnic composition and resources and in assessing the needs of the patient; this remains an essential feature of any assessment. Based on the pressures in the environment, it is not uncommon for social workers to feel that they are forced to only treat patients who have a formal mental health diagnosis (Pomerantz & Sergist, 2006). Or to reduce services to patients, treat only those who are covered by insurance or can pay privately or terminate patients because the services are too costly (Ethics meet managed care, 1997). This makes the role of assessment and diagnosis critical for the health care social worker as it not only opens the door for services but also determines which ones will be provided. It also makes knowledge of the rules and professional expectations that govern the profession of social work a necessity (Reamer, 2009).

For the health care social worker, the definition of *assessment* involves the reasoning process that leads from the facts to tentative conclusions regarding their meaning (Sheafor & Horejsi, 2008). Assessment is viewed as the professional (as opposed to lay person) interpretation depicting what is viewed as the problem. It is the process that controls and directs all aspects of patient care including the nature, direction, and scope. This assessment process also takes into account recognizing how behavioral health is influenced by the complexity of the human condition and the factors related to a specific patient's situation (Pearson, 2008).

Given that health care social work is such an eclectic field with many different duties, it is not unusual that the assessment process reflects this diversity. There are numerous health care settings in which social workers provide service. This makes the process of assessment dependent on a multiplicity of factors, including patient need, agency function, practice setting, service limitations, and coverage for provision of service.

Considering this explanation, Dziegielewski (2010a) warns that although assessments completed today may appear to have a narrower focus, it is essential that utility, relevance, and salience be maintained. Therefore, for the health care social worker, the process of assessment must continually be examined and re-examined carefully to ensure quality of the practice provided. If the process of assessment is rushed in the health care setting, observed mental health features may not be clearly related to physical health factors and vice-versa. This can lead to important psychosocial factors being de-emphasized or overlooked. Health care social workers are tasked with establishing that the practice provided is quality driven, no matter what the administrative and economic pressures may be. This means focusing on quality service rather than compelling demands to address practice reimbursement (Davis & Meier, 2001). This is no easy task as the formulas that surround reimbursement differ and this complicated patchwork system can involve out-of-pocket consumer expenses as well as insurer and policy limitations as well as tax revenues that support public-funded programs (Darnell & Lawlor, 2012).

To support this further, social workers remain active in reviewing changes in health care and making recommendations for consumer protection and health care quality (Steps taken to watchdog managed care, 1997). The time is ripe for social workers to step forward and assume the vital role in all aspects of health care including advocacy for the consumer and public policy and other leadership roles (Darnell & Lawlor, 2012). Therefore, health care social workers are expected not only to provide assistance in developing a comprehensive strategy to help patients but also to ensure that quality service is made available and obtained (Dziegielewski & Holliman, 2001). In the assessment process, they can also ensure that the needs of the patient are recognized, thereby increasing adherence and consistency (Auslander & Freedenthal, 2012).

CLINICAL ASSESSMENT: A SYSTEMATIC APPROACH TO ASSESSMENT

In health care practice today, there are many forms of formal assessment that can support and assist in the development of an intervention plan. One system of assessment designed by social workers is that of the PIE classification system. The PIE was developed through an award given to the California chapter of the National Association of Social Workers (NASW) from the NASW Program Advancement Fund (Whiting, 1996).

This system was designed to focus on psychosocial aspects, situations, and units larger than the individual (Karls & Wandrei, 1996a, 1996b). The foundation is built around two major premises: recognition of social considerations and the PIE stance. Knowledge of the PIE is relevant for all mental health social workers regardless of educational level because of its emphasis on situational factors (Karls & O'Keefe, 2008, 2009).

According to Karls and Wandrei (1996a), the PIE system calls first for a social work assessment that is translated into a description of coding of the patient's problems in social functioning.

> Social functioning is the patient's ability to accomplish the activities necessary for daily living (for example, obtaining food, shelter and transportation) and to fulfill major social roles as required by the patient's subculture or community. (p. vii)

The PIE was formulated in response to the need to identify the problems of patients in a way that health professionals can easily understand (Karls & Wandrei, 1996a, 1996b). As a form of classification system for adults, the PIE provides:

- A prescribed format and common language for all social workers in all settings to describe their patients' problems in social functioning.
- A way to capsulate the description of social phenomena that could facilitate intervention or ameliorate problems presented by patients.
- A way to gather the data needed to measure services and to design human service programs to evaluate effectiveness.
- A mechanism for clearer communication among social work practitioners as well as practitioners, administrators, and researchers.
- A basis for clarifying the domain of social work in human service fields (Karls & Wandrei, 1996a).

The PIE system breaks down patients' problems into four distinct categories or "factors" and originally was designed to supplement the *DSM-IV-TR* and the previously used multiaxial diagnostic system, not replace it. An abbreviated version of these factors is presented in this chapter. The first area is termed *Factor I*. Here the social role within each problem is identified and explored. Factor I has five categories. The first, social role, is divided into four subcategories: family roles, the role a person performs within the family (e.g., parent role, spouse role, child role, sibling role, other family role, and significant other role); other interpersonal roles where interpersonal relationships between individuals who are not family members are considered (e.g., lover role, friend role, neighbor role, member role, and other interpersonal role); occupational roles, which are either paid or unpaid roles that a patient fills (e.g., worker role—paid economy, worker role—home, worker role—volunteer, student role, and other occupational role); and special life situation roles that patients assume that are time limited and situation specific (e.g., consumer role, inpatient/patient role, outpatient/patient role, probationer/parolee role, prisoner role, immigrant role—undocumented, immigrant role—refugee, and other special life situation role) (Wandrei & Karls, 1996).

The second category to be considered under Factor I is the type of social problem that is being experienced. In the first category, emphasis is placed on identifying the social role that is causing difficulty; in this second category of Factor I, emphasis is placed on the kind of problem experienced. When dealing with problems, it is believed that there are nine types of interactional difficulties that represent the areas that social workers most often encounter and must assist in the negotiation: power, ambivalence, responsibility, dependency, loss, isolation, victimization; and the categories of mixed, and other. Because oftentimes problems interact and are not mutually exclusive, Wandrei and Karls (1996) recommend using the mixed category, if needed, to describe these types of problems. When the interactional difficulty cannot be related to any of these types, the category of "other" is used.

The third, fourth, and fifth areas or categories under Factor I were designed to help social workers decide if intervention was needed, the severity of the impairment, the level of impairment, and how quickly services needed to be provided. Therefore, the following three indexes were developed: the severity index, the duration index, and the coping index.

In the severity index, the prospect of change is measured. Generally, change factors are a necessary and functioning part of life; however, when the change factors get too extensive or rapid, problems can occur in adaptation and adjustment for the patient. Wandrei and Karls (1996) proposed six levels for rating severity. In scaling, the higher the number given, the higher the degree of problem noted. The six levels identified by Wandrei and Karls (1996) are (a) no problem, (b) low severity, (c) moderate severity, (d) high severity, (e) very high severity, and (f) catastrophic. In (a) no problem—both patient and practitioner perceive the problem as nondisruptive, and no intervention is needed. In (b), low severity—there are some changes noted, but the patient sees the problem as nondisruptive. It is important to note, however, that although the patient notes no disruption, the practitioner may note some disruption occurring. In this case, intervention is desirable but not necessary. In category (c), moderate severity—intervention would be helpful. Here the problem is viewed as disruptive to the patient's level of functioning, but the level of distress does not impair function. In (d), high severity—the patient is in a clear state of distress, and early intervention is indicated. In (e), very high severity—the patient is in a high state of distress and *immediate* intervention is probably necessary. Here the patient is subjected to significant and multiple changes in the environment that must be addressed. Lastly, in (f), catastrophic—immediate intervention is needed because the patient's problem is characterized by sudden, negative changes that have devastating implications.

In the *duration index*, the length or recency of the problem is noted. This can also help in assessing the chronicity of the problem, and how this length of time may be related to prognosis. The duration index has six levels: (a) more than 5 years, (b) 1 to 5 years, (c) 6 months to 1 year, (d) 1 to 6 months, (e) 2 to 4 weeks, and (f) 2 weeks or less.

In the *coping index*, the degree to which a patient can handle a problem within his or her internal resources is noted. The coping index is reflective of "the social worker's judgment of the patient's ability to solve problems, capacity to act independently, and his or her ego strength, insight and intellectual capacity" (Wandrei & Karls, 1996, p. 33). There are six levels in the coping index: (a) outstanding coping skills, which reflects the patient's ability to solve problems and act independently using intellectual capability and insight to cope; (b) above-average coping skills, which is similar to level one, and several coping skills are generally expected from the average individual; (c) adequate coping skills, where the patient is able to function adequately in the earlier stated areas; (d) somewhat inadequate coping skills, where the patient has a fair problem-solving ability but has major difficulty in addressing and solving current problems; (e) inadequate coping skills, where the patient has some skills but is unable to solve current problems and ego strength, insight, or intellectual ability are impaired when applied to the problem solving process; and (f) no coping skills, where the patient shows little or no ability to solve problems or act independently. At this level, ego strength, insight, and intellectual ability are impaired (see Table 8.1).

The second area for consideration in the PIE is *Factor II*. In Factor I, consideration was given to explaining the problem of the patient in conjunction with interpersonal relationships. Factor II goes beyond the interpersonal and looks at issues and forces that are beyond this that can affect the patient. Six social system environmental problem areas are delineated. These areas are the economic/basic needs system, the educational/training system, the judicial/legal system, the health safety and social services system, the voluntary association system, and the affectional support system. Once the areas to be considered have been established, the specific type of problem within each social system is identified. Each of the major six categories listed previously

Table 8.1 PIE Factor I: Structural Breakdown

Type	Definition
Social role	Where each problem is identified (four categories)
Type of problem	Clarifies the interactional difficulty within the social role (nine types)
Severity of the problem	Where the problem is rated for severity based on change factors on a scale from one to six
Duration	Identifies the length and frequency of the problem (six categories)
Coping index	Measures the patient's ability to cope with the problem (six levels)

have numerous subcategories that can further describe them. The last two considerations for Factor II involve assessing a measure for the severity of the problem and recording the duration of the problem (similar to Factor I).

Factor III of the PIE classification system looks specifically at mental health problems. Clinical syndromes as recorded in the *DSM-IV* classification system on Axis I are recorded on Factor A. This codification system is discussed later in this chapter, and special attention should be given to Axis I and its application here. Category B of Factor III deals with personality and developmental disorders that an individual might have. In the *DSM-IV* classification, most of these (except the developmental disorders) were generally recorded on Axis II and would be listed here.

Factor IV of the PIE classification scheme looks at physical health problems. Factor IV, category A, deals with diseases that are generally diagnosed by a physician. Factor IV, category B, looks at other health problems reported by the patient and or other individuals (e.g., family, significant others) that may be important to the assessment process.

Using the PIE in the health care setting is similar to use in mental health; however, greater emphasis needs to be placed on Factor IV (the physical health problems). Adkins (1996) believes that this makes knowledge of the health and medical conditions patients suffer from essential for social work professionals. Establishing Factors I and II can help social workers get a clear sense of the relationship the problem has to the environment—in a friendly and adaptable way.

As with any coding scheme, learning to use the PIE will take time. The book and manual with its practical application guidelines make the PIE a viable and practical method for assessment. However, it is important to stress that the PIE is not an independent classification system. Similar to *DSM-IV* and *DSM-IV-TR*, when it comes to billing it uses the diagnostic classification system of the *International Classification of Diseases Ninth Revision, Clinical Modification (ICD-9-CM)*. For diagnostic support PIE relies heavily on the *DSM-IV* and the *DSM-IV-TR* classification system. This means that health care social workers must also know these two other codification systems. Actually, this may be positive for the health care social worker because it incorporates the methods used within the health care and mental health setting, which most often governs reimbursement patterns.

Usage of the PIE allows health care social workers a way to categorize the numerous factors regarding the patient's environment that must be considered. Classification systems like the PIE offer health care social workers a systematic way to address the patient and his or her social factors in the context of the environment (see Tables 8.2–8.4).

CLINICAL DIAGNOSIS IN THE HEALTH CARE SETTING

The concept of formulating and completing a diagnosis is richly embedded in the history and practice of the clinical health care social worker (Dziegielewski, 2010a). In health care practice today, compelling demands to

Table 8.2 PIE Factor II: Structural Breakdown

Type	Definition
Environmental systems	Six types of system difficulties usually beyond the individual control of the patient
Economic/basic needs system	Refers to the production, distribution, and consumption functions of the economic system (e.g., food, shelter, and employment)
Education/training system	Refers to the ability of the community to meet the goals of the educational system (e.g., access to education, nurture intelligence, and provide quality education programs)
Judicial/legal system	Refers to factors related to the criminal justice system of social control (e.g., lack of adequate prosecution, inadequate defense, and insufficient police services)
Health/safety and social services system	Refers to the factors in the community regarding health, safety, and so on that are beyond the direct control of the patient (e.g., absence of support services impairing use of mental health services and the occurrence of a natural disaster)
Voluntary association system	Refers to the ways patients meet needs through the community by participating in social or religious groups, and so on (e.g., lack of patient's preference for religious affiliation)
Affectional support system	Refers to patients who have under-involved or over-involved support systems in the marital family, extended family, friends, acquaintances, and so on
Specify type of problem in each system	Clarifies the system difficulty
Severity of the problem	Where the problem is rated for severity based on change factors on a scale from 1 to 6
Duration	Identifies the length and frequency of the problem (six-point indicator)

Table 8.3 PIE Factor III: Structural Breakdown

Type	Definition
Clinical	Refers to *DSM-IV* Axis I classifications
Personality and developmental disorders	Refers to most of the mental health conditions that are coded on Axis II

address practice "reimbursement" has clearly emphasized this rich tradition. Numerous types of diagnostic and assessment measurements are currently available—many of which are structured into unique categories and classification schemes. As stated earlier, the health care social worker to be familiar

Table 8.4 PIE Factor IV: Structural Breakdown

Type	Definition
Physical health diagnoses	Refer to diseases that are actually diagnosed by a physician. These are related to Axis III of *DSM-IV* or the *ICD-9*.
Other health problems	Refers to conditions that are noted, that may impair functioning, and that are reported by patients and others by a physician.

with the major formal methods of diagnosis and assessment—especially the ones used and accepted in the area of health service delivery. Social workers need this information to (a) choose, gather, and report this information systematically; (b) to be aware and assist other interdisciplinary team members in the diagnostic process; (c) to interpret and assist the patient to understand what the results of the diagnostic assessment mean; and (d) to assist the patient to choose empirically sound and ethically wise modes of practice intervention. Because most fields of practice in the health care area subscribe to the medical model, the *DSM* and its latest version is examined as a formal diagnostic system. This will later need to be applied to the changes that are forthcoming in *DSM-5* which is due in May of 2013.

The *DSM-IV-TR* and *DSM-5*

Since its inception in 1995, few professionals would debate that the most commonly used and accepted sources of diagnostic criteria are the *Diagnostic and Statistical Manual for Mental Disorders, Fourth Edition, Text Revision (DSM-IV-TR)* and the *International Classification of Diseases, Tenth Edition (ICD-10)*. As of May 2013, the American Psychiatric Association will launch its newest edition called the *DSM-5*. This book will be expected to relate directly to the *ICD-10-CM* for billing purposes. These books are generally considered reflective of the official nomenclature in all mental health and other health-related facilities in the United States.

Since the *DSM* has historically been used as an educational tool, it was felt that recent research might be overlooked if a revision was not published prior to *DSM-5*, which was released in 2013. Surprisingly however, even with the addition of much new research and information, the *DSM-IV* (published in 1995) continued to be relatively up-to-date. Therefore, in formulating the text revision published in 2000, none of the categories, diagnostic codes, or criteria from the *DSM-IV* were changed. However, what was changed is that more supplemental information was provided for many of the edition's categories (American Psychiatric Association, 2000). In addition, more information is provided on many of the field trials that were introduced in the *DSM-IV* but were not yet completed or required updated research findings to be applied. Furthermore, special attention was paid to update the sections in terms of diagnostic findings, cultural information, and other information to clarify the diagnostic categories (American Psychiatric Association, 2000).

In the *DSM-IV* and the *DSM-IV-TR*, the billing codes are very similar to the *ICD-9-CM* and the *ICD-10*; however, this wasn't always the case. As late as the 1980s, clinical practices often used the *ICD* for billing but referred to the *DSM* to clarify diagnostic criteria. It was not uncommon in the past to hear psychiatrists, psychologists, social workers, and mental health technicians "moan and groan" about the lack of clarity and uniformity in both of these texts (Dziegielewski, 2010a). This professional discontent became so pronounced that the message for revamping was received. Therefore, later versions of these texts clearly responded to the professional outcry of dissatisfaction over the disparity between the two texts; this was achieved by using similar criteria in the *DSM* and the *ICD* when outlining descriptive classification systems that cross all theoretical orientations.

The *DSM-5*, similar to previous versions of the *DSM* before *DSM-IV* and *DSM-IV-TR*, is falling under similar scrutiny as the billing codes do not appear to match the *ICD-10-CM* or prepare for the *ICD-11*, which is scheduled to come out in 2015. Historically, while most clinicians are knowledgeable about both books, the *DSM* appears to have gained the greatest popularity in the United States and is the resource most often used by psychiatrists, physicians, psychologists, psychiatric nurses, social workers, and other mental health professionals throughout the United States. In terms of licensing and certification of most social workers, a thorough knowledge of the *DSM* is considered essential for competent clinical practice. Since all professionals working in the area of health and mental health need to be cognizant and capable of completing what is needed for service, it is not surprising that the majority of mental health professionals support the use of this manual (Corey, 2001).

Nevertheless, some professionals such as Carlton (1984) questioned the choice of this path. Carlton believed that all health and mental health intervention needed to go beyond the traditional bounds of simply diagnosing a patient's mental health condition. From this perspective, social, situational, and environmental factors are considered key ingredients for addressing patient problems. Therefore, to remain consistent with the "person-in-situation" stance, utilizing the *DSM* as the path of least resistance might lead to a largely successful fight—yet would it win the war? Carlton, along with other professionals of his time, feared the battle was being fought on the wrong battlefield and advocated for a more comprehensive system of reimbursement that took into account environmental aspects.

Furthermore, research findings have suggested that when engaging in clinical practice many professionals did not use the *DSM* to direct their interventions at all. Rather, the focus and use of the manual was primarily limited to ensuring third-party reimbursement, qualifying for agency service, or to avoid placing a diagnostic label. For these reasons, patients could be given diagnoses not based solely on diagnostic criteria, and the danger of connecting diagnostic labels to unrelated factors such as the social stigma and the loss of other opportunities for the patient became obvious (Moses, 2009). Social stigma and concerns related to reimbursement became obvious.

Therefore, some health and mental health professionals were more likely to pick the most severe diagnoses so that their patients could qualify for agency services or insurance reimbursement. However, other mental health professionals engaged in the opposite behavior by assigning patients the least severe diagnoses to avoid stigmatizing and labeling them (Kutchins & Kirk, 1986, 1988, 1993). Avoidance of this label could increase patient empowerment by avoiding the personal and social stigma attached to such a label (Hinshaw & Stier, 2008).

Historically, although use of the *DSM* is clearly evident in mental health practice, some professionals have contested its use. The controversy centers on whether it is being utilized properly. Yet, regardless of the controversy in mental health practice, the continued and increased popularity of the *DSM* makes it the most frequently used publication in the field of mental health. In addition, each previous version of the *DSM*, including *DSM-5*, highlights the importance of taking into account the medical condition and how the medical condition can indeed affect the mental health of the individual patient served.

For some professionals such as social workers, however, the controversy over using this system for diagnostic assessments remains. Regardless of the school of thought or specific field of training that a mental health practitioner ascribes too, most professionals would agree that there is no single diagnostic system that is completely acceptable by all. Furthermore, it is the opinion of this author that some degree of relative skepticism and questioning of the appropriateness of the use of this manual needs to continue and should remain unabated. Since placing a diagnostic label needs to reach beyond ensuring service reimbursement, and can have serious consequences for the individual patient knowledge of how to properly use the manual is needed. In addition, there must also be knowledge, concern and continued professional debate about the appropriateness and the utility of certain diagnostic categories since those with professional experience are well aware of the fertile ground that exists for abuse.

Factors Suggestive of a Mental Disorder

- Previous psychosocial difficulties not related to a medical or neurodevelopmental disorder.
- Chronic unrelated complaints that cannot be linked to a satisfactory medical explanation.
- A history of object relations problems such as help-rejecting behavior, co-dependency, and other inter-relationship problems.
- A puzzling lack of concern on the part of the patient as to the behaviors he or she is engaging in with a detached attitude and tendency to minimize or deny the circumstances.
- Evidence of secondary gain where the patient is reinforced by such behaviors by significant others, family, or other members of the support system.
- A history of substance abuse problems (alcohol or medication abuse).

- A family history of similar symptoms and/or mental disorders.
- Cognitive or physical complaints that are more severe than what would be expected for someone in a similar situation.

In explaining assessment from either the older multiaxial system utilized in the *DSM-IV* and *DSM-IV-TR* and comparing it to the changes that occur with *DSM-5*, which no longer uses the multiaxial system, is beyond the scope of this chapter. To learn more about the diagnostic system itself it is suggested that the reader go to the original source, the *DSM-5*. For a further description and in-depth application of this information, Dziegielewski (2010a) and for the application and treatment aspects related to *DSM-5*, (Dziegielewski, in press) is suggested. Generally, all clinical syndromes are coded on Axis I (e.g., mood disorders, schizophrenia, dementia, anxiety disorders, substance disorders, disruptive behavior disorders). In addition, all other codes that are not attributed to a mental disorder but are the focus of intervention are also coded here.

In completing the diagnostic assessment, the following questions may be helpful in formulating the diagnosis.

1. What are the major psychiatric symptoms a patient is displaying?
2. What are the frequency, intensity, and duration of the symptom?
3. Have environmental factors, such as cultural and social factors, been considered as a possible explanation?
4. Do these identified patterns tend to cause difficulty in intimate, social, or work relationships?

In completing the diagnostic assessment utilizing the *DSM-5*, the general medical condition currently referred to as "another medical condition" should always be considered. This aspect of the diagnostic assessment is particularly important for the health care social worker as often medical and mental health conditions overlap. To prepare for properly noting the medical condition that affects the mental health one, the health care social workers should become familiar with the signs and symptoms of these conditions and assist in understanding the relationship of this medical condition to the assessment and planning process that will evolve.

To assist the health care social worker, Pollak, Levy, and Breitholtz (1999) suggested several factors that can help a practitioner to separate mental health clinical presentations that may have a medical contribution. First, give special attention to patients that present with the first episode of a major disorder. In these patients, particularly when symptoms are severe (e.g., psychotic, catatonic, and nonresponsive), close monitoring of the original presentation, when compared with previous behavior, is essential.

Second, note if the patient's symptoms are acute (just started or relative to a certain situation) or abrupt with rapid changes in mood or behavior.

Examples of symptoms that would fall into this area include both cognitive and behavioral symptoms such as: marked apathy, decreased drive and initiative, paranoia, lability, or mood swings, and poorly controlled impulses.

Third, the practitioner should pay particular attention when the initial onset of a problem or serious symptoms occurs after the age of 40. Although this is not an ironclad rule, most mental disorders become evident before the age of 40. Thus, onset of symptoms after 40 should be carefully examined to rule out social, situational stressors, cultural implications, and medical causes.

Fourth, note symptoms of a mental disorder that occur immediately before, during, or after the onset of a major medical illness. It is very possible the symptoms may be related to the progression of the medical condition as well as the possibility that it could be medication or substance related (Dziegielewski, 2010b, 2005). Poly-pharmacy can be a real problem for many individuals who are unaware of the dangers of mixing certain medications and substances that are not considered medications by the individual (i.e., herbal preparations) (Dziegielewski, 2006).

Fifth, when gathering information for the diagnostic assessment, note whether there is an immediate psychosocial stressor or life circumstance that may contribute to the symptoms the patient is experiencing. This is especially relevant when the stressors present are so minimal that a clear connection between the stressor and the reaction cannot be made. One very good general rule is to remember that anytime a patient presents with extreme symptomology of any kind and with no previous history of such behaviors, attention and monitoring for medical causes is essential.

Sixth, pay particular attention in the screening process when a patient suffers from a variety of different types of *hallucinations*. Basically, a hallucination is the misperception of a stimulus. In psychotic conditions, *auditory hallucinations* are most common. When a patient presents with multiple types of hallucinations such as *visual* (seeing things that are not there), *tactile* which pertain to the sense of touch (e.g., bugs crawling on them), or *gustatory*, pertaining to the sense of taste or *olfactory* relative to the sense of smell, this is generally too extreme a hallucination to be purely a mental health condition.

Seventh, note any simple repetitive and purposeless movements of speech (e.g., stuttering or indistinct or unintelligible speech), the face (e.g., motor tightness or tremors), and hands and extremities (e.g., tremor, shaking, and unsteady gait). Also note any experiential phenomena such as derealization, depersonalization, and unexplained gastric or medical complaints and symptoms such as new onset of headache accompanied by physical signs such as nausea and vomiting.

Eighth, be sure to note and document any signs of cortical brain dysfunction such as *aphasia* which is a disturbance in the production of language; apraxia which is related to movement; *agnosia* which constitutes a failure to recognize familiar objects despite intact sensory functioning, and *visuo-constructional deficits* which occurs when a patient is unable or has difficulties drawing or reproducing objects and patterns.

Lastly, note any signs that may be associated with organ failure such as jaundice related to hepatic disease or dyspnea (difficulty breathing) associated with cardiac or pulmonary disease. For example, if a patient is not getting proper oxygen he or she may present as very confused and disoriented. When oxygen is regulated, the signs and symptoms would begin to decrease and quickly subside. Although mental health practitioners are not expected to be experts in diagnosing medical disorders, being aware of the medical complications that can influence mental health presentations are necessary to facilitate the most accurate and complete diagnostic assessment possible (Dziegielewski, 2010a).

Questions to Guide the Health Care Social Worker

* Has the patient had a recent physical exam? If not, suggest that one be ordered.
* Does the patient have a summary of a recent history and physical examination that can be reviewed?
* Are there any laboratory findings or tests or any diagnostic reports that can assist in establishing a relationship between the mental and physiological consequences that result?

Lastly, the social worker should carefully assess the severity of the psychosocial stressor(s) that have happened in a patient's life over the past year. Here, we are reminded of the importance of the environment. If a stressor(s) is considered great when a mental health disorder develops—the prognosis for recovery is better. Carefully accounting for the stressor(s) involved that may affect the patient's response and the level of disability that is experienced is an important part of a comprehensive assessment. Generally, both the stressor and the severity are assessed.

To rate the patient's psychosocial and occupational functioning in the past year. To complete this task, a scale known as the Generalized Assessment of Functioning (GAF) is used. In *DSM-IV-TR*, the scale of the GAF had been extended to 100 points. If scales such as this are used in *DSM-5*, similar to before, the lower the number, the lower the level of functioning (1 = minimal functioning; 100 = highest level of functioning). The scale is listed in the *DSM-IV-TR*, and most professionals are not expected to memorize what each of the numbers mean. The GAF assesses both symptomology and level of functioning. Generally, the *highest* level of functioning is determined and rated.

With the pressure in the health care field for measurement of competent and professional service, some social workers and other professionals are now turning to the GAF and other forms of additional measurement to provide rating scores for each patient that they see (Dziegielewski, 2010a).

Generally, in the health setting, functional ratings are assigned as patients enter therapy and again upon discharge. This allows for a comparison of scores that can be viewed as representing the achievement of increased patient functioning.

Also, in the *DSM-IV* "Criteria Sets and Axes Provided for Further Study," there are two scales that provide a format for ranking function that might be particularly helpful to social work professionals. The first relational functioning scale to be considered is the Global Assessment of Relational Functioning (GARF). This scale is used to address family or other ongoing relationship status on a hypothetical continuum from competent to dysfunctional (American Psychiatric Association, 2000). The second scale is the Social and Occupational Functioning Assessment Scale (SOFAS). This scale measures the individual's level of social and occupational functioning, especially the behaviors that are not directly influenced an individual's psychological symptoms (American Psychiatric Association, 2000). The use of all three of these tools can help social workers to employ concrete measurements that help establish increased levels of functioning from the individual (GAF), family (GARF), and social (SOFAS) perspectives.

SPECIAL CONSIDERATIONS FOR HEALTH CARE SOCIAL WORKERS

When completing the diagnostic assessment, there are two medical conditions that are often overlooked and neglected, yet their importance is critical to a well-rounded comprehensive diagnostic assessment. The first falls under Diseases of the Eye and has to do with *Visual Loss* or *Cataracts*. Visual loss is related to a decrease in vision (sight) yet the apparent loss of vision acuity or visual field is not related directly to substantiating physical signs. This problem may be best addressed with patient reassurance.

Cataracts relate to the loss of transparency in the lens of the eye. Both of these conditions result in vision impairment. For the health care social worker assessing for problems with vision is critical because decreased or impaired vision may lead individuals to interpret daily events incorrectly. For example, a patient sitting by a window could be easily startled by his or her own reflection and may misinterpret what he or she sees, causing misperceptions and subsequent confusion. Patients might even be shocked and frightened, believing that someone is watching them. If patients do not have their glasses with them it may be easy to become lost and confused. This lack of vision can be very frustrating for the patient, especially when they cannot distinguish the shape in the window as their own. Imagine how frightened these patients might become and how easy it could be for that individual to become convinced a stranger is watching their every move? The frustration with the present situation alone can lead to symptoms being misperceived or misinterpreted. For health care social workers, the most salient issue to identify once the vision difficulty is recognized or corrected is whether the problem resolves itself. Regardless, as part of the general assessment, special attention should always be given to screening for vision problems that may cause distress to the individual in terms of individual and social functioning.

The second medical area that is often overlooked in the mental health and health assessment process is related to Hearing Loss. A patient with hearing impairment or hearing loss will experience a reduction in the ability to perceive sound that can range from slight impairment to complete deafness (*Physician's Desk Reference*, 1995). Many times a patient who is having hearing difficulty may not want to admit it. At times, when an individual does not hear what is said he or she may try to compensate by answering what he or she thought was asked or refusing to respond at all. In addition, many individuals may rely on hearing enhancement devices such as hearing aids, which amplify sound more effectively into the ear. Such hearing aids may not be able to differentiate among selected pieces of information as well as the human ear. Furthermore, as a normal part of aging high-frequency hearing loss can occur. Most noises in a person's environment, such as background noise, are low frequency. Therefore, an individual with the high-frequency loss may not be able to tune out background noise such as television sets or side conversations. He or she may get very angry over distractions that other people who do not have a similar hearing loss do not perceive. Special attention should always be given during the diagnostic assessment process to ask very specific questions with regard to hearing and vision problems as these medical problems can be misinterpreted as signs of a mental health problem.

In the assessment process, Dziegielewski (2010a) suggests that the social worker ask the following questions:

* Do you have any problems with your hearing or vision?
* How would you rate your current ability to hear and see?
* Can you give examples of specific problems you are having?
* When did you have your last vision or hearing check-up?
* Have you ever worn glasses or contact lenses?

BEGINNING THE ASSESSMENT PROCESS

In assessment, there are five expectations or factors that need to guide the initiation of the clinical assessment in the health care setting.

1. *Patients need to be active and motivated in the intervention process.* As in almost all forms of intervention, the patient is expected to be active. Furthermore, patient motivation for participation in intervention planning in the

health area is essential. Generally, the issues that the patient must face often require serious exertion of energy in attempting to make behavioral change. This means that patients must not only agree to participate in the assessment process but must be willing to embark on the intervention plan that will result in behavioral change.

2. *The problem needs to guide the approach or method of intervention used.* Health care social workers need to be aware of different methods and approaches for clinical intervention; however, the approach should never guide the intervention chosen. Sheafor and Horejsi (2008) warn against social workers becoming over-involved and wasting valuable clinical time by trying to match a particular problem to a particular theoretical approach, especially because so much of the problem identification process in assessment is an intellectual activity. The health care social worker should never lose sight of the ultimate purpose of the assessment process. Simply stated, the purpose is to complete an assessment that will help to establish a concrete service or intervention plan to address a patient's needs (see Table 8.5).

Table 8.5 Areas for Consideration in the Diagnostic Assessment

Area	Explanation
Biomedical factors	
General medical condition	Describe the physical illness or disability from which the patient is suffering.
Overall health status	Patient is to evaluate his or her own self-reported health status and level of functional ability.
Maintenance of continued health and wellness	Measurement of the patient's functional ability and interest in preventive medical and intervention.
Psychological factors	
Life stage	Describe the developmental stage in life in which the individual appears to be functioning.
Mental functioning	Describe the patient's mental functioning. Complete a mental status measurement.
	Can the patient participate knowledgeably in the intervention experience?
Cognitive functioning	Does the patient have the ability to think and reason? What is happening to him or her?
	Is he or she able to participate and make decisions regarding his or her own best interest?

(continued)

Table 8.5 (*continued*)

Level of self-awareness self-help	Does the patient understand what is happening to him or her?
Is the patient capable of assisting in his or her level of self-care?	Is the patient capable of understanding the importance of and being educated about health and wellness information?
	Is the patient open to help and services provided by the health care team?

Social factors

Social/societal help-seeking behavior	Is the patient open to outside help?
	Is the patient willing to accept help from those outside the immediate family or the community?
Occupational participation	How does a patient's illness or disability impair or prohibit functioning in the work environment?
	Is the patient in a supportive work environment?
Significant other support	Does the significant other understand and show willingness to help and support the needs of the patient?
Ethnic or religious affiliation	If the patient is a member of a certain cultural or religious group, will this affiliation affect medical intervention and compliance issues?

Functional/situational factors

Financial condition	How does the health condition affect the financial status of the patient?
	What income maintenance efforts are being made?
	Do any income efforts need to be initiated?
	Does the patient have savings or resources from which to draw?
Entitlement	Does the patient have health, accident, disability, or life insurance benefits to cover his or her cost of health service?
	Has insurance been recorded and filed for the patient to assist with paying of expenses?
	Does patient qualify for additional services to assist with illness and recovery?
Transportation	What transportation is available to the patient?
	Does the patient need assistance or arrangements to facilitate transportation?
Placement	Does the patient have a place to return or a plan for continued maintenance when services are terminated?
	Is alternative placement needed?

(*continued*)

Table 8.5 Areas for Consideration in the Diagnostic Assessment (*continued*)

Area	Explanation
Continuity of service	If the patient is to be transferred to another health service, have the connections been made to link services and service providers appropriately?
	Based on the services provided, has patient received the services he or she needs during and after the intervention period?

3. *The influence and effects of values and beliefs should be made apparent in the process.* Each individual, professional or not, is influenced by his or her own values and beliefs. It is these beliefs that create the foundation for who we are and what we believe. In the practice of health care social work, it is essential that these individual influences do not directly affect the assessment process. Therefore, the individual values, beliefs, and practices that can influence intervention outcomes must be clearly identified from the onset of treatment. For example, an unmarried patient at the public health clinic tested positive for being pregnant. The social worker assigned to her case personally believes that abortion is "murder" and cannot in good conscience recommend it as an option to her patient. The patient, however, is unsure of what to do and wants to explore every possible alternative. The plan that evolves must be based on the patient's needs and desires, not the social worker's values. Therefore, the social worker is advised to tell the patient of her prejudice and refer her to someone who can be more objective in exploring abortion as a possible course of action. Patients have a right to make their own decisions, and health care social workers must do everything possible to ensure this right and not allow personal opinion to impair the completion of a proper assessment.

In addition to the social worker and patient, the cultural constructions of reality such as the beliefs and values of the members of the interdisciplinary team must also be considered (Gehlert, 2012). Social workers need to be aware of value conflicts that might arise among the other team members. These team members need to be aware of how their personal feelings and resultant opinions might inhibit them from addressing all of the possible options with a patient. For example, in the case of the unmarried pregnant woman, a physician, nurse, or any other member of the health care delivery team who did not believe in abortion would also be obligated to refer the patient. This is not to assume that social workers are more qualified to address this issue, or that they always have an answer. Social workers should always be available to assist these professionals and always advocate for how to best serve the needs of the patient. Values and beliefs can be influential in identification of factors within individual decision-making strategy and remain an important factor to consider and identify in the assessment process.

4. *Issues surrounding culture and race should be addressed openly in the assessment phase.* The social worker needs to be aware of his or her cultural heritage as well as the patient's to ensure the most open and receptive environment is created. Dziegielewski (2012) suggested the following: (a) the social worker needs to be aware of his or her own cultural limitations; (b) the health care social worker needs to be open to cultural differences; (c) the social worker needs to recognize the integrity and the uniqueness of the patient; (d) use the patient's learning style including his or her own resources and supports; and (e) implement the biopsychosocial approach to practice from an integrated and as nonjudgmental a format as possible. For example, when completing a mental health assessment, cultural factors are identified and addressed before any type of assessment or intervention. These factors can clearly influence and mitigate mental health and medical illness, recognition and bringing these concerns to the attention of the team can help to identify and in some ways negate the power these influences can have on the assessment and treatment context (Heller & Gitterman, 2011). How much the social worker attends to these issues will depend clearly on how obvious they tend to be. Regardless, the importance of being aware of these similarities and differences should be noted and attended to clearly in the assessment and treatment process (Frankel & Gelman, 2011).

5. *The assessment must focus on patient strengths and highlight the patient's own resources for providing continued support.* One of the most difficult tasks for most individuals to complete is to find, identify, and plan to use their own strengths. People, in general, have a tendency to focus on the negatives and rarely praise themselves for the good they do. With the advent of behavioral managed care, health care social workers must quickly identify the individual and collectively based strengths that each patient possesses. Once this has been achieved, these strengths must be stressed and implemented as part of the intervention plan. Identifying an individual's strengths can be directly linked to self-determination and the individual's support networks. In this time-limited intervention environment, individual resources are essential for continued growth and maintenance and can continue as a sign of wellness long after the formal intervention period has ended.

COMPLETING THE ASSESSMENT PROCESS

To initiate the process, it is assumed that the assessment begins with the first patient–social worker interaction. The information that the health care social worker gathers will provide the database that will assist in determining the requirements and direction of the helping process. In assessment, it is expected that the social worker will gather information about the patient's present situation and history regarding the past, and anticipate service expectations for the future. This assessment should be multidimensional and always include creative interpretation of perspectives and alternatives for service delivery. In starting this process, clear expectations are needed in terms of patient confidentiality and obtaining patient consent as it may relate directly to ensuring continuity of care (NASW, 2011).

Generally, the patient is seen as the primary source of data. This information gathered can come from either a verbal or written report. Information about the patient is often derived through direct observation of verbal or physical behaviors or interaction patterns between other interdisciplinary team members, family, significant others, or friends. In recognizing that a problem exists, the patient or someone in the family/support system becomes aware that something is wrong and although they might not be able to concretely identify the problem it becomes clear that something is wrong. Once this recognition takes place there will be some type of reaction with varying degrees of uncertainty and feelings of vulnerability (Webb & Bartone, 2012).

Once the problem is recognized, viewing and recording these patterns of communication can be extremely helpful in later establishing and developing strength and resource considerations. In addition to verbal reports, written reports are also employed. Oftentimes, background sheets, psychological tests, or tests to measure health status or level of daily function may be used. Although the patient is perceived as the first and primary source of data, social work's traditional emphasis of including information from other areas cannot be underestimated. This means talking with the family and significant others to estimate planning support and assistance. It might also be important to gather information from other secondary sources, such as the patient's medical record and other health care providers. Furthermore, to facilitate assessment, the social worker must be able to understand the patient's medical situation. This is where the connection between the medical concerns and mental health concerns cannot be separated. The social worker, although not expected to act as a physician or nurse, needs to be aware of what medical conditions a patient has and how these conditions can influence behavior (Dziegielewski, 2010a, 2010b).

In completing a multidimensional assessment, there are four primary steps for consideration that can be well adapted into the health care setting. First, the problem must be recognized. Here the health care social worker must be active in uncovering problems that affect daily living and engaging the patient in self-help or skill-changing behaviors. It is important for the patient to acknowledge that the problem exists because once this is done and the problem is identified, clearly it sets the stage for further exploration and examination (Hepworth et al., 2010).

Second, the problem must be clearly identified. The problem of concern is identified as what the patient sees as important; after all, the patient is the one who is expected to create change behavior. In the health care field, it is common to receive referrals from other health care professionals. These same referrals often provide the basis for reimbursement as well. Caution needs to be exercised to prevent the referral source from determining how the problem is viewed, and what should constitute the basis of intervention. It is a good idea clinically and from a cost-effectiveness stance for the health care social worker to look at each individual case and process this referral information. In addition, when striving to help the patient, referral information and suggestion should always be part of your discussion with the patient.

Third, problem strategy and a plan for intervention must be developed. According to Sheafor & Horejsi (2008), the plan of action is the basis for that links the assessment and the intervention. Here the health care social worker must help to clearly focus on the goals and objectives that will be followed in the intervention process. In the initial planning stage, emphasis on the outcome to be accomplished is essential.

Lastly, once completed an assessment plan must be implemented. The outcome of the assessment process is the completion of a plan that will guide, enhance, and, in many cases, determine the course of the intervention to be implemented. With the complexity of human beings and the problems that they encounter, a properly prepared multidimensional assessment is the essential first step for ensuring quality service delivery.

In selecting the type of service delivery, increased attention is being given to the provision of mental health services that utilize *peer-provided services*. These services are delivered by individuals who identify as being delivered by recipients of the same mental health services. These services are considered to be empowering and emphasize individual strengths and self-determination. Solomon, Schmidt, Swarbrick, and Mannion (2011) describe this type of treatment as a way that individuals can identify common problems and concerns, and when used to promote recovery, this method has been recognized as an emerging best practice.

CHAPTER SUMMARY AND FUTURE DIRECTIONS

The helping relationship is a complex one that cannot be measured completely through the information gathered, through either the systematic approach as used in the PIE or the more diagnostic approach presented with the *DSM* diagnostic system. The PIE represents an environmentally sensitive tool that supplements the *DSM*, bringing to the forefront the importance of recognition of the human condition through a humanistic and pluralistic approach rather than the medical foundational basis within the *DSM* (Satterly, 2007).

In May of 2013, the American Psychiatric Association released its new version of the *DSM* tilted "*DSM-5*." This new volume of the *DSM* brings many changes, including replacement of the categorical approach used in the *DSM-IV* and the *DSM-IV-TR*. For example, this new volume changed the entire diagnostic system of recording moving away from establishing discrete categories of symptoms related to a diagnosis to a cross-cutting of symptoms across diagnostic categories. It also directly formulates the diagnostic criteria, moving away from a categorical system to a dimensional assessment approach (Helzer et al., 2008). The changes with this edition (*DSM-5*) are significant and will clearly have a direct effect on all aspects of diagnostic assessment. Since assessment provides the groundwork for the intervention strategy its impact should not be minimized. Since assessment and treatment are based primarily on the practitioner's clinical judgment and interpretation, a thorough grounding of these new changes is highly recommended as it will help the practitioner to make relevant, useful, and ethically sound evaluations of patients. For more information on *DSM-5*, the reader is referred to the American Psychiatric Association website: www.dsm5.org

Regardless of what type of assessment is used and the changes announced in *DSM-5*, the process used to gather information from these diagnostic schemes will continue to support and assist the assessment process. These assessment schemes are meant to support and serve as the basis for the development of intervention strategy. After all, the *DSM* is a diagnostic and statistical manual and it clearly does not intend to change this focus and suggest treatment.

The future will continue to hold the expectation that gathering information through a diagnostic impression or assessment be intervention friendly, thereby outlining and providing the ingredients for the treatment planning and strategy to follow. The practitioner should always consider incorporating a number of evidence-based tools such as direct behavioral observation techniques and self-anchored rating scales as mentioned in the chapter highlighting documentation.

Since the concept of formulating a diagnosis is richly embedded in the history and practice of the clinical health care social worker, demands for practice reimbursement cannot be underestimated. Whether social workers truly subscribe to or support this distinction between assessment and diagnosis, they still must be able to relate to other professionals and/or service providers who do. In the current health care profession, social workers must be able to show clearly that they are able to complete the task at hand—no matter what it is called. Regardless, all diagnostic or assessment activity in the health care field should be related to the needs of the patient.

The social work profession has embraced the necessity for diagnosis in practice; however, this need has been recognized with caution. In accepting the requirement for completion of a diagnosis, much discontent and dissatisfaction still exists. Some social workers feel that diagnosis, when linked to the traditional definition of a medical perspective, is inconsistent with social work's history, ethics, and values. Today, however, this view is changing. Many health care social workers, struggling for practice survival in this competitive cost-driven health care system, disagree. They think that practice reality requires that a traditional method of diagnosis be completed to receive reimbursement. Their argument rests within the practice reality that it is this capacity for reimbursement that influences and determines who will be offered the opportunity to provide service (Dziegielewski, 2010a).

To compete in today's current social work environment, the role of the social worker is threefold: (a) to ensure that quality service is provided to the patient; (b) to ensure that the patient has access to services and is given an opportunity to see that his or her health needs are addressed; and, (c) to advocate for changes on a macro level within the current existing system and helping to develop a system, within a realistic framework of limited resources, that can benefit all. None of these tasks is easy or popular in today's environment. The push for health care practice to be conducted with limited resources and services and the resultant competition to be the provider have really changed and stressed the role of the health care social work professional. However, amid this turbulence, the role and the necessity of the services the social worker provide in the area of assessment, intervention, and advocacy remain clear. Social workers must know the tools for assessment and diagnosis that are being used in the field, and must be familiar and able to use them. Assessment and diagnosis are often viewed as the first step in the intervention hierarchy, a step that social work professionals should become well versed in.

In the practice of health care social work, there are numerous tools and methods of diagnosis currently being used. The PIE, the *ICD-10*, and the *DSM* represent only a small portion of what is available. These forms of systematic assessment can help to provide social workers with a framework for practice. Particularly, the *ICD-9-CM* and the *DSM-IV* are most reflective of the dominant view in the United States, which is rooted in the medical model. Many social workers fear that these methods may result in a label being placed on patients that is difficult to remove and can end in social stigma and the loss of other opportunities (Moses, 2009). Regardless, social workers have a unique role in assessment and diagnosis that cannot be underestimated. As part of the interdisciplinary team, the social worker brings a wealth of information regarding the environment and family considerations essential to practice strategy. Social workers, with a focus on "skill building" and "strength enhancing" of the patient, are well equipped not only to provide a key role in the psychosocial assessment of the patient, but also to establish the intervention plan that will guide and determine the course and quality of service delivery that will be received by the public.

In closing, health care social workers can also play an important role in policy advocacy (Darnell & Lawlor, 2012). As changes in reimbursement are unfolding such as the 2010 Affordable Care Act, social workers are at a pivotal point where advocacy and change can result. Understanding the culture and in many cases using the terminology that creates a shared language will improve communication and give social work a seat at the table where these changes will be determined.

Glossary

Agnosia   This constitutes a failure to recognize familiar objects despite intact sensory functioning.

Aphasia   In the assessment process, this is recognized as a disturbance in the production of language.

Apraxia   In the assessment process, this is recognized as related to movement.

Assessment   The process of determining the nature, cause, progression, and prognosis of a problem and the personalities and situations involved therein; it is the thinking process by which one reasons from the facts to tentative conclusions regarding their meaning.

Axis I   This is the first level of coding with the *DSM* multiaxis diagnostic system. According to the *DSM-IV* classification system, the following diagnostic categories are included: pervasive developmental disorders, learning disorders, motor skills disorders, communication disorders, and other disorders that may be focus of clinical treatment.

Axis II   This is the second level of coding with the *DSM* multiaxis diagnostic system. According to the *DSM-IV* classification system, the following diagnostic categories are included: personality disorders and mental retardation.

Axis III   This is the third level of coding with the *DSM* multiaxis diagnostic system. According to the *DSM-IV* classification system, general medical conditions that can affect the mental health condition of the patient are recorded.

Axis IV   This is the fourth level of coding with the *DSM* multiaxis diagnostic system. According to the *DSM-IV* classification system, the psychosocial and environmental problems/stressors, such as problems with primary support, problems related to social environment, educational problems, occupational problems, housing problems, economic problems, problems with access to health care services, problems related to interaction with the legal system, and other psychosocial problems, are recorded here.

Axis V   This is the fifth level of coding with the *DSM* multiaxis diagnostic system. According to the *DSM-IV* classification system, the level of functioning a patient has is recorded on this axis.

Coping index   A coding classification within the PIE considering the degree to which a patient can handle a problem within his or her internal resources.

Diagnosis   The process of identifying a problem (social and mental as well as medical) and its underlying causes and formulating a solution.

Diagnostic process   Examination of the parts of a problem to determine the relationships between them and the means to their solution.

Diagnostic product   This is generally identified as what is obtained after the health care social worker uses the information gained in the diagnostic process.

DSM-IV-TR   The *DSM-IV-TR* is a manual that presents a classification system designed to assist professionals in assigning a formal diagnostic pattern.

Duration index   A coding classification within the PIE where the length or when the problem last occurred is noted.

Factor I   This is the first of the four levels for problem classification used in the PIE. This constitutes a measurement of social functioning.

Factor II   This is the second area for classification used in the PIE. Emphasis here is placed on the identification of environmental problems.

Factor III   This is the third area for classification using the PIE. This category deals with mental health problems and uses the codification of the *DSM-IV* to describe it.

Factor IV   This is the fourth category of the PIE classification system. This area explores the physical problems and diagnoses that can affect the patient.

Generalized assessment of functioning   A scale used on Axis V of the *DSM-IV* to incorporate a recording measure for a patient's highest level of functioning over a certain period.

Global assessment of relational functioning   This assessment is used to address family or other ongoing relationship status on a hypothetical continuum from competent to dysfunctional.

Labeling   The process of assigning a clinical diagnosis to a patient that will stay with that patient indefinitely.

Person-in-environment (PIE)   This is a formal method of codification that was designed by and for social workers to assist in the assessment process.

Social and occupational functioning assessment scale   A scale that can be used to address an individual's level of social and occupational functioning that is not directly influenced by overall severity of the individual's psychological symptoms.

Visuo-constructional deficits   This is assessed when a patient is unable or has difficulties drawing or reproducing objects and patterns.

Questions for Further Study

1. Based on the current trends and reimbursement patterns for assessment and diagnosis, what do you see as the future role for health care social workers regarding this process?

2. Do you believe that the PIE will continue to gain in popularity in the health care professions, other than social work?

3. Do you believe health care social workers will abandon the use of the *DSM-IV* diagnostic categories in the future because of the potential problem that labeling can cause the patients it is designed to serve?

4. Do you believe that a diagnostic, assessment, and intervention planning framework to guide social work practice is required for reimbursement of social work services to increase?

5. Identify what you believe are the major strengths and weaknesses in diagnostic and assessment process used today in health care service delivery.

6. What changes do you predict the *DSM-5* will have in regard to diagnostic assessment?

Websites

Mental Health Net
Guide to mental health online, featuring over 6,000 individual resources; winner of several awards.
www.mentalhelp.net

Psychiatric Times
Full text of news and clinical articles for mental health professionals.
www.psychiatrictimes.com/home

American Psychiatric Association
www.psych.org

The Mental Health Social Worker
A site dedicated to the field of social work that pulls items from many sources. Topics include practice, advocacy, education, careers, ethics, research, and new developments.
www.mhsw.org

Today's Health Care Social Worker

Name:	Lisa "Todd" Graddy, MSW
Title of Current Position:	Mental Health Therapist
Where You Practice:	Kentucky
Professional Job Title(s):	Mental Health Therapist, Hospice Social Worker, and Lifestyle/Behavioral Management Therapist

Describe briefly what your duties are in a typical day.
1. I am a therapist for families of the terminally ill. I perform suicide risk assessments, drug diversion assessments, and provide grief counseling to those who are involved in the patient's life.
2. In my position as a wellness/lifestyle therapist, I assess patients for their ability to change their current lifestyle. I use a model to predict success for their ability to change.

What do you like most about your current position?
I like to work with the Individual as a whole. I am able to perform a psychosocial assessment that includes both their mental capabilities as well as their physical limitations. This ability gives me a broader framework to assist the patients and their families.

What do you like least?
The perception of what others see as the role of social work and the limits it places on what I can do to help others.

What is your favorite health care social worker story?
The chaplain and I look alike. We are the same age and have the same haircut. One time she was working with a terminally ill man who wanted to give his confession. They spent a long time working on this issue together. A few days later I was in the mans' home and he leaned over to me and said, "Now I sure feel better about telling you all of that stuff, so just make sure that no one else knows about it." I reported this to the chaplain and she asked if I had written up her note for visiting the patient that day since she did not have to go to make her weekly visit, having already been there that day!

What "words of wisdom" do you have for the new health care social worker who is considering working in a similar position?
Get a variety of education and experience. Try not to specialize in the established areas of medical social work. The medical arena is changing rapidly and there is much room for medical social workers to expand their expertise and skills in these new areas.

Today's Medical and Psychiatric Hospital Social Worker

Name: Halim Faisal, LCSW
List State of Practice: Georgia

Experiences in Hospital Social Work:
I have been practicing social work in hospital settings since 1987.
I started off working with AIDS hospice in the late 1980s at a large
public hospital in Atlanta, Georgia. From there I went to inpatient/
outpatient neurology and orthopedic services. I also worked in
inpatient physical rehabilitation. I did all of this between 1987
and 1997. In 1998, I worked in a partial hospitalization setting
for chronically mentally ill. And, from 2000 to 2010, I worked in
outpatient hospice and community mental health. I have worked
in a private inpatient psychiatric hospital since 2010.

Today what are your duties in a typical day?
In the private psychiatric hospital, where I work today, on a typical
day I facilitate at least two groups, and I do individual therapy, family
sessions, and discharge planning. And case management, of course.

What do you like most about your current position?
I like facilitating groups, and I think this is the most effective
therapy for the patients. I prefer process groups over psychoeducational groups. The unit that I like the best is the locked unit
where the patients with serious mental illness or crises are. I like
the challenges and the level of skills I am able to use with these
patients with such complex problems.

What is most challenging about your current position?
This is probably across the board for many social workers, but
being managed by people who have expertise in business, and
how to make money, but who don't have expertise in or appreciation for what social workers can do. Also, in our setting, I don't
think we are encouraged to see things the way patients see things.
We are not encouraged to have empathy for patients. There is a
dissociation between the patients and professionals.

**What words of wisdom do you have for social workers who are
considering a similar position?**
You may not be appreciated in your setting for your skills and
what you bring to the table, but use your position as an opportunity to develop your skills and learn how to be a good social
worker. Let the patients teach you. Get supervision from an LCSW,
stay in touch with other social workers, join and participate in

(continued)

(continued)

---

the NASW. You also have to take responsibility for your own development in the absence of having supervision at work. Think about what you are doing, why you are doing it, and what you are learning. Learn how to identify patient strengths and resources and teach the patients to access them. The patients may not be with you long. Treat every session with a patient as if it was your last session with the patient.

How do you see case management?
The problem with case management in health care is that it has been taken over by nurses. But, learn from the nurses and develop your relationships with the nurses. You will need them and they will need you. They will call you when there are cases that they cannot handle. Remember this.

What is your favorite hospital social work story?
There are several from my medical hospital social work. I can remember being snowed into the hospital during a blizzard and being the only social worker there. It was very exciting. I would go from floor to floor and case to case. I really felt like a part of the team.

Another thing I enjoy is working with the patients that the other hospital staff does not want to work with, especially the patients who are angry, complaining all the time, or breaking the hospital rules. Often the nurses and doctors don't know what to do with them or want to get them out of the hospital as soon as possible. It is a challenge to build rapport with these patients, and they usually have a point about what they are saying or complaining about.

What do you see as the difference between medical and psychiatric hospital social work?
In my opinion, comparing the medical and psychiatric hospitals is like comparing apples and oranges. Medical settings are far more structured, and usually in medical settings, there is a presenting acute problem and protocols for how to treat the problem. In psychiatric settings, there is the *DSM*, but the categories keep changing. Mental health is more subjective in defining and treating the problem. And, in medicine, the treatments like medications are more exact, whereas in psychiatric settings even with medications sometimes they work and sometimes they don't.

In medical settings, you want to readily see the patient get functionally better and the health care interdisciplinary team will need to function as an integrated team supporting the patient in

---

(continued)

Today's Medical and Psychiatric Hospital Social Worker (*continued*)

this process. In mental health, there is still the stigma, and often the responsibility for getting better falls solely on the patient. If there is a sense that the patient will not get better, the staff in psychiatric hospitals can distance themselves from patients and show less empathy when the person suffers from chronic mental illness as opposed to suffering from a medical condition such as cancer.

Another concern when placed in a psychiatric hospital is that the patients are away from their work, family, and lives. For some patients with limited contacts in the environment, this can seem like vacation. The patients in this setting will see other patients that they know from other mental health settings and these contacts provide comfort as they too understand what it is like to live with mental illness. Therefore, the inpatient hospital needs to recognize the importance of the PIE and the family and other support systems that will be needed for successful return to the community.

PART III

Fields of Clinical Social Work Practice in Health Care Settings

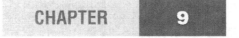
Acute Health Care Settings

Sophia F. Dziegielewski and Diane C. Holliman

The history of health care social work, traced earlier in this book, lends credence to the role of the health care social worker as an integral part of health care service delivery. Throughout history, social work has been at the forefront in providing health care services to patients/clients/consumers (hereafter referred to as patients) in the acute care setting. Furthermore, in a national survey of licensed social workers, Whitaker, Weismiller, Clark, and Wilson (2006) reported that general and acute care medical facilities are the most common employment settings for health care social workers. Therefore, as the number of practicing health care professionals continues to rise (Jansson, 2011), the role and influences the health care social worker has on the acute practice setting will remain pronounced.

The skills and tasks of the acute care social worker are varied. This chapter will seek to identify the actual tasks completed by the acute care social worker and the expectations within the field of practice. To facilitate this description, three popular and prominent areas where acute health care social workers are employed will be explicated. Case exemplars are provided to highlight acute care social work and the processes that are involved in assessment, intervention, and treatment and areas of strength and concern in the present state of practice delivery will be explicated.

HEALTH SERVICE PROVISION IN ACUTE CARE SETTINGS

The importance of acute care social work intervention was first highlighted in 1903 at Massachusetts General Hospital when Dr. Richard C. Cabot appointed Garnet Isabel Pelton, a trained nurse, to act as a clinic social worker. Dr. Cabot, as did many other physicians of his time, realized the importance of psychosocial factors in medical illness and understood that as the role and responsibilities of the physician grew, psychosocial responsibilities would have to be delegated to other helping professionals. The medical social worker was assigned duties focusing on the economic, emotional, social, and ecological needs of patients and families and was expected to relay all information gathered back to the physician (Cabot, 1919). To accomplish the assigned tasks in the late 1800s and early 1900s, the health care social worker was required to have adequate medical knowledge, an understanding of disease and factors that affected mental health, as well as a firm comprehension of public health. For social workers in the acute health setting, responsibilities initially included reporting problematic domestic and social conditions to the physician, assisting and ensuring treatment compliance with the established medical regime, and providing linkages between the acute care setting and the appropriate community agencies.

With the medical advances of the late 1950s came the promotion of cardiac surgery, transplant surgery, dialysis, and neonatal intensive care. The medical social worker was identified not only as an instructor for sick patients and their families, but also developed challenging roles as educators of interdisciplinary health care professionals. In the 1960s, the nation's interest in health care increased dramatically when Medicaid and the Community Mental Health Projects were developed. With the public's resurgent regard for health matters in the United States, social work in health care began its own rebirth. "The medical social worker is in the best position of anyone on the hospital staff to bridge the gap between the hospital bed, the patient's home and the world of medical science" (Risley, 1961, p. 83).

Today, in the area of acute health care social work, there are numerous roles and services that social workers provide. Subsequently, there are also numerous areas or fields of practice where they are employed. Three major areas of practice for the health care social worker that will be discussed in this section are acute care medical hospitals, acute care mental health hospitals, and social work in the nephrology setting.

Areas of service provision in these acute health care settings include case consultation, case finding and screening, case planning, comprehensive psychosocial assessment and intervention, helping patients and families understand illness, collaboration with other members of the interdisciplinary team, treatment team planning, group therapy, supportive counseling, crisis intervention, organ donation coordination, health education, providing education on the health care system and treatment process, advocacy and policy practice, case management, discharge planning, information and referral, quality assurance, and research (Holliman, 1998; Judd, 2010, National Center for Workforce Studies & Social Work Practice, 2011a). Table 9.1 provides a definition and brief description of the role social work professionals in the major acute clinical practice settings such as hospitals and medical centers, psychiatric hospitals, health clinics and outpatient health care settings which includes nephrology settings.

These acute care settings are often where elder abuse, neglect and elder self-neglect (Dong, Simon, & Evans, 2012), domestic violence (Power,

Table 9.1 Acute Care as a Field of Practice for Social Workers

Social workers in hospitals and medical centers	Social workers in hospitals and medical centers provide direct services to patients and their families with conditions from the entire health care continuum. Functions of social workers in hospitals and medical centers include initial screening and evaluation of patients and families, comprehensive psychosocial assessments, helping patients and families understand illness and treatment options as well as the consequences of the treatment and refusal of treatment, helping patients and families adjust to hospital admission and possible role changes due to illness, educating patients on the role of team members, assisting patients and families in communicating with each other, educating patients and families on discharge options and resources, employing crisis intervention, educating hospital staff on psychosocial issues, coordinating patient discharge, promoting patient navigation services, arranging resources for medications, durable medical equipment and other services, advocating for the patient and family in the hospital and community, and championing health care rights of the patient through advocacy at the policy level.
Social workers in psychiatric hospitals	Methods and services provided to patients and their families to ensure that a patient's illness, recovery, and safe transitions from one care setting to another are considered. Psychosocial factors are highlighted that include living arrangements, developmental history, economic, cultural, religious, educational, and vocational background that may impinge on the understanding, treatment, and relapse prevention of the psychiatric disorder. Functions and services provided include intake or admission evaluation, psychosocial assessment and treatment planning, high social risk case finding, education and advocacy, individual, group, family treatment and counseling, crisis intervention, consultation, expert testimony, discharge and after-care planning, and so on.
Nephrology settings	Methods and services provided to improve the quality and appropriateness of psychosocial services for patients with end-stage renal disease. Major services provided include psychosocial evaluations, casework, group work, information and referral, facilitation of community resources, team care planning and collaboration, and advocacy for patient and family education.

[a]All definitions taken from NASW, Center for Workforce Studies and Social Work Practice (2011). Social Workers in Hospitals and Medical Centers [Brochure] (2011a). Social Workers in Psychiatric Hospitals [Brochure] (2011b). UNC Kidney Center, www.unckidneycenter.org/hcprofessionals/nephsocialworkers.html#guidelines

Bahnisch, & McCarthy, 2011), and suicidal behaviors are first identified. Acute care social workers have played important roles in the identification, assessment, intervention, and referral of these individuals and their family systems. In acute care settings, the results of substance use, misuse, and abuse are often clear because of their physical and acute components. With substance abuse, domestic violence, elder abuse and neglect, suicide, mental illness, self-neglect, and dementia, there is often denial among the patients and their families. However, when a patient presents to an acute care setting and the effects of these events are evident, this critical incident needs to be identified and clarified in terms of how it is affecting the patient and his or her family system.

Social workers will need to intervene by carefully assessing the situation and helping those affected understand what is happening, and then, once the problem has been clearly and concretely identified, proceed with the necessary and appropriate treatment strategy whether it be supportive counseling or simply information and referral.

The first case exemplar, from Chapter 1 of this book, highlights the situation related to Ms. Martha Edda. Ms. Edda's involvement in acute care settings includes when she was admitted to the hospital after being discovered in her apartment filled with rotted food, urine, and feces. During this hospitalization, she was diagnosed with moderate to advanced vascular dementia. After deliberation with her health care team consisting of the hospital social worker and the medical staff, Ms. Edda was discharged to her daughter Joan's home. The placement with Joan was not without complications as home health services stopped after 2 months. The loss of the nurses' aid caused Joan's husband to have to help to get Ms. Edda in and out of the bath tub. This created an embarrassing and uncomfortable situation for both Ms. Edda and her son-in-law. The lack of spots available in the local adult day care center left the family responsible for helping with all Ms. Edda's activities of daily living. Her daughter later ended up quitting her job to care for her mother which put further financial strain on the family system.

The second hospitalization occurred when Joan found Ms. Edda lying face down in bed, incontinent of bowel and bladder, unable to speak, and unresponsive. Ms. Edda was transported to the emergency department by ambulance and tests were begun. Unfortunately, there were no available beds in the hospital, so Ms. Edda spent the night in the emergency department before she was admitted in the morning. During this admission, Ms. Edda was incontinent, refused to eat, and became so confused that she was restrained. Despite these changes, her medical tests came back negative, her vital signs were stable, and the social worker was notified that she was cleared for discharge. The family said that they could not accept Ms. Edda at home because of her care needs, and she was referred for nursing home placement. This was problematic because Ms. Edda did not have private insurance and she was 62 years old, making her too young to qualify for Medicare. An application for Medicaid was made, although there were no nursing home beds available. The time was also a consideration as it was after 4:00 p.m., when most administrative offices were closing in the hospital and at nursing homes. The social worker planned to secure an out-of-area placement the following day. The physician, however, wrote an order for an immediate discharge for Ms. Edda as medically she was stabilized. With no other options available, she was discharged home to the care of her daughter. Since she was still incontinent, the social worker promised to help arrange for home health care the next day.

This series of complications surrounding illness, hospitalization, and discharge planning is not uncommon. The effects of these medical, physical, emotional, social, organizational, economic, community and larger system, or macro (city, state, national, and international) difficulties coupled with a lack of resources, programs, and services becomes a reciprocal, systemic, and intertwined process. This is a difficult case and the decisions that must be made are not easy. In this case, none of the available choices, services, or courses of action was ideal or optimal for the patient, family, organization, or community. To best assist the patient, social workers in this setting will always require creative, critical, and complex thinking and actions as well as flexibility. The NASW *Code of Ethics* and the knowledge, skills, and values of generalist social work practice are a foundation for the specialization of hospital social work.

In summary, to explore this case further examine the following statements and answer the subsequent questions:

1. Apply the six core values of the NASW *Code of Ethics* (service, social justice, dignity and worth of the person, importance of human relationships, integrity, and competence) to this case. Which sections and subsections from the NASW *Code of Ethics* apply to this case?
2. Which direct practice theoretical perspectives can be used to describe and intervene with Ms. Edda? With her daughter and daughter's family?
3. What macrointerventions (organizational, community, policy, funding, state, national, and international) could be utilized or developed to improve the quality of services for patients like Ms. Edda and her family?

Case Study (Walter and James)

Walter (age 60) and James (age 44) had been a couple for over 20 years. Walter was African American and a history professor at a small liberal arts college in Mississippi. His partner, James, was Caucasian American and a professional musician who directed adult and youth choirs and taught voice to high school and college students. The couple lived and worked in Mississippi where same-sex marriage and civil unions are not recognized. Because Walter was 16 years older than James, Walter had completed a living well and a durable power of attorney (including a health care power of attorney) with James designated as his principal agent who could make decisions for Walter if he were unable to do so for medical or other reasons. James had often said that he too was going to get around to completing a living will and durable power of attorney with Walter as his principal agent or decision maker, but the time always seemed to slip away and one was never completed. James also had clearly told Walter and other friends that he did not want to be kept alive by artificial means if there was not a chance of recovery. James was in relatively good health and was very active. He did have what Walter termed "unusual eating habits" and was constantly dieting and voicing concern about his weight. He felt that because of his work and public performances that he needed to look his best. James's primary care physician had suspected that James had bulimia or another eating disorder, but it had never been diagnosed.

On July 20, 2010, James was exercising at the gym and went into a full cardiac arrest. Cardiopulmonary resuscitation was done at the gym, but James could not be revived. The Emergency Medical Service was called and from the gym James was transported to the emergency department of a local hospital. This incident resulted in massive brain damage due to lack of oxygen. From the emergency department, James was admitted to the intensive care unit (ICU) and was in a *coma* and unable to respond to anyone. When James had this incident, the staff at the gym called Walter, who was also a member of the gym and listed as James's emergency contact. However, as James was being admitted to the hospital, the medical staff would not communicate with Walter because he was not a legal relative of James even though they had lived together and been a couple over 20 years. James did not have children, but his mother and father were alive and were his next of kin. His parents knew Walter and about their son's relationship with him. Both of his parents did not approve of this union, but over the years had grown to be cordial to Walter. However, Walter was never invited to family gatherings and was referred to as James's roommate rather than his life partner.

When the hospital social worker did the initial psychosocial assessment with James's parents, they said that James lived alone as far as they knew and did not mention Walter as a significant other, friend, roommate, or any other contact. James's parents restricted visitation to only family, again excluding Walter. James's parents were prominent in the community and James was known throughout the region as a choir director, voice teacher, and performer. Because of his work, James had connections with several churches and other faith-based groups who may have objected to James being gay, so his personal life was always kept private in those settings. Members of the hospital board of directors and a hospital administrator knew James's parents and supported the wishes of his parents.

Two days after James was admitted to the hospital, the social worker received a frantic phone call from Walter insisting to meet with her as soon as possible. At first, the social worker did not make the connection that Walter was James's partner until Walter came in he introduced himself as James's significant other and life partner. Walter was in a panic and stated he had to see James. When he tried earlier to enter the ICU, the nursing staff would not allow him near Walter. Walter exclaimed that when he asked to talk to James's physician, he was told him that she could not give him any information. The physician referred him to James's parents who were his next of kin. Walter said that he then left at least 20 messages in 2 days for James's parents, but they would not return his calls. Walter then received a very brief e-mail from James's brother telling him to stop trying to contact his parents. The message warned him that if he did not stop and continued to try to communicate with them, the family would have to take legal action against him. As Walter shared this, he was sobbing and visibly shaken. He stated that he felt so guilty for not pushing James harder to get his living will and durable power of attorney completed. Walter also believed that James's parents did not know his wishes and would probably want James to have the most aggressive life-saving measures because of their religious beliefs. Walter then stated that he could not live without James and he always thought that he would die first. Walter shared with the social worker that this entire situation was so upsetting that he had not eaten or slept since James's incident and continued to sob and shake.

The hospital social worker could see the pain that Walter was experiencing; the social worker found his concerns very credible and wanted to help him. However, she realized that the hospital board and administration would probably be displeased that she had even met with him. The social worker also was concerned about how distraught Walter was and the fact that he reported he could not eat or sleep he was so filled with distress and grief. Her professional judgment told her that she needed to intervene to provide support for Walter during this time of crisis. She asked Walter if there was a friend or relative that he could call right now to be with him. She also asked him if he had a social worker, therapist, counselor, clergy, health care provider, or other professional that he could talk to. From these questions, the hospital social worker sat with Walter as he contacted his friend, Loretta, who was willing to pick him up at the hospital social worker's office and spend the rest of the day with him. Walter also told the hospital social worker that he and James had seen a social worker in private practice several years ago because James's anxiety about his job and his appearance were interfering with their relationship. As Walter was sitting in the hospital social worker's office, he made an appointment to meet with this social worker for later in the day. The hospital social worker discussed Walter's feelings with him and assessed for suicide as well as helped him to come up with a plan to identify these feelings of extreme distress and hopelessness when they come up, and how Walter can address these feelings in a proactive way rather than in a way that would be destructive for him and others. Walter sat in the hospital social worker's office until Loretta came to pick him up.

James's condition and this case example have some similarities to the very public Terri Schiavo case. In 1990, 27-year-old Terri Schiavo had a full cardiac arrest, was in a coma for several months and then was diagnosed to be in a *persistent vegetative state* (ABC News, 2006). A persistent vegetative state is diagnosed when there is severe brain damage, but the person may appear to be in a wakeful yet still unconscious state (The Multi-Society Task Force on PVS, 1994). The Terri Schiavo case involved a legal battle between Terri's husband and parents from 1998 to 2005 about whether or not to remove life supports and Terri's artificial feeding tube. Terri did not have a living will and was not able to communicate her wishes after 1990. Terri also was suspected of having an eating disorder before her cardiac arrest (Schiavo case highlights eating disorders, 2005).

Obviously, a difference between the case of James and Walter and that of Terri Schiavo is that James and Walter are a gay couple rather than a heterosexual couple. And, with James it is still early in his treatment, his condition could improve, he could come out of the coma and be able to respond and even complete a living will and power of attorney. In this case of James, the hospital social worker developed a plan to meet with the interdisciplinary care team that consisted of the physician, ICU charge and specialty nurses, physical therapist, speech language pathologist, dietician, and herself to discuss the situation involving James's parents and Walter. Then the hospital social worker would meet with James's family and broach the subject of involving Walter in the discussions of James's care, and how involving Walter could be beneficial for James and helpful for the rest of the family as well. The hospital social worker is aware of how James's medical condition could quickly change along with the responses and positions of the interdisciplinary care team, James's family, and Walter. These changes would lead to further assessment and planning by the hospital social worker.

Unfortunately, situations similar to the case of Mrs. Edda and James and Walter are becoming all too often and can continue to occur within the acute care setting. Acute care social workers often report that they feel torn among what is best for their patient, the needs of the agency, and the restrictions placed on them as part of service delivery. It is clear that in situations such as this, the price of this seemingly "cost-effective" coordinated care strategy far exceeded the dollar emphasis placed on it (Aronson et al., 2009; Dziegielewski & Holliman, 2001; Golden, 2011; Unger & Cunningham, 2002). Mrs. Edda, Walter and James, and their families became silent victims, making the role of the acute care social worker as broker and advocate an essential one. For hospital social workers and many other professionals working in these types of short-term health care facilities, reports of such cases are becoming increasingly more common. Today, attending physicians are pressured to seek quick or early discharges for patients. In addition, the traditional roles of couples, relationships, and partners are changing rapidly and traditional definitions are strained when new situations are taken into account (Bell, Bern-Klug, Kramer, & Saunders, 2010; Wheeler, & Dodd, 2011).

In this pressured environment, the press for time can limit the "humanistic" aspects of patient care which may include listening and supportive counseling. These important ingredients for success can be sacrificed for maintaining the more "technical" ones such as stabilizing the patient's medical condition and prescribing medications. In this type of environment, no matter how good is the medical care delivered, the patient and his or her family will always be left at a loss.

ACUTE CARE MEDICAL HOSPITALS AND SOCIAL WORK PRACTICE

The current state of practice in the health care setting mirrors the turbulence found in the general health care environment (Darnell & Lawlor, 2012; Dziegielewski & Holliman, 2001; Lens, 2002; Mizrahi & Berger, 2005). For those who work in hospitals, this setting for social work has always been considered a place of fast pace with repeated and continuous access to emotionally charged areas of practice where, when cost cutting is considered central, the behavioral, social, and environmental components of health care are not given high priority (Ferguson & Schiver, 2012; Haber, 2010).

Today, in this turbulent environment, acute care social workers are forced to face numerous situations such as declining hospital admissions, and reduced lengths of stay, along with numerous other restrictions and methods of cost containment that do not directly affect direct patient care. Struggling to resolve these issues has become necessary based on the inception of prospective payment systems, managed care plans, and other changes in the provision and funding of health care (Lens, 2002; Saleh, Freire, Morris-Dickinson, & Shannon, 2012). To complicate this situation, research has linked not receiving services to higher rates of high-risk patient relapse (Duffy & Healy, 2011; Hudson, 2001).

In most hospitals, the goal of discharge planning is the arrangement of an appropriate follow-up service plan for return to a lesser level of care. The role of the social worker does not end once the patient is discharged from the facility. Hospital social workers often report that they are being forced to discharge patients from services more quickly, and patients are being returned to the community in a weaker state of rehabilitation than ever before. Also, discharge plans need to take into account what will happen postdischarge and use the patient's own resources as much as possible.

Acute care hospital social workers also may have different expectations of what they perceive as their role in the practice environment (Blumenfield & Epstein, 2001; Duffy & Healy, 2011). These different expectations may lead to blurring and overlap of the services that these health care professionals provide. When health care administrators are forced to justify each dollar billed for services, there is little emphasis placed on the provision of what some deem to be expendable services. These services include mental health and wellness services, as well as thorough discharge planning, in the hospital setting. Unfortunately, the services that the hospital social worker provides are often placed in this category, and as a result, they have been forced to adjust to the brunt of initial dollar-line savings attempts (Judd, 2010).

As discussed earlier, just the sheer numbers of allied health care professionals who are moderately paid provide an excellent hunting ground for administrators pressured to cut costs. These administrators may see the role of the hospital social worker as adjunct to the delivery of care and may decide to cut back or replace professional social workers with nonprofessionals with less training in human behavior, advocacy, research and evaluation, and critical thinking or essential medical personnel, such as nurses, simply to cut costs. These substitute professionals do not have either the depth or breadth of training when compared with the hospital social worker, and the services provided may be reflective of a different and possibly substandard level of care. For example, a trained paraprofessional such as an

LPN or an administrative professional in hospital discharge planning may simply facilitate a placement order. Issues, such as the individual's sense of personal well-being, ability to self-care, or level of family and environmental support may not be considered. All of these issues were evident in the cases of Mrs. Edda, James and Walter, and even the highly publicized case of Terri Schiavo. Therefore, the employment of this type of paraprofessional can be cost effective but not quality care driven.

If these personal/social and environmental issues are not addressed, patients may be put at risk for harm. The patient who is discharged home to a family that does not want him or her is more at risk of abuse and neglect. A patient who has a negative view of self and a hopeless view of their condition is at greater risk for depression or even suicide. Many paraprofessionals or members of other professional disciplines can differ from social work professionals because they may not recognize the importance of cultural, and social and environmental factors as paramount to efficient and effective practice. Other examples of situations when cultural, and social and environmental factors play a part in patient care is when a patient's family objects to a blood transfusion for religious reasons, or when an elderly wife who has never driven a car is devastated that her husband is being placed in a nursing home over 50 miles away from their home, or when a Mexican family seems reluctant to talk to the treatment team because of language barriers or immigration statuses. The de-emphasis or denial of this consideration can result in the delivery of not only "cheap" but also substandard care.

FUTURE OF ACUTE CARE HOSPITAL-BASED SOCIAL WORK

Today's health care environment is filled with attempts to ensure behavioral health care, capitation, and fee for service, while decreasing the number of hospital inpatient beds. The traditional roles and tasks that are ascribed for social workers in this area, however, will continue to change. Acute medical care in the hospital setting needs to combine humanitarian objectives with efforts toward cost control and rationing of resources.

In the 1990s, hospital social work departments were moving away from traditional linear management and the result was fewer structured administrative positions (Mizrahi & Berger, 2005). There appeared to be much activity in the area of managing social work services from restructuring of departments (putting these departments under nursing or as part of nursing) to maintain independent social work departments to other various forms of decentralization. This has happened in VA hospitals, for example, where Social Work Services were originally decentralized and forced out of social work and into other service lines such as mental health or long-term care. Today, however, these departments seem to be revitalizing and social work departments do appear to be returning (Ferguson & Schriver, 2012).

In addition, several social work programs have now begun to enter areas and provide services that are not considered traditional to increase marketability. For example, a program in Oregon had hospital social workers assist as financial assistance workers by helping to facilitate the efficiency and accurate identification of Medicaid and other eligibility assistance programs. By providing this service, it was hoped that hospital revenues would be directly supplemented. In addition to developing new avenues for emphasis, each program is pressured to address the cost and benefits. As new programs and services are being considered, cost–benefit ratios are also being calculated as part of development and service evaluation. Cost–benefit information is of interest to administrators and hospitals because these programs must be viewed as viable and cost enhancing to get the initial support needed to be considered for implementation (Saleh et al., 2012).

Along with calculating the cost–benefit ratios, acute care hospital social workers can prioritize research and look at outcomes of their interventions with patients and families. This evidence can be collected through documentation that includes recording more specifically about the interventions that are done. For example, when recording that counseling was conducted on the emotional aspects of the illness the social worker would cite the specific tasks and interventions that were completed. This would include activities such as communicating with the patient and having her verbalize her concerns. It also involves planning and facilitating a meeting with the patient, her husband, and adult children where she can verbalize her concerns, and the other family members can listen and then respond to her as well (Simons, Shephard, & Munn, 2008). If the medical record does not allow this elaborate documentation, a separate note can be added that highlights data collection. If trends are to be measured, patient names can be removed to protect the privacy of the patient and the results can be aggregated and analyzed for general trends in interventions and outcomes.

Social workers in acute hospital settings are often only evaluated on their performance as discharge planners which include patient length of stay and patient satisfaction. Other measures to look at are patient quality of life and quality of care (Simons et al., 2008). The Centers for Disease Control and Prevention (2012b) provides federal guidelines for how health-related quality of life can be measured. Today acute care social workers and all social workers need to be proactive in evaluating their practice as well as their own professional development. Social workers must seek out specialized continuing education and mentoring to better their skills in acute care social work (McAlynn & McLaughlin, 2008; Simons et al., 2008). Learning more about evidence-based interventions, recording outcomes, and providing comprehensive assessments along with serving as part of a professional organization and receiving social work supervision can lead to more systematic and reflective practice as well as stronger networks for advocacy, policy making, and leadership in acute care social work in hospital settings.

SOCIAL WORK IN THE ACUTE MENTAL HEALTH SETTING

Since the inception of social work the care and treatment of the mentally ill in hospitals and institutional settings has been a prominent part of social work history. In the nineteenth century, Dorothea Dix's campaign for more humane treatment of the mentally ill resulted in the construction and improvement of mental institutions throughout the United States (Karger & Stoesz, 2010). In the middle 20th century with the enthusiasm for civil rights and community mental health reform, deinstitutionalization occurred, and many individuals who were seriously mentally ill were discharged from institutions to their communities. This was also during the advent of psychiatric medications that allowed individuals with mental illness to live more safely and enjoy a better quality of life (Holliman, 1998). However, the mental health problems experienced by these individuals were often too serious to be handled in the community and with the pressure to return for inpatient stabilization a "revolving door" phenomenon occurred. Acute inpatient stabilization became necessary repeatedly as outside of the facility the community system remained underdeveloped and ill prepared. Many of these mentally ill also became homeless or part of the prison population or criminal justice system (Auslander & Freedenthal, 2012; Barker, 2010; Corcoran & Walsh, 2011; Draine & Solomon, 2001).

When examining health care social work service provision in the inpatient acute psychiatric center, the short duration of stay cannot be overlooked. These acute services provided are clearly time limited and are generally reserved for those in crisis who are in need of immediate stabilization related to either suicidal or homicidal behavior. After stabilization, these patients are generally transferred as quickly as possible to less intensive and expensive outpatient settings (Auslander & Freedenthal, 2012; Biancosino et al., 2009; Lyons, Howard, O'Mahoney, & Lish, 1997). These can be programs that meet on weekdays where individual and group therapy are offered or outpatient behavioral health programs where the patient has appointments with a psychiatrist and therapist on a routine basis. Working in inpatient mental health can be challenging for social workers because of the rapid pace of admissions and discharges, and working with high-risk populations. Many of the patients who are there are hospitalized because they are a threat to themselves or others, and physical security is often a concern for inpatient psychiatric social workers and other staff. Psychiatric social workers in hospitals have to take responsibility for developing their own support networks and self-care activities (Badger, Royse, & Craig, 2008).

FUTURE OF ACUTE INPATIENT MENTAL HEALTH SERVICES

Behavioral health care and an emphasis on health promotion and disease-preventing activities are expected in health care delivery (Haber, 2010; Ruth & Sisco, 2012). The effect this emphasis has had on the acute care setting, as in all areas of health care, is pronounced. Managed care strategies and managed health benefit programs are now considered a part of most U.S. corporations (Coleman et al., 2005; Karger & Stoesz, 2010; Kongstvedt, 2012). The current focus on health and wellness and the decreased stigma associated with the treatment of mental health problems has clearly created and increased in service requisition (Druss, 2010; Epstein & Aldredge, 2000; National Alliance on Mental Illness, 2012). Before the onset of managed care service delivery, most mental health services were operated on a fee-for-service basis. This meant that fee negotiations occurred between the consumer and the provider. In today's health care environment, this has changed. Today, one basic concept of managed care intervention is that the managed care provider now serves as the gatekeeper, overseer, and advocate for the services the patient will be eligible to receive (Coleman et al., 2005; Kongstvedt, 2012). Because inpatient mental health treatment is considered the highest level of care and the most costly for mental health disorders, case managers for managed care organizations are reluctant to approve it.

Considering the primary purpose of managed care, which is cost-containment strategy, one learns that "shorter" acute inpatient mental health treatment has become practice reality. The actual cost of inpatient mental health treatment, by history, is known to be variable. Thus, emphasis on cost containment is expected to continue to grow, along with the increased acceptability and desire for mental health services. Health care social workers in practice over the last 30 years have witnessed unprecedented service curtails and cutbacks—which will continue to occur. Inpatient facilities are being forced to become creative in the way they deliver services. Many of these facilities are now offering intermediate-level care programs, where less expense is associated with the treatment. Oftentimes, mental health and substance abuse programs are developing service associations, and in many cases, offering interventions to address both problems under the same agency auspice.

In addition, most programs are continuing to develop more community-based systems where medication management and compliance are the primary service issues. In this managed system of health care, service delivery care within the formal acute inpatient setting will continue to decrease. This decrease will result in the direct increase of more home-based service systems, hospital care day programs, or other inpatient diversion programs. Outpatient detoxification programs and intensive outpatient substance abuse treatment programs will become more common. Considering the severe degree and unpredictability of certain mental health problems, it is not believed that acute psychiatric services will ever stop completely; however, services of this nature are sure to be more tightly controlled and severely curtailed in the future.

SOCIAL WORK IN THE NEPHROLOGY SETTING

Kidney dialysis (artificial kidney treatment) and organ transplant are two medical treatments designed to help individuals who suffer from permanent kidney failure. In some cases, dialysis may also be used for acute kidney failure. Basically, the kidneys are bean-shaped organs that provide three primary functions necessary for life: (a) to help remove waste; (b) to filter the blood; and (c) to help regulate blood pressure (National Kidney Foundation, 2012). When neither of these organs is capable of working adequately, severe and often fatal illness may result.

Individuals require kidney dialysis when they develop end-stage renal disease (ESRD) where about 85% to 90% of the normal kidney function is lost. Others, who are considered good candidates, may elect to have a kidney transplant where the goal is to replace current kidney function with another human kidney that can improve the overall quality of life for the patient (National Kidney Foundation, 2012). However, finding a family member who is a match or enduring the transplant waiting list is sometimes tedious and difficult. Generally, kidney dialysis services are offered in a hospital, in a dialysis unit or clinic that is not part of the hospital, or at home.

There are two types of dialysis: hemodialysis and *peritoneal dialysis.* In hemodialysis, where the patient's blood is pumped through an artificial kidney machine, it can be completed either in the acute care setting or at home. Oftentimes, treatments are done three times a week and last 3 to 4 hours. This procedure can be given at home; however, it is essential that a family member or friend is standing by to assist. In peritoneal dialysis, a solution called dialysate flows from a bag into the peritoneum, and waste products and excess fluids pass from the blood into this solution. The used solution is later removed from the body by gravity or machine. Oftentimes, when using the machine, this procedure can be done at night by connecting the tube to the machine before going to bed and disconnecting it in the morning. If it is done by gravity, the patient usually changes the bag solution several times throughout the day (National Kidney Foundation, 2012).

The process of dialysis is an intensive, tedious, and time-consuming one, and those on dialysis must increase their protein intake while limiting fluids and salt from their diets. For those with end-stage renal disease, the kidneys cannot get rid of waste products or fluids on their own so adhering to this diet is critical (National Kidney Foundation, 2012). The resulting health care intervention for the nephrology patient is generally considered a team effort. Interdisciplinary team members often include the *nephrologist* (physician), transplant surgeon, nephrology nurse, renal nutritionist, patient care technicians, financial counselors or billing personnel, donor coordinators (when waiting for a transplant), clinical transport coordinator (link for transportation to treatments), and the nephrology social worker. The nephrology social worker is considered an essential and service-reimbursable part of this health care delivery team (Browne, 2012a; Rocha, 2010). Because these treatments are expensive and can be draining on the social and emotional well-being of the patient and their family, the social worker is expected to help provide direct counseling and referral to help patients and their family members cope. The rates of depression are higher for patients on dialysis than those in the general population, and because the dialysis and diet regimen for end-stage renal disease patients is so strict, noncompliance is common (Blades, 2010). Social workers are also designated to help the patient develop treatment plans and sources of emotional support to improve quality of life. In addition, the nephrology social worker must be aware of what services are available to the patient within the federal, state, and community agencies and help link the patient to them whenever necessary (Dobrof, Dolinko, Lichtiger, Uribarri, & Epstein, 2001). Sledge et al. (2011) developed a symptom-targeted intervention for patients on dialysis which is implemented by nephrology social workers, and at this point the outcomes of this social work intervention are promising.

Dialysis treatment was approved for Medicare reimbursement with the passage of Public Law 92603 (Sec. 2991) in 1972. In these earlier years, there was little coordination of service, and most dialysis programs were run autonomously with no coordination from the Medicare system. In 1978, however, this changed, and the ESRD network was formed (Forum of ESRD Networks, 2012). This body was to provide an oversight system to unite and regulate the care given by dialysis providers. The goal of the ESRD networks is to (a) provide immediate access to treatment; (b) treat patients with quality medical care standards of practice; and (c) help individuals to maintain a quality of life that enables them to remain functioning members of the community (Forum of ESRD, 2012). In today's managed care environment, because these expensive treatment services, including those provided directly by the social worker, remain Medicare reimbursable, coordination and control to minimize excess waste and expenditures are considered essential.

To help maintain quality of life, the role of the social worker is considered integral. The functions of the nephrology social worker can include psychosocial evaluations (assessment for the treatment plan), casework (counseling and supportive intervention), group work (education and self-help); information and referral, facilitation of community referrals, team planning and coordination, patient and family education, as well as advocacy for patients on their behalf within the setting or beyond that with local state and federal agencies (UNC Kidney Center, 2012). In addition, with the numerous service cutbacks and cost-effectiveness strategies, many nephrology social workers are now being required to expand their duties. Many are being asked to serve as financial counselors to ensure that the patient and the service agency will receive adequate reimbursement for services needed. These services can involve assisting patients to apply for Medicare disability—to seeking outside insurance carriers to cover additional services not directly covered under Medicare guidelines (medicines, eye glasses, transportation, etc.).

COMPLETION OF THE PSYCHOSOCIAL ASSESSMENT

For the nephrology social worker in today's managed care environment, the completion of the outcomes-based psychosocial assessment can be the most difficult and time-consuming task that must be faced. However, its completion is essential to the present and future care that the nephrology patient will receive. When tasked with the completion of an outcomes-based psychosocial assessment, the social worker should first ask him- or herself the following questions: Why am I gathering this information (be clear about the purpose)? What will this psychosocial assessment tell me about the patient? How will I best use this information in the establishment of specific outcome-based objectives that will help my patient once collected? In gathering information, key areas to be noted include pertinent family history, family history of illness, important people and significant others in the patient's life, impact of the illness, physical functioning, occupational functioning, and emotional factors that are related to functioning level. In addition, it is important for nephrology social workers to assess social factors related to whether a person could have a kidney transplant, social support, adherence to medications and diet regimen, and the person's substance use and mental health history. See Table 9.2 for an outline that lists factors to be considered in the development of an outcomes-based assessment.

Table 9.2 Nephrology Outcomes-Based Psychosocial Assessment

Assessment category and information to be gathered:	
Family of origin, nuclear family, and other information	
Family Information	List and briefly describe the following: • Incidence of family illness • Myths, attitudes, beliefs about condition • Myths, values, and beliefs about health care system • Previous education about the illness • Religious, ethnic, cultural beliefs about condition • Coping strategy for dealing with illness • History of alcohol or other substance abuse • History of previous psychiatric problems
	Outcome indicators developed should include • Recommendations for specific education and prevention services needed • Recommendations for "ethnic sensitive" practice

(continued)

Table 9.2 (*continued*)

Family presence and level of involvement	List and briefly describe the following: • All family members active within the family system. • Dependence and interdependence patterns of involvement. • Family members viewed as helpful to the patient • Family members viewed as essential to patient functioning • Family members the patient cares the most about
	Outcome indicators developed should include • Identify available family supports • If limited support, make concrete recommendations on how to increase family support network

Level of physical functioning

List and briefly describe the following:
• Pre-dialysis level of functioning
• What is different now in level of functioning
• Present level of functioning
• patient's perception of long-term effects and illness complications
• What does patient want to achieve?

Outcome indicators developed should include
• Establish a baseline level of functioning
• Identify return to a desirable level of functioning
• Educate about advanced directives
• Educate regarding realistic outcomes of disease

Level of social functioning

List and briefly describe the following:
• Pre-dialysis level of social functioning (church, school, clubs, friends, hobbies, etc.)
• Present level of social functioning (what can and cannot be done?)
• Long-term effects of the illness on social functioning

Outcome indicators developed should include
• Establish a baseline of social functioning
• Determine a desirable level of functioning
• Determine ways to increase patient involvement

Level of emotional functioning

List and briefly describe the following:
• Pre-dialysis level of functioning
• Previous coping skills (acceptance, understanding)
• Level of self-esteem and contentment
• Unresolved grief and loss issues
• Ability to appropriately express feelings
• Suicidal ideation and intent
• Spirituality beliefs
• Identify problems with intimacy, sexuality, sensuality, body image, etc.
• Long-term effects of the illness on emotional functioning

Outcome indicators developed should include
• Establish a baseline for emotional functioning
• Identify emotional issues that need to be addressed
• Educate and assist in development of appropriate coping skills as needed

(*continued*)

Table 9.2 Nephrology Outcomes-Based Psychosocial Assessment (*continued*)

Occupational level of functioning

List and briefly describe the following:
• Pre-dialysis level of functioning
• Employment history
• Current employment status
• Present level of occupational functioning
  • As perceived by patient
  • As perceived by family members
  • As perceived by health care team
• Understanding of long-term effects of illness
• Future employment expectation

Outcome indicators developed should include
• Establish a baseline level of functioning
• Factors that will help patient return to a satisfactory level of functioning
• Outline future career considerations for enhanced functioning (education, change of job area, etc.)

Other considerations

Financial
• Identify present financial situation
• List insurance and income availability

Transportation issues
• Identify transportation barriers or service limitations

CHAPTER SUMMARY AND FUTURE DIRECTIONS

The role of the health care social worker in the acute care setting remains essential. Regardless of the acute care setting, health care social workers are integral in providing assistance with treatment plans and compliance issues; assisting patients and families with discharge planning and referral; providing counseling and support for patients and significant others in the areas of health, wellness, mental health, bereavement, and so on; assisting patients and their families to make ethical and morally difficult decisions that can affect health and mental health; educating patients, their families, and significant others to psychosocial issues and adjusting to illness; assisting in resolving behavioral problems; assisting in identifying and obtaining entitlement benefits; securing nonmedical benefits; assisting with risk management and quality assurance activities; and lastly, advocating for enhanced and continued services to ensure continued patient well-being. In working with clinical social workers in the acute care setting, the practice issue that seems to cause the most concern can most simply be stated as: The pressure remains great to prove (with outcomes-based interventions) that more can be done with less and that all this can be accomplished in the least restrictive environment using the most time-limited strategy possible (Duffy & Healy, 2011; Ferguson & Schriver, 2012). The role of the health care social worker with the emphasis on the total person will continue to facilitate the continuity of care whether it is in the acute care inpatient setting or facilitating a smooth transition back into the community.

Glossary

Acute care medical hospitals   The provision of services that include problems related to completion of daily activities; environmental problems; patient and family adverse reactions or dysfunctional adjustment to illness and changes in functional status; problems related to physical, sexual, and emotional maltreatment; vocational and educational problems; legal problems; and so on. Major functions include psychosocial assessment, high-risk case finding and screening, preadmission planning, discharge planning, psychosocial counseling, financial counseling, health education, postdischarge follow-up, consultation, outpatient continuity of care, patient and family conferences, patient and family advocacy, and so on.

Acute care nephrology settings   Methods and services provided to improve the quality and appropriateness of psychosocial services for patients with end-stage renal disease. Major services provided include psychosocial evaluations, casework, group work, information and referral, facilitation of community resources, team care planning and collaboration, advocacy for patients, and family education.

Acute care psychiatric facilities   Methods and services provided to patients and their families to ensure that a patient's illness, recovery, and safe transition from one care setting to another is considered. Psychosocial factors are highlighted that include living arrangements, developmental history, economic, cultural, religious, educational, and vocational background that may impinge on the understanding, treatment, and relapse prevention of the psychiatric disorder. Functions and services provided include intake or admission evaluation, psychosocial assessment and treatment planning, high social risk case finding, education and advocacy, individual, group, family treatment and counseling, crisis intervention, consultation, expert testimony, discharge and after-care planning, and so on.

Acute care setting   A restrictive inpatient setting that is generally of a short time-limited nature.

Advance directive   Legal documents that allow a person to convey his or her decisions about end-of-life care such as the use dialysis, ventilators, feeding tubes, and other interventions and treatments prior to the time they meet the requirements for these treatments. Advance directives are completed when a person is of sound mind and are most often utilized when the person cannot speak or make these decisions for them. Living wills and the durable power of attorney (especially the health care power of attorney) are advance directives.

Artificial kidney   A device that removes waste products and excess fluids from the human body when the kidneys are unable to do so.

Caregivers   Individuals who assist family members to stay in the least restrictive environment possible.

Coma   A deep state of unconsciousness where a person is alive, but unable to respond to their environment. A coma rarely lasts more than 2 to 4 weeks.

Dialysate   A solution used in dialysis to remove excess fluids and waste products from the blood.

Dialysis   Process of maintaining the chemical balance of the blood when an individual's kidneys are not able to do so.

Durable power of attorney   An advance directive and legal document completed when a person is of sound mind that designates an agent or principal person to handle his or her affairs and make decisions if he or she is unable to. The durable power of attorney includes the health care power of attorney, who is someone designated to make health care treatment decisions for a person if they are incapacitated, and the durable power of attorney for property and finances, who can make financial decisions and manage property for the person in these incidences. The health care power of attorney and property and finances power of attorney can be the same person or different people. This decision is up to the person completing this advance directive.

End-stage renal disease   (ESRD) The stage at which permanent kidney failure has occurred, and dialysis or a kidney transplant is needed to maintain life.

Hemodialysis   A form of dialysis using an artificial kidney machine to remove fluids and waste products from the bloodstream.

Living will   An advance directive and legal document that a person completes when they are of sound mind that provides specific instructions about the person's wishes for end-of-life treatments such as dialysis, feeding tubes, and artificial breathing machines.

Medicaid   A federal–state supported program that pays for medical services for those who meet certain means-tested criteria.

Medicare   Medical insurance provided by the federal government under the Social Security Act.

Nephrologist   A physician who specializes in dealing with patients who suffer from kidney diseases.

Peritoneal dialysis   A form of dialysis that uses the patient's abdominal cavity or peritoneum for dialysis treatment.

Persistent vegetative state   An ongoing state of severely impaired consciousness where severe brain damage is present, but the person may appear to be awake from for periods of time.

Questions for Further Study

1. Do you believe that the role of the hospital social worker will continue to change? If so, what future changes do you anticipate happening?

2. How can a cost–benefit ratio be computed for social workers in the acute care setting? How can revenue be produced in acute care settings (medical, mental health, and nephrology) by social workers?

3. Do you believe that services presently offered to nephrology dialysis patients will increase or decrease in the future? Why?

4. How can outcome studies of social work be implemented in acute care settings (medical, mental health, and nephrology)? What research questions would you begin your outcome studies with?

Websites

Centers for Disease Control and Prevention (CDC)
Online directory of information and tools for health promotion, disease prevention, injury and disability, and preparedness for new health threats.
www.cdc.gov

Centers for Disease Control and Prevention
Guidelines for measuring health-related quality of life.
www.cdc.gov/hrqol/wellbeing.htm#/four

Health Resources and Services Administration (HRSA)
HRSA directs national health programs for vulnerable and in-need populations.
www.hrsa.gov/index.html

Med Help International
Helping those in need find qualified medical information and support for patients.
www.medhlp.netusa.net

Medline Plus
The National Institutes of Health's website produced by the National Library of Medicine. This website provides information on health treatments, drugs, and supplements as well as health and medical definitions, videos, and illustrations.
www.nlm.nih.gov/medlineplus

National Alliance on Mental Illness (NAMI)
NAMI is the largest grassroots mental health organization. NAMI advocates for access to services and treatment, supports research, and is committed to fighting stigma and building communities of hope.
www.nami.org

National Cancer Institute (NCI)
The NCI is the federal government's principal agency for cancer research and training.
www.nci.nih.gov

National Institutes of Health (NIH)
The NIH website provides material on consumer health, federal grants and institutes, and the latest science and health research findings and conclusions.
www.nih.gov

National Kidney Foundation (NKF)
A major voluntary nonprofit organization dedicated to preventing kidney disease, improving the well-being of those with kidney disease and increasing the availability of organs for transplantation.
www.kidney.org

National Registry of Evidenced-Based Programs & Practices (NREPP)
A searchable registry of more than 230 intervention programs for mental health and substance abuse prevention and treatment.
www.nrepp.samhsa.gov

UNC Kidney Center
Website describes nephrology and social work services in this setting
www.unckidneycenter.org/hcprofessionals/nephsocialworkers.
html#guidelines

The American Medical Association (AMA)
The AMA promotes the art and science of medicine and the betterment of public health.
www.ama-assn.org

Today's Health Care Social Worker

Name: Michele Saunders, LCSW
List State of Practice: Florida
Title of Current Position: Vice President, Community Relations
                                 Licensed Clinical Social Worker

Duties in a Typical Day:
I represent an acute care facility where I am involved with community organizing and planning for the improvement of the service system for people with mental illnesses and/or substance use disorders. This involves strategic planning meetings with other providers, key stakeholders, and funders of services. I am also involved with program development for our organization, exploring new service opportunities to help our clientele and writing business plans or grants for funding.

I provide education through workshops, resource fairs, and community forums to the community about mental illnesses, the efficacy of treatment and the need for the community to support these programs. I do a variety of training around mental illness issues. I also participate in legislative advocacy to impact improving policies and financial appropriations to people with mental illnesses and/or substance use disorders.

1. **What do you like most about your current position?**
    I enjoy being involved with so many of the other community providers and stakeholders for system change and improvements. I enjoy working on the macrolevel of social work to impact policy decisions. I find it very rewarding to help bring around changes and improvements that will help many people. I also enjoy the advocacy and education components.

2. **What do you like least?**
    Sometimes the politics involved with policy changes and system improvement can create barriers that slow down progress. Also, I have learned that not everyone involved plays fairly and there are many different (and sometimes opposing) agendas to deal with.

3. **What "words of wisdom" do you have for the new health care social worker who is considering working in a similar position?**
    I would suggest they have good communication skills, learn good negotiation skills, get to know their community and its needs and be able to build good relationships and sustain good relationships across the board. Have lots of energy and passion

(*continued*)

Today's Health Care Social Worker (*continued*)

and be optimistic, yet realistic. Know how to separate out the issues from what is agency based and don't allow the issues to become personal.

4. **What is your favorite health care social worker story?**
My favorite health care social worker story related to my current position is when I was able to convene a group of providers, family members, and law enforcement officers to develop an crisis response model (based on one in Memphis, TN) called Crisis Intervention Team (CIT). Through my facilitation and direction, the group developed an effective police-based crisis response system in which specially trained officers are diverting people with mental illnesses and/or substance use disorders into treatment and away from jail when they are in crisis. It is very rewarding to see all groups working together for the betterment of the consumer, their family, and the community as a whole.

Today's Health Care Social Worker

Name: Kenna TrenKamp
List State of Practice: Georgia
Professional Licensure: Licensed Master Social Worker

1. **The chapter states that the social workers tasks includes *psychosocial evaluations, casework, counseling, supportive intervention, group work (education and self-help), information and referral, facilitation of community resources, team planning and coordination, patient and family education, financial counseling, connecting patient with resources, advocacy.* Do you do anything that is not on the list? Or, is there something on the list that you do not do? Do you want to elaborate about anything on this list?**
I don't do any formal psychosocial evaluations, but I know that in Texas they are mandated to do them. I think each state dictates what the social worker is required to do, and at this time, Georgia doesn't require us to do them. I don't provide much counseling except for crisis counseling (i.e., when people are arrested, about to get kicked out of their home, etc.). One of our nurses does all of the educational requirements that GA has set for dialysis patients, so I don't provide much of

(*continued*)

(continued)

that either. I do complete the KDQOL, which is a yearly survey emphasizing positive decision making and self-help strategies.

I also work with community resources to get patient food supplies or have ramps built to facilitate independence. I generally am called upon to do a variety of supportive services. I have also helped people create budgets for them to be able to meet their insurance co-pays, so that their medication costs will go down. Today, however, a lot of the transplant hospitals have social workers that help patients with financial planning for obtaining the post-transplant medications and other medical needs. We also work closely as a team and have licensed meetings where the RNs, I, and the dietician all meet to discuss patient needs and care support changes that need to take place. I schedule transportation and oversee the creation of the care plans, which could be considered a type of psychosocial evaluation. It is a state requirement that each *stable* patient (i.e., haven't been in the hospital more than 10 days, etc.) has to have a plan every 3 months. The *unstable* patients get one every month until they are no longer unstable. It provides information about transplantation (interested or not), living situation, any mental health problems, and other psychosocial factors. It is a modified psychosocial evaluation.

2. **As a nephrology social worker, what are your duties on a typical day?**
   A typical day is scheduling Medicaid transportation, getting appointments made for specialty doctors, completing prior authorizations for procedures, working on transient paperwork when patients want to go out of town, completing care plans, and talking with all of the patients to determine whether or not there are any new needs to be addressed.
   A. **What do you like the most about nephrology social work?**
      The patients become like family, and you really learn to care about them.
   B. **What do you like the least about nephrology social work?**
      Transportation is a real need for this group and scheduling transportation daily—it's a headache.

3. **What "words of wisdom" do you have for new social workers who are considering taking a position in nephrology social work?**
   Go into it with an open mind. At first, these patients may not seem receptive to help and appear "rough around the edges" and difficult to work with. When you feel frustrated try to think

(continued)

Today's Health Care Social Worker (*continued*)

of what it is like for them as they spend anywhere from 2 to 4.5 hours in a chair at a minimum 3 days a week and can't do anything about it. Of course, they are going to have bad days sometimes. When they need to be left alone give them space. Always try, however, to check on them and let them know that you are there and willing to help. Just make yourself visible to them—it goes further than you know.

4. **What is your favorite story about your work as a nephrology social worker?**
   One of our patients was transplanted about 3 months after I started. She was so humble and so sweet. It was so nice to see someone try and take charge of her situation despite the fact that she was dealing with ESRD. She always had positive things to say and was always checking on the other patients. She made a difference in the lives of the other patients and made me really think about what they go through on a day-to-day basis.

CHAPTER 10

Restorative Health Care: Long-Term and Home Care

George A. Jacinto
and Sophia F. Dziegielewski

This chapter reviews the basic concepts related to the delivery of social work services and the many roles of the social worker in traditional and nontraditional long-term care (LTC) settings such as the LTC facility and home care settings. Whether we call patients *clients*, or *consumers*, the efforts of the social worker generally involve assisting patients/clients/consumers (hereafter referred to as patients) and their families in these transitional restorative settings. According to the National Association of Social Workers (NASW, 2003a), there has been significant changes in the way LTC services are provided, and these services can cross a spectrum of care. These services and programs now cross institutional and noninstitutional modalities. In the LTC setting and in home care, many of the same concerns are noted, and although this chapter will focus mainly on the needs of older adults in these settings, other population such as children, adolescents, and persons with disabilities may also receive services.

This chapter will discuss the important role of health care social workers, stressing the importance of being knowledgeable of chronic conditions, by knowing the signs and symptoms and the expected progression of various diseases in regard to the population served. The issues related to providing services in these settings and the availability of affordable health care insurance will also be addressed. The need for system revision is stressed based on the recent passing of the Patient Protection and Affordable Care Act (ACA) (U.S. Department of Health and Human Services, 2012). For LTC and especially home care, increased utilization of these services, while enhancing affordability, will also need to increase.

In LTC, similar to other areas of health care, balancing quality of care while utilizing best practices that are effective and cost efficient will continue to be the expectation for standard practice. The current services provided in these settings will be presented along with the historical context for funding for LTC facilities and home care. The implications of the current health care debate in regard to LTC and home care along with issues related to the transition from LTC to home care will be outlined. With a shortage of professional social workers in this area (NASW, 2008b), a future plan for attracting new social workers to this area and providing comprehensive health care services is recommended.

LONG-TERM TRANSITIONAL CARE

It is clear in today's environment that there are numerous fields of practice for health care social workers. Clinical health care practice in long-term residential care and rehabilitative home care cannot be simply defined as it refers to a wide range of clinical settings and services that can include rehabilitative efforts from maintenance to coordinated care. Care in these settings can include transitions from hospitals to skilled facilities such as nursing homes or direct home care supported by community-based services such as home health care and other rehabilitative services. Ensuring continuity of care from one transitional setting to another will also need to change accordingly as the patient's condition and situation also changes (Diwan, Balaswamy, & Lee, 2012). The use of transitional care options continues to gain in popularity especially if hospital or acute or short-term costs can be defrayed by a less-expensive residential option such as LTC or home care. Transitional facilities such as LTC and community-based home care can help to save money for hospitals by reducing acute care services such as those provided in the emergency department.

This is especially important in cost reduction as historically the emergency room is often the place where increasing numbers of individuals who are homeless, poor, and uninsured often receive care. What complicates this further is that many of the individuals receiving emergency department care lack the means or ability to adhere to medical advice making their health conditions worse (Ross & Mirowsky, 2000). Respite or LTC programs can also assist with diversion from hospital admissions or decrease hospital stay by offering individuals with medical problems alternative options to inpatient acute care (Respite Conference Notes, 2000). Yet, this type of patchwork continuum requires a level of comprehensive and interrelated care that requires collaboration from an interdisciplinary perspective (Rivers, McCleary, & Glover, 2000).

This intensive coordination can leave patients with unmet needs and increased controversy between local, state, and federal government regarding who bears the responsibility for funding these services (Feder, Komisar, & Niefeld, 2000). Further, the lack of adequate and timely health care, lack of available drugs, lack of health professionals, and unaffordable user fees can have a negative impact on disease outcomes. These circumstances can escalate the problems for those who require these types of services (Amoah et al., 2000; Bassili, Omar, & Tognoni, 2001; Bjork, 2001). Without resources for medical or social services, a remediable health problem can become a permanent condition.

In 1995, Poole stated several guiding principles for transitional care that still remain essential such as (a) services should be provided in the least restrictive environment possible; (b) services should help and support patients in autonomous decision making; and (c) services should maximize a patient's optimal level of physical, social, and psychological function and subsequent well-being. These services can be delivered in numerous settings such as rehabilitative hospitals and clinics, nursing homes, intermediate care facilities, and supervised boarding homes as well as services provided in home care such as home health care agencies, hospices, hospital home care units, and so on.

Just as the settings in this area are variable, so are the services that these health care social workers provide. The Murray Alzheimer Research and Education Program (2007) outlined the importance of staff participation in this process, outlining the need for providers to create a welcoming environment, act as a resource for the family, and facilitate communication about the resident with all care providers including those in the facility. There also needs to be development of a culture that supports patient *re-enablement* where from this perspective the patient viewed as a person with abilities that is empowered to regain abilities lost as a result of illness or injury (NursingTimes.net. [Practice Comment], 2012).

THE SKILLED LTC FACILITY

As part of the Social Security Act, Section (1819, 42.U.S.C. 13951-3), a *skilled nursing facility* (SNF) is an institution that primarily provides skilled nursing care and related services for residents and is not primarily for the care and treatment of mental diseases.

Silverstone (1981) defined LTC as "one or more services provided on a sustained basis to enable individuals whose functional capacities are chronically impaired to be maintained at their maximum levels of health and well-being" (p. 85). The U.S. Department of Health and Human Services (2006) defined LTC similarly, stressing the need for the services to help those with chronic health problems that limit their ability to perform everyday activities. Providing a full array of services, some facilities offer short-term services where patients require extra care and rehabilitation that do not need to be provided in an inpatient hospital setting. This could occur after an accident or surgery allowing time for the patient to regain their health and independence. It could also be utilized for patients where the family member in home care needs a personal time that allows the primary caregiver to get rest and take care of his/her own needs without having to worry about the care of the loved one.

Other facilities offer LTC services that allow the patient who can no longer be cared for at home access to a physician, nurse, and supportive care that would not be available or extensive enough in the home setting. For all these facilities, they are quick to advertise the specialized rehabilitation services they offer as well as the complex continuous 7 days a week and 24-hour service provision. The term often advertised to represent supportive services is "personal support services." These services are provided by *professional support workers* who are available to assist with increasing quality of life by providing all the supportive care a patient needs, such as assistance with mobility, personal hygiene and care, and providing emotional support and physical satisfaction. The need for these supportive services is so strong that it is clear that what is needed by the patients in these 24-hour care facilities goes beyond direct rehabilitation and nursing care. According to the Centers for Disease Control and Prevention (CDC, 2012a), there are 16,100 nursing homes in the United States, with 1.7 million beds that have an occupancy rate of 86% (CDC, 2012c).

The sheer utility of placement in an LTC facility is the provision of 24-hour care and support. The majority of the individuals served in these facilities will be older adults and, therefore, will provide the bulk of the discussion in this chapter. This emphasis is clear as due to the sheer numbers of older adults, many of these facilities have decided to become specialists in geriatric care and focus their care provision services in this area (Temkin, 2009). This makes it essential to be aware of the services a facility provides, and the majority of patient needs will most likely determine the level of services provided. Other populations served can also include persons with disabilities and children with serious medical illnesses who require 24-hour care.

For people with a disability, being placed in an LTC facility meets the standard of care and provides a safe physical care environment. Temkin (2009), however, identifies that when serving this population, the following areas are in need of improvement. First is looking at possible deficiencies with the direct care staff and professional support providers who provide basic services. These staff members may lack knowledge of disabilities or may be deficient in the specific skills needed when working with persons with a disability. This lack of awareness and experience may limit the services available to persons with disabilities, and the inexperienced care provider may not know what is missing or whom to ask.

The second concern relates directly to the age of the person with a disability. He or she may be the youngest person in the facility, and when services are geared toward the older adult for all younger patients, including those with disabilities, the social milieu may fall short. Third is the social isolation that can result related to the patients in the facility that may not understand what the person is experiencing, or special attention to important social connection needs may be ignored. Finally, the facility may be limited in direct services and may fall short of what is actually needed, as in the area of persons with disabilities, since although no best practices have been clearly defined yet, there is a body of knowledge developing that allows facility services to become specialists in caring for both the young person with a disability and older adults (Temkin, 2009).

For children with chronic illness who requires 24-hour care, most professionals would agree that traditional LTC facilities can fall short as placement options for a variety of reasons. Whether in children or adults, chronic physical conditions can place extreme psychological and social burdens on the family system. When the needs of the child are so pronounced that parents and other family members cannot handle the child in the home setting or group home, and foster care options are not available, seeking the need of a 24-hour facility could be a possibility. Placement of these children in these types of facilities can be problematic for many reasons. First, careful assessment is needed as the medical, behavioral, and psychosocial needs of the patient need to be comprehensively identified. Similar to the young persons with a disability, staff may not be trained to recognize these needs and the young person may be the youngest person in the facility. Again when services are geared toward the older adult rather than the younger patient, the social milieu will be deficient. School and other services this population group needs are different from the services needed by older patients. Finally, the social isolation that can result as he or she may be the only person of that age in the entire facility.

One disturbing trend that seems to be occurring is the placement of children in these LTC facilities where foster homes are not available to meet the needs of these children. This is particularly concerning as these facilities are not equipped to deal with such a young population, and in these facilities, they may be denied such basic rights as going to school and receiving other essential services that constitute their own rights as human beings (Elder, 2012).

Knowledge of Chronic Conditions

For older adults, as well as persons with disabilities, the fear of continued activity loss is often of great concern. Because many of the patients initially placed in these 24-hour care facilities may suffer from chronic conditions, the probability of the condition getting better is unlikely. This may be further complicated by family members and other interdisciplinary team members telling the patient that the condition will get better rather than helping the individual develop ways to cope with the existing condition and empower him or her to maximize existing skills. Health care social workers working in the LTC need to be knowledgeable of these chronic conditions, knowing the signs and symptoms and the expected progression of various diseases. They also need to be keenly aware that when patients served in this facility are not older adults, the services that are needed will need to be customized to the patient.

One area in need of further research is that of the LTC needs of older adults who are also persons with a disability. The development of a disability profile that outlines the services required by this population is needed to address the changing preferences of family members who may have a say in the care the person receives (Temkin, 2009). Staff will also need to be trained to address these unique needs with the caveat that not "one size of care" will fit all.

Table 10.1 Definition of Services in the Long-Term Care Setting

Long-term care health care social worker services	A method of providing services of assessment, treatment, rehabilitation, supportive care, and prevention of increased disability of people with chronic physical, emotional, or developmental impairments. These areas of practice are generally multidisciplinary and involve a number of intuitional and noninstitutional modalities. Facilities can include general hospitals, chronic disease hospitals, nursing homes (skilled nursing facilities and intermediate care facilities), rehabilitation centers, hospices, residential centers for the developmentally disabled, day care programs, home health care programs, and so on.

Source: Definition taken from NASW standards for the practice of *NASW Standards for Social Work Services in Long-Term Care Facilities* (2003a).

Further, there is considerable evidence to support the importance of the involvement and support shown to patients by family members in creating a general sense of well-being and maintaining a home-like atmosphere. A definition of the methods and roles of the health care social worker in the long-term setting is provided in Table 10.1. However, the role of the health care social worker in educating patients and family members to cope with and understand changes that will occur cannot be underestimated. A comprehensive assessment is needed that takes into account the age of the patients, the medical condition, and family and supportive factors important to the patient.

Accreditation in Skilled Nursing Facilities

In accordance with legislation, all LTC facilities need to be licensed and operate under contract with the accrediting bodies that govern the services they provide. The Joint Commission (TJC) accredits LTC facilities and assesses nursing homes based on four criteria: patient care, communication, on-site visits and interviews, and documentation. Nursing homes are eligible for accreditation if they meet the state licensing requirements for the amount of patient beds. The facility must also be accredited to accept reimbursement from Medicare and Medicaid. The mission of TJC is "to continuously improve health care for the public, in collaboration with stakeholders, by evaluating health care organizations and inspiring them to excel in providing safe and effective care of the highest quality and value" (The Joint Commission, 2012). Although the services can vary at each level of care identified, in the provision of LTC, resident quality of life must be maintained.

The SNF provides important services that could not be given at home such as providing oversight and monitoring of medicines given orally or when provided by injection; professional services such as facilitating tube feeding; and wound care and other professional nursing services that cannot be delivered without the oversight or direct application of a trained professional. Ancillary services also include physical, occupational, and speech therapy services. Personal care services can include helping patients with their activities of daily living (ADL) such as walking, bathing, dressing, and eating. Overall the skilled facility can serve in the provision of residential services that result in increased safety through assistance and supervision. It also assists by providing direct access to physician visits where the provider will visit the facility. All professionals in the facility are accessible and able to respond directly to the need for special diets and restorative and rehabilitative procedures.

To ensure that each resident receives the benefit of enhancement and maintenance of the quality of life, a comprehensive quality assessment is completed on each individual on admission. All certified nursing homes under Medicare and Medicaid guidelines must receive a comprehensive assessment within the first 14 days of admission (Diwan et al., 2012). This admission to the facility involves a comprehensive, accurate, standardized, reproducible assessment of the resident's functional capacity. As specified, the standardized minimum data set (MDS) version 2.0 (2000), form 1721ORNH will need to be completed on all residents within the 14-day time frame.

The assessor must represent a coordinated effort on the part of all health professionals involved in the resident's care, and to insure accuracy, the resident must have had periods of interaction with the assessor(s) within the last 7 day as stated in the MDS version 2.0. This is an extensive evaluation that takes into account both subjective and objective information in regard to cognitive patterns, mood and behavior patterns, and psychological well-being. Changes are noted every 3 months thereafter. This makes the evaluator's capacity to interpret, assess, and understand the residents individualized needs critical. Based on differences between differing assumptions and commitments to resident care, keeping the assessment as objective as possible is important.

All professionals directly involved in the resident's care are encouraged to participate. This means that the resident's physician not only needs to participate in the medical care of the patient, but also needs to stay active in the continuum of care identifying resident's needs. Conversely, Robinson, Barry, Resnick, Bergen, and Stratos (2001) warn that for physicians, this can be a problem because many physicians currently in practice were not exposed to specific topics in geriatric medicine in medical school or during residency training. Therefore, some professionals are concerned that there may not be a lot of interest leading to creative initiatives on the part of these physicians.

In an attempt to measure physician's confidence and interest in geriatric topics and assessment, Robinson et al. (2001) surveyed 242 North Carolina community physicians. As a result, only 53% of the physicians in practice claimed that at least half of their caseload was constituted with seniors, although interest in learning more about this population was high. According to the study results, the highest area of interest was in learning more about dementia, urinary incontinence, and completing functional assessments. What is interesting about this study is that the senior physicians in practice showed a higher confidence in geriatric care, in comparison to recent graduates, but less interest in learning more about geriatric topics. To assist physicians to be better prepared to work with geriatric population, Robinson et al. (2001) discussed the need for continued efforts to improve geriatric education in medical school and residency.

Addressing Health and Mental Health Problems

In the SNF, one topic of concern for most professionals is how to best address health conditions such as stroke and psychiatric mental health problems. Medical conditions such as stroke are considered one of the leading causes for the transfer of older patients to nursing homes (Heart and Stroke Foundation, 2011). A study by Stolee, Hillier, Webster, and O'Callaghan (2006) warned that the transition from acute care facilities to LTC facilities is crucial for making sure that coordinated care is provided consistently, and in too many cases, they are found to be lacking.

In the area of mental health, Snowdon (2001) reported the prevalence of residents with psychiatric disorders in skilled nursing homes at 80% to 91%. The author referred to clinical data that suggested that the most common mental health condition was dementia at approximately 80%, with 25% to 50% of residents with dementia also displaying psychotic symptoms. Similarly, significant depressive symptoms were reported in 30% to 50% of nursing home patients who could be assessed, and major depression was found in 6% to 25% of those who were not cognitively impaired (Snowdon, 2001). However, Snowdon (2001) warned that this attribution for the prevalence could be inadequate because of problems in the assessing process, and once admitted to a nursing home, there was no encouragement to recognize or treat the patient's psychiatric problems.

Problems with how to best assess and treat residents who suffer from mental disorders in the LTC facility is not a problem unique to the United States. For example, the results from a survey of Canadian nursing homes suggested that administrators reported that there were no psychiatrists available for consultation in the nursing home setting. In addition, 36.8% reported that residents received no psychiatric care, and 88.2% of responders who needed psychiatric care were likely to get less than an estimated 5 hours per month (Meeks, Jones, Tikhtman, & LaTourette, 2000).

In an attempt to address the unavailability of psychiatric services in U.S. nursing homes, the Omnibus Reform Act of 1987 required preadmission screening and annual review of nursing home residents. Unfortunately, some authors believe this reform act was more of a cost-saving measure designed to restrict resident access to nursing home and not to solve the existing problem of unmet mental health needs (Snowdon, 2001). This type of cost-reduction strategy is not a surprise as establishing a cost–benefit ratio for providing care to residents in a SNF has been the concern of legislators and community residents for years. The provision of comprehensive mental health services that enhance availability could increase the utilization and effectiveness of all services offered. Also, providing ongoing consultation-liaison services could help nursing home staff to recognize psychiatric problems more readily (Meeks et al., 2000).

Issues for Social Workers in the Long-Term Care Setting

LTC services are provided in an environment that is characterized by the medical model and a funding system that continues to be impacted by budget cuts (NASW, 2012b). Both government agencies and private institutions have not successfully addressed the need to coordinate among the many providers to this population. LTC recipients lack access to care, and there are great disparities between urban and rural residents seeking long-term health care. In response to the passage of the Patient Protection and Affordable Care Act (ACA) of 2010, social work will need to re-examine its function in the every shifting environment of managed care. As the ACA is implemented, social workers may need to act as advocates for their patients to insure high-quality LTC (NASW, 2012b).

The optimal system would offer a full range of care including acute medical services such as rehabilitative care and skilled home care; LTC services such as a nursing home, adult day treatment, meals-on-wheels, and personal care attendants; social and economic services such as Medicare and Medicaid; and social events (NASW, 2012b). For health care social workers, the need for supportive intervention in these facilities has never been greater. The services provided can be both cost effective and timely, especially when it comes to linking these patients to the resources they need. In addition, it is essential to stress *re-enabling*, where a patient is taught and empowered to regain as many of the abilities that were lost before the accident, illness, or event that resulted in the current condition (NursingTimes.net, 2012). Ensuring confidence that some level of previous independence can be regained and then be maintained is essential to hope and improvements in the patient's continued physical health and mental health.

In summary, it appears that most residents admitted to the SNF require more than just direct medical care. Oftentimes, the services require multiple and extensive rehabilitative efforts. In general, rehabilitative services include physical therapy, occupational therapy, and speech therapy, and do not include any types of mental health therapy. This lack of recognition for mental health services in the SNF is unfortunate because oftentimes the exclusion of mental health therapy may directly affect the patient's progression when engaged in other rehabilitative services. To fund these services, Medicare or Medicaid or private pay remains the main source of payment.

Data from the Health Care Financing Review (2010) reported distribution of Medicare SNF program payments increased from less than $2 million in 1983 to over $25,530 million in 2009 (Health Care Financing Review, 2010). A large portion of these increased charges reflect the increase in rehabilitative services offered to incoming residents. This crisis is expected to continue to grow when providing Medicare coverage for LTC placement as the latest government census continues to support that the fastest growing population in need of this service are adults aged 65 years and older. This age group consumes the highest medical cost, and most often this is the population group in need of LTC facility placement; the major funding sources for this type of service continue to be Medicaid, Medicare, private policies, or policies with LTC coverage options.

HOME CARE

If there is one trend that is increasing, it is the recent effort to navigate away from inpatient long-term and rehabilitative inpatient settings to home and community-based services (Benjamin & Fennell, 2007). *Home care* refers to health care and the social services that are provided to individuals and families in their home or in community and other home-like settings. Home care includes a wide array of services including nursing, rehabilitation, social work, home health aides, and other services.

This rapidly expanding area of health care social work roots can be traced back as far as the early 19th century (Cowles, 2000; National Association for Home Care & Hospice, 2010).

The profession of social work has a strong history grounded in home visitation with most notably the friendly visitors from the Charity Organization Societies. Traditionally, home visitation provided one way to offer services to nonvoluntary patients and those less likely to frequent agency offices because they were socially isolated, ostracized, ill, incapacitated, or homebound (Norris-Shortle & Cohen, 1987). Home visitation enabled social workers to intercede with populations who otherwise would be less likely to receive interventions and services.

In 1955, the U.S. Public Health Services endorsed a physician-oriented organized home health care team designed to provide medical and social services to patients within their home. The team consisted of a physician, nurse, and social worker (Goode, 2000). Since that time social workers have continued to provide social services in the home care setting, and this area of health care social work remains a diverse and dynamic service industry. When the Community Mental Health Act of 1963 shifted care toward the community, the government mandated that local communities provide services to meet the basic mental health needs of residents. Title XVIII amendments to the Social Security Act inspired Medicare services in 1965. Medicare mandated service delivery within the home and reimbursed social work services offered through certified home health agencies (Axelrod, 1978).

Home Care: Family as Caregiver

Hospital discharges often present challenges to family caregivers who care for frail, older individuals (Bauer et al., 2009). Discharge planners need to take into account the caregiver's needs and the level of caregiving experience of the caregiver when engaging in discharge arrangements for the patients. Mindful discharge planning is directly associated with the quality of care offered after discharge from the hospital and prevention of readmission to the hospital (Bauer et al., 2009). Most times these discharges involve frail older adults, and when these patients cannot access formal, community support systems, not only are they put at enormous risk (for readmission to the hospital, long-term institutionalization, and extreme emotional consequences) but also family/friend caregivers then bear the burden of inadequate discharge planning.

The profile of the caregiver depicts family members and friends, most often women, usually a spouse, daughter, or daughter-in-law, likely to accept responsibilities to the detriment of their own work and families, who must juggle their own commitments when adding caregiver responsibilities to other roles and functions (Robison, Fortinsky, Kleppinger, Shugrue, & Porter, 2009). Spouse caregivers are more likely to be older, unemployed, and view provision as a normative expectation of marriage. They provide a greater number of care hours and a higher number of services. Child providers encounter a greater degree of role strain showing interesting gender patterns of care provision and experiencing the effects of stress associated with other responsibilities such as family and work demands (Robison et al., 2009; Wang, Shyu, Chen, & Yang, 2011). Men are more likely to assist with home repairs, household chores, and driving functions, whereas women cook, clean, shop, and become involved in the more intimate operations (e.g., bathing, personal care). In the study by Wang et al. (2011), male caregivers reported more role strain, experienced less affinity with the care receiver, had more children younger than 18 years living in the household, spent more time in caregiving activities, were employed full time, experienced problems balancing work and caregiving tasks, and the care receiver demonstrated more memory deficits.

Several important factors impact caregiving including the number and level of patient demands, additional caregiver responsibilities, the physical condition of the caregiver, and whether the caregiving function is temporary or permanent, the amount of social support available (e.g., respite), and the number of family conflicts surrounding the caregiving situation (e.g., one sibling assuming major caregiving responsibilities). Clearly, professional help can only benefit overburdened informal systems.

Research also demonstrates that caregiver burden, caregiver strain, caregiver inner emotional conflict, and a lack of community support greatly impact family/friend and older adult well-being (Etters, Goodall, & Harrison, 2008; Limpawattana, Theeranut, Chindaprairst, Sawanyawisuth, & Pimporn, 2012). Because people are being discharged from hospitals "quicker and sicker," as has been stated previously, caregivers are being asked to know and do more in a greatly technologically advanced, medical environment. As a result, families can be left to feel coerced into caregiving because of economic and moral pressures, and these pressures may be so great that they do not take into account their caregiving abilities that could result in inadequate care.

Family burden may be great when insufficient discharge planning involves the lack of family participation in the process, lack of knowledge, and insufficient communication about home health services (Bull, Hansen, & Gross, 2000). When caregivers feel excessive burden, feelings of desperation can lead to seeking what is perceived to be a simpler solution such as inpatient or other institutionalized settings.

The importance of well-coordinated, excellent home health service, capable of providing caregiver respite and training, is critical to the containment of emotional and financial burdens. This must be a collaborative effort involving the community system where staff and family/friends can be invited to be part of this process. However, this involvement will require evaluation of caregiver capabilities with great sensitivity on the part of the professional, to assess the level of "ownership" of the caretaking tasks. Assessing how to involve the support system is inherent in social work training and our focus on the person in environment stance.

Restorative Home Care and Community-Based Case Management

Understanding coordinated care has typically been defined as a method of providing services whereby a professional social worker assesses the needs of the patient and the patient's family. When appropriate, the social worker can also arrange, coordinate, monitor, evaluate, and advocate for services. In coordinated care agencies, the traditional definition has been modified as case managers (many of which are not social workers) can serve as gatekeepers, capable of referring, initiating, or disallowing service provision. Therefore, the primary role of the coordinate care case manager is to link the patient to the most cost-effective and efficacious service possible.

The medical conditions and factors that generally trigger a home health referral include the need for a diagnostic profile; the patient's case meets the use review referral criteria; or there are unmet discharge planning needs. Home health care social workers need to be aware of the role of the case manager and keep open the lines of communication.

Being accessible by telephone, fax, and mail are just some of the ways that communication between the two can be highlighted. Each case manager will expect that the referral source is accredited by The Joint Commission and that an understanding of these principles will be inherent. For example, the social worker must be aware of the importance of coordination of care while implementing the basic standards for a continuum of quality care. He or she must also be able to outline the service area that will be provided with specific objectives that ensure that insurance benefits are understood, and outcome data highlight treatment effectiveness as intended whether the health care social worker deals directly with the managed care case manager or not; many times the case manager will be the entry point for service delivery. When working in the restorative health care setting, the social worker needs to familiarize her or himself with the individuals serving in this role and the influence that these communications can have on service referral and delivery.

Restorative Home Health Care and the Social Worker

Social work roles in home health care can be varied as well as demanding and relevant. These include dealing with parent/child relations; recognizing, reporting, and intervening with elder abuse; counseling regarding family/marital issues; assisting with personality adjustment and adjustment to diagnoses and consequences of medical illness; advocating in legal and housing predicaments; and obtaining community resources and material assistance. It can also include facilitate "home-care re-ablement or 'restorative' services" that are intensive and short term (Rabiee & Glendinning, 2011). Features that contributed to "effectiveness of re-ablement services included: service user characteristics and expectations, staff commitment, attitudes and skills; flexibility and prompt intervention, thorough and consistent recording systems; and rapid access to equipment an specialist skills in the team" (Rabiee & Glendinning, 2011, p. 495). External factors also had implications for effectiveness: "these included: a clear, widely understood vision of the service; access to a wide range of specialist skills; and capacity within long-term home care services" (p. 495).

Assessment, a primary social work function, requires a thorough comprehension of the medical, emotional, mental, social, and environmental factors impacting a patient. These elements are essential in formulating decisions as to whether the patient will adjust and adequately function at home. Goode (2000) identifies the major functions of home health social workers to include problem areas for clinical assessment and intervention, various staffing models that include both bachelor's and master's level social workers, policy implications associated with the home health care setting, standards of practice, and a review of social work literature relevant to home health care practice. This takes on both a macro and micro approach to care. From a macro perspective, skills of advocacy and program coordination remain central. From a micro perspective, the health care social worker duty expectations will often start with a complete assessment and lead to the development and implementation of a treatment plan. Through this comprehensive approach, both family/caregiver and patient can receive therapeutic interventions that will enable them to develop skills of coping and independence, while addressing some of the greater needs relevant to the service provision and availability.

Home care visits are short term and time limited in nature, necessitating proper referrals and interdisciplinary cooperation. Many social workers in home care have assumed the role of program coordinator and have had to subsequently assume supervisory responsibilities. When they are accountable to the agency for assurance that service is being delivered, this expectation cannot interfere with the ultimate goal, which is to provide services for patients and caregivers that will maximize the ability for patients to perform ADL and experience a higher quality of life.

The social work supervisor in home care has additional responsibilities of training and consultation and the ongoing provision of support to staff. Interdisciplinary team members must coordinate efforts to optimize patient recovery and movement toward independent function. Development and organization of new programs, such as volunteer training and activation of volunteer units, can be a primary role of the home health social worker. From the macro perspective, the supervisor needs to take the lead in writing grants, locating funding sources, and advocating through legislative testimony. This makes the role of the home care supervisors critical as they have the supplementary obligation to ensure that efficient discharge planning from home care services occurs.

Discharge planning from home care services is as critical as discharge planning from the hospital. It entails teaching caregivers and patients to manage independently. The home health social worker is crucial to this process maximizing patient/caregiver abilities. As demonstrated earlier, family and friends may not be properly trained and can provide only so much in the way of caregiving assistance. These gaps in service often reflected a failure of family and friends to provide all that the discharge planner hoped might be available through these sources. Home health services alleviate caregivers' stress, a necessary element in the equation of maximizing recovery for older home health patients.

Health care social workers help patients and their families cope with chronic, acute, or terminal illnesses and handle problems that may stand in the way of recovery or rehabilitation. In addition to the focus on patient and family, social workers are impacted by the restructuring of the health care and the increased workloads that involve case management, interdisciplinary collaborations, and discharge planning (NASW, 2012a). The demands incurred with the increased workload have resulted in a decrease in clinical services offered by social workers (Mizrahi & Berger as cited in NASW, 2012a). Evidence-based studies regarding the efficacy of services with a decrease in psychosocial interventions provided to patients as they adjust to serious medical diagnoses are needed to determine the outcome of this shift in practice focus.

The home care social worker and his or her duties can be varied. Rossi (1999) described home care social workers' duties as the following: "(1) helping the health care team to understand the social and emotional factors related to the patient's health and care; (2) assessing the social and emotional factors to estimate the caregiver's capacity and potential, including but not limited to coping with the problems of daily living, acceptance of the illness or injury or its impact, role reversal, sexual problems, stress, anger or frustration, and make the necessary referrals to ensure that the patient receives the appropriate treatments; (3) helping the caregiver to secure or utilize other community agencies as needs are identified; and (4) helping the patient or caregiver to submit paperwork for alternative funding" (p. 335).

Goode (2000) believed that the obstacles to providing social work services consisted of three major areas: "lack of knowledge on the part of physicians and the public about the benefits of social workers—reported by five agencies; lack of knowledge among agencies—reported by ten agencies; and no reimbursement for social work visits, which prevented many patients from obtaining services—reported by all twelve agencies" (p. 25). Goode's findings indicated that all 12 agencies identified no reimbursement for social work visits as the same major obstacle to providing social work services. This is significant in that it could support the possibility that changes in Medicare reimbursement could affect utilization of social workers in home care because social work visits are no longer reimbursable by Medicare.

Egan and Kadushin (1999) have done extensive research on home care social workers. They believe that "empirically based research on social work practice in home health agencies is essential to help the profession explain its function to other disciplines, to educate practitioners for community-based practice, and to serve as the basis for the development and measurement of outcomes for social work practice in home health" (p. 44). Initially their focus was to identify types of services provided and agency auspice. Through their research, they were able to "identify a high degree of consensus that the respondents performed functions such as coordination of services, assessment, counseling, interagency collaboration and home visits" (Egan & Kadushin, 1999, p. 46). Additional social work functions included advocating for patients and providing health education. Over 80% of the social workers also spent time educating coworkers about social work. An interesting finding was that the "auspice of the social workers' agencies were associated with practice activities" (Egan & Kadushin, 1999, p. 51). It appears that social workers in proprietary settings provide more advocacy and health education to patients than those social workers in a nonprofit setting. This can be attributed to reimbursement criteria. This means that social workers in proprietary settings advocated for patients for needed visits. Social workers in proprietary settings also had more opportunity to experience denials for requests for services and identified this barrier to services as an ethical dilemma.

Kadushin and Egan (2001) later expanded on their previous research and targeted the ethical dilemmas experienced by home care social workers. Their survey examined several factors related to the frequency and difficulty of resolving four ethical conflicts in a national sample of 364 home health care social workers (Kadushin & Egan, 2001). Eligible participants rated four ethical conflicts: (1) assessing patients' mental competence, (2) patient self-determination, (3) implementation of advance directives, and (4) patient access to service.

The findings indicated that social workers rated assessing patient's mental competence, patient access to service, and patient self-determination as similarly frequent and difficult to resolve. They rated patient self-determination as moderately frequent. On average, respondents reported rarely having to compromise their ethics. When faced with ethical dilemma, social workers identified social work colleagues and consulting nurses as being helpful in resolving conflicts (Kadushin & Egan, 2001).

The research also identified reimbursement restrictions as "creating pressures for social workers to restrict services or prematurely terminate care to patients who require a higher intensity of services" (Kadushin & Egan, 2001, p. 15). Social workers are ethically obligated to advocate for their patients; yet it is an ethical dilemma when trying to stay within the guidelines of the agency's expectations of social work services and yet not abandoning a patient when they have continued needs.

It is apparent that research has defined the ongoing need for social work in the home care setting. It is also evident that social workers do encounter ethical dilemmas when working in home care (Barber & Lyness, 2001). What is not known at this time is how the changes in Medicare reimbursement have impacted the utilization of home care social workers.

Home Care Funding

The majority of home care services are considered third party and reimbursable by Medicare, Medicaid, private pay, private insurance policies, health maintenance organizations, and group health plans. Other than private pay, these types of payments are determined by several factors, including patient diagnosis and the types of services required. Medicare and rapidly rising numbers of private pay recipients remain the largest group of patients needing home health care services.

On October 1, 2000, home care entered a new era of reimbursement when the Medicare Prospective Payment System (PPS) took effect in all home health agencies. Previously, home health agencies received payment from Medicare under a cost-based reimbursement system subject to limits referred to as the *Interim Payment System*. This per-visit cost allowed as many visits by skilled nurses, therapists, and social workers as deemed necessary for patient recovery. Payments under the PPS are based on a 60-day "episode" of care, instead of the "per-visit" reimbursement that Medicare had formerly paid. This episodic reimbursement system is based on a national payment rate that is adjusted to reflect the severity of the patient's condition (Grimaldi, 2000; Moore, 2000).

With the passage of the ACA, the challenge has become to maintain quality care while reducing health care costs (Huckfeldt, Sood, Escarce, Grabowski, & Newhouse, 2012). Recent changes related to reimbursement for services support identification of an episode-based system that aims at improving efficiency and accountability. This shift from a fee-for-service approach will allow the patient to pay significantly less for the services rendered in many situations. Huckfeldt et al. (2012) applaud this change but stress the importance of clearly defining what constitutes a treatment episode and whether there are any adverse consequences based on these evidence-based reimbursement rules.

The Health Care Financing Administration (HCFA) developed the *outcome and assessment information set (OASIS)*, which is a core standard assessment data set for home care. OASIS data are federally mandated assessment questions that must be collected every 60 days. On the basis of responses to items on the OASIS assessment, the patient will fall into 1 of the 80 *home health resource groups (HHRGs)*. Each HHRG has its own weighted score intended to result in a payment that reflects the intensity of care required (Health Care Financing Administration 2000; Moore, 2000).

Each payment is based on the episode experienced by the individual beneficiary. An agency is paid for a 60-day period of care without regard to the amount of services it provides in the 60-day period. Therefore, an agency receives incentive to provide short-term, service-limited care in the most cost-effective way for the agency possible. It is believed that this system has seriously jeopardized patient's access to home health care benefits, especially for social work.

Each agency must manage their utilization of services to keep expenses down. As the number of older individuals grows, so does the number of individuals who require home care. Because the sheer numbers of older adult individuals are growing so rapidly, this population group is making the greatest demand on home care services. More frequently than not, the services they need often involve social and medical supports, making the role of social work crucial in the field of home care. "When psychosocial needs go unmet whether through lack of detection or lack of treatment, older adult patients are at risk of further health problems that can lead to physical deterioration, reduced independence, and eventually to the need for more intensive and expensive services" (Berkman et al., 1999, p. 9).

For many years, NASW has encouraged the HCFA to acknowledge the importance and grant skilled status to social work services. This would require that each social worker provide for each patient an evaluation to assess for psychosocial needs. Studies have shown that the increased services of mental health practitioners has been associated with improved quality and outcomes for nursing home residences diagnosed with mental illness (Grabowski, Aschbrenner, Rome, & Bartels, 2010). The Medicare Improvements for Patients and Providers Act of 2008 provides parity for medical and mental health services, thus harkening a positive shift in the provision of mental health services that was lacking under previous legislation (Grabowski et al., 2010). Little research has been done to date that explores how these changes have impacted the role of the home care social worker.

Case Example: The Helgados

Mary Helgado is 73 years old. Her husband Jack Helgado is 78 years and has recently suffered a stroke. Mr. Helgado and his wife retired to Florida from New York and have been living there for the past 5 years. They have no family in the state; however, they do have several friends and acquaintances who live nearby. Ms. Helgado also has had several health problems and is recovering from an episode of shingles that surfaced after a recent episode of the flu. She has repeatedly told the health care team members working with her husband in the hospital that she wants him home but worries whether she can handle all of his needs without extensive 24-hour assistance.

On discharge from the hospital, Mr. Helgado was released home with the assistance of home health care services. Services that he was assigned include speech therapy, physical therapy, and nursing assistance. Supportive direct care services where he is assisted with his ADL such as bathing are not permanent nor do they assist 24 hours a day. Mr. Delgado's need for physical therapy has been met, and this service will be discontinued shortly. With the stop of the physical therapist going to the home, there will also be a withdrawal of the home health aides that have been going to the home and assisting with bathing and so on. Ms. Delgado has requested to see a social worker for an appointment, after calling the home health care agency in tears, stating that she does not know what she will do because she cannot possibly handle her husband without this support.

Ms. Delgado remembered how helpful the social worker was in implementing the treatment services at discharge from the hospital and felt comfortable for a social worker to assist her once again with advice and support. Yet, in her response, the social worker will feel limited as many of the services that would make this patient and his spouse most comfortable may be available, but figuring out how to pay for them may be the hardest task. Her discussions will most probably start with explaining what personal care or personal assistance services (PAS) are available in her area that can assist with many of the ADL such as bathing, dressing, food preparation, shopping, and housekeeping. A social worker not working directly with a PAS may need some help in finding out what services are available and how they can be covered. These types of services may need to be paid for through private pay or possibly through other public programs, so exploration of the options will be needed.

Today, the popularity of home-based services has grown rapidly because of the personal care that can be provided as well as the emphasis on cost savings over institutionalized care (Benjamin & Fennell, 2007). One reason cited for the increase in demand for home care services is that hospital stays have decreased through the years. Other reasons for the increasing demands for home care services include (1) the aging of the population with a high rate of functional disabilities; (2) the shift from acute infectious diseases to chronic diseases as major health problems; (3) the increase in technology that allows people to be cared for at home in spite of the need for medical equipment such as IVs, catheters, suction machines, portable oxygen, and infusion pumps; (4) the fear of nursing home placement, which prompts people to choose home care instead; (5) the AIDS epidemic; and (6) the increase in medically fragile children (Cowles, 2000).

Based on these factors, it is easy to see why home health care has experienced enormous growth over the last 20 years. Providing in-home services provides a humane and compassionate way to deliver health and supportive services. The transformation of hospital reimbursement into the coordinated care setting continues to necessitate the swift discharge of patients from the hospital setting to home. In addition, they are likely to be more acutely ill on discharge from the acute care facility. This had led many to think that older adult patients are being discharged from hospitals rapidly, and at times this occurs when services in the home setting can be limited. One major drawback with this trend is that home care services are limited in providing around the clock nursing and monitoring similar to inpatient extended rehabilitative facilities. Regardless, the resultant movement toward the incorporation of home health services has created and re-created meaningful roles for health care social workers.

To bring this literature up to date, in a systematic review of home and community care service models for older people, Low, Yap, and Brodaty (2011) observed that case management services lead to improvement in functioning and compliance with medication, fewer nursing home admissions, and growth of community services. In today's coordinated care milieu, with continued focus on cost containment and expense reduction, home social work visitation provides an economical, viable option in service delivery. In fact, home health care often serves as a mechanism to offset institutionalization, such as rehospitalizations, rehabilitative hospital stays, and skilled LTC placements.

THOSE IN NEED OF TRANSITIONAL CARE

Any discussion of LTC facilities and restorative home care services would be incomplete without a discussion of older adults, as they are the primary recipients of such services in the United States (Kayel, Harrington, & LaPlante, 2010; Resnick et al., 2009; Tinetti, Charpentier, Gottschalk, & Baker, 2012). The number of older persons is projected to grow to 19.3% of the population by 2050 (Low et al., 2011). The increased number of older persons is accompanied by the demand for more long-term services. For many frail older individuals who need LTC, the cost will be prohibitive. Therefore, because of increasing inpatient health care costs, the movement is strong toward placing individuals in home care settings offering community care services to assist older individuals to live independently (Tinetti et al., 2012).

With the increased emphasis on cost-effective approaches to enhance health and well-being outlined in the Patient Protection and Affordable Care Act of 2010, there is concern about the increased healthy life span. It is further predicted that death rates will continue to decline, leaving more aged individuals in society, especially among the "old" or those older than 75 years. Growth within the older adult population combined with strides within the scientific community have led to increased interest in promoting holistic wellness counseling approaches that integrate mind, body, and spirit (Smith, Myers, & Hensley, 2002). Recognition of these factors presents an area for clinical social work advocacy and intervention in the long-term and restorative settings that cannot be ignored.

In general, older adults are now seeking and, in many cases, expecting relief from their health care concerns. Currently, LTC services in the United States are needed by 10.9 million persons, and approximately half of that number are older adults (Kayel et al., 2010). Ninety-two percent of community residents who receive unpaid assistance, while approximately 13% require some form of paid assistance. There is a large disparity in pay between community residents and nursing home residents. The use of acute hospital services, physician services, and LTC services for older adults have increased more than any other age group. This is an interesting development, as in 2011, 40 million people were older than 65 years and this number is expected to reach 89 million by 2050 (Jacobsen, Kent, Lee, & Mather, 2011). The percentage ranges from 13% to more than 20% of the population in certain counties across the United States. This service use trend has made older individuals the focus of much discussion in the managed health care environment.

Older Adults: Unique Needs of the Patient

When working with older patients in transitional care settings whether it is restorative home care or LTC settings, health issues considered important can generally be divided into two types: chronic physical impairment and mental health concerns. The number of years individuals expected to live free of disability has risen during the past three decades (Jacobsen et al., 2011). The decrease in the incidence of disability of aging individuals and increase in recovery from illness due to health care advances have been a positive factor. Many individuals fear the chronic loss of unaided activity or perceived independence. A chronic illness is a condition generally defined as an illness that is of 3 months duration or longer (MedicineNet.com, 2012). An acute illness, conversely, generally has an abrupt onset that lasts for a short duration (MedicineNet.com, 2012).

Although people are living longer due to advances in medicine, the health care system effectively treats short-term illnesses; however, treating chronic diseases is costly (GlaxoSmithKline, 2012). To date, there are many studies relating the financial costs of chronic diseases to the quality of life of ill people and their families. The costs related to the chronic conditions continue to grow. Obesity is associated with higher risk for diabetes, heart and lung diseases, and Alzheimer's disease (GlaxoSmithKline, 2012). The number of adults who are obese has doubled in 20 years, and the number has tripled among children 2 to 11 years of age. Currently, the cost for health care for someone with one or more chronic conditions is five times greater than individuals in good health (GlaxoSmithKline, 2012). The costs directly related to chronic illnesses include charges for medical care or self-treatment that are borne by the patient, government, organized health care providers, or insurance companies. Thrall (2005) estimates that chronic illnesses account for over $1.5 trillion dollars and that 90 million people in the United States are diagnosed with a chronic health condition. The direct cost of people with chronic illnesses was $659 billion in 1990 (Thrall, 2005). Examples are inpatient care, emergency visits, physician services, ambulance use, drugs, devices, outpatient, and diagnostic tests. The burden of any chronic disease weighs not only those who are ill. It also has a significant indirect cost that amounted to $234 billion in 1990 (Thrall, 2005). Unfortunately, the older or disabled individual is often affected by chronic physical or mental conditions, as opposed to acute ones. From a psychosocial perspective, suffering from a chronic condition is generally the older adult's worst fear. A systematic review of the literature on aging and its association with multimorbidity found that half of the older adult population is diagnosed with more than one illness (Marengoni et al., 2011). Further, physical and mental health conditions are often related and interdependent. For example, a physical (physiological) condition, such as a stroke, may develop into a mental health (psychological) condition known as dementia.

Older Adults: Needing–Receiving Services

In this environment of deliberation as to the financial solvency of Medicare, the well-being of our aged population may stand in the balance. Health care organizations are intensifying efforts to coordinate appropriate discharge plans for older adults, in an effort to link this population with the services needed to maintain within the community. It has always been expected that this relevant linkage with community resources will result in decreased hospital readmission rates. In the United States, the average readmission of Medicare patients who are discharged from hospitals within 30 days is 20% (Thorpe & Cascio, 2011). The incidence of readmissions may be due to poor quality of care and could have been potentially preventable. The cost to the Medicare program averages $12 billion a year. Thorpe and Cascio (2011) observe that Medicare reimburses hospitals based on diagnosis related groups (DRGs). The DRGs pay one fee per specific diagnosis and not for the services that might be incurred when working with a specific patient. In addition, when a patient is readmitted, there is frequently a breakdown in communication between physicians and associated health professionals providing services and the Medicare beneficiary's primary care physician. This lack of communication can potentially result in conflicting care or conditions that require readmission.

It is obvious that those patients 60 years and older often exhibit a greater need for home health care, display longer hospital lengths of stay, and suffer from a greater number of chronic medical conditions. Therefore, several social variables appear to play an important role in hospital readmission especially those that involve skilled-care placement due to the inadequacy of community social support systems. Ironically, these groups were not only the most likely to experience hospital recidivism but also those most in need of appropriate home health services. Those needing services are often unaware of exactly what community resources exist and may not comprehend how to access such services. Recognizing that many hospital readmissions are due to inadequate supportive services in the home is essential to starting the process for improving care. Home health social workers serve a critical need both before hospital discharge and most certainly afterward.

Under the current reimbursement systems, skilled home care needs are more likely to be reimbursable through insurance than custodial care needs. Those needing home health aides to assist with ADL may find themselves ineligible in the absence of skilled service needs, and with recent cutbacks in funding of social services, community resources are not always readily available. Therefore, the time-limited home health assistance of intensive post-hospital care administered to older adult patients resulted in decreased hospital lengths of stay and decreased hospital readmissions and assisted the older adult population served in maximizing their levels of independence. Integration of adequate home care services has the potential to reduce hospital readmission rates greatly, simultaneously maximizing the potential recovery and independence of the older adults.

Ingoldsby, Kumar, Cohen, and Wallack (1994) employed a three-division classification system to depict home health care participants. Their study delineated individuals who are postacute, medically unstable, and primarily chronic. Postacute was defined as individuals receiving recuperative care (e.g., recovering from a stroke, fracture, and recent surgery). Medically unstable was defined as individuals with a medical condition, making them vulnerable to additional medical complications (e.g., diabetes, respiratory problems, and congestive heart failure). The third group was defined as those with chronic long-term illnesses that resulted in a steady decline in function (e.g., dementia, Parkinson's disease, and general frailty) (Ingoldsby et al., 1994, pp. 27–28). These three groups of identified home health patients offer a comprehensive representation of the population most likely to obtain home health care services.

MANAGING COST IN LONG-TERM AND HOME CARE SETTINGS

In 1965, Title XVII (Medicare) was implemented to provide health insurance for older adults, a high-risk group in terms of vulnerability to illness and poverty (Jansson, 2011). Medicare was one of the amendments to the Social Security Act of 1935. It was found that an increase in service use, primarily health care admissions of older adults, did occur once the Medicare program was implemented. With the implementation of the Medicare program, there was an increase in older adult hospital usage. Medicare allowed many older adults and disabled individuals to access health care who could not afford it previously. Physicians and hospitals also benefited, as greater flexibility in providing needed health care services was secured. In the original system that was "fee for service," Medicare paid what hospitals charged for a particular service. This resulted in cost differences charged by various providers for the same services.

It is clear that since its inception, Medicare has contributed greatly, supporting the medical needs of our older adults and people with disabilities. There are significant gaps; however, as Medicare is not designed to pay for LTC. Rather Medicare is designed to pay for the treatment of short-term illness. The services offered through Medicare in the long-term setting are often time limited and rest in providing skilled nursing care and certain therapies designed for rehabilitation. For example, one of the concerns with the continuum of care is that there is a high rate of rehospitalizations from SNFs that vary greatly across the United States (Mor et al., 2010). From 2000 to 2006, the rate of SNF rehospitalizations increased by 29%. In 2006, 23.5% of hospital discharges to SNFs were readmitted to the hospital from the SNF, costing Medicare $4.34 billion per year. Over a 2-year period, Mor et al. (2010) discovered that the tendency to rehospitalize and use other Medicare services was a local trend.

With that said, Medicare spending is estimated at roughly 20% of the national spending on LTC (Georgetown University Long-Term Care Financing Project, 2007). For low-income Medicare recipients, the means tested Medicaid programs are often called on to supplement LTC costs. Nursing homes and other facilities clearly represent a large percentage of Medicaid expenditures. See Georgetown University Long-Term Care Financing Project (2007) for more information on LTC policy options and ways for improvement.

As health care expenditures continue to grow, it has become obvious that more serious efforts are needed to address affordable health care including those who need transitional health care services. In support of this contention, during 2008, the amount of money for health care spent by citizens of the United States exceeded $2.3 trillion (Sunier, 2011). The increased costs are "attributed to such factors as technological advances, inflation, increased needs of a growing older adult population, longer life spans, and the cost of medical liability" (Sunier, 2011, p. 22).

As stated in Chapter 1, history related to the DRGs and managed care, with all good intentions health care expenses continued to rise at inconceivable rates. As of 2012, health care spending has continued to grow at 1.5%, the rate of the gross national product, and is already 20% of the economy (Hixon, 2012). This continues to be of such serious concern that Hixon (2012) and others remain quick to point out that the United States continues to spend far more on health care than any other country in the world (Hofschire, 2012).

In 2010, there were 49.9 million people who were uninsured in the United States (Smith & Stark, 2012). Morgan (2012) reported that one in four Americans are without health care. Waananen (2012) reports that in 2022, there will be 27 million uninsured with ACA, and the number would increase to 43 million without the individual mandate and to 60 million without the ACA. The large number of people without health care poses challenges for social workers who are trying to work with the uninsured in an environment where resources are scarce and many times unavailable.

Related specifically to LTC, the incredible amounts of health care expenditures related to Medicare and Medicaid in LTC continue to create a blaring call for action. Furthermore, with these burgeoning expenses, it is no surprise that LTC is embracing *coordinated care*, which emphasizes the use of primary care physicians and specialists, as well as technology, enhancing diagnostic centers within LTC and restorative care settings. This type of care coordination involves focused attempts to assist the patient utilizing independent providers that integrate patient care services and activities, while trying to eliminate health care fragmentation of services (Bodenheimer, 2008). Efforts have been strong to intervene, providing services that support transitional care, thereby reducing rehospitalizations while ensuring continuity of care (Kanaan, 2009). Although many SNF rehospitalizations are necessary, previous research indicates that a significant number of rehospitalizations occur for preventable conditions. The five conditions for which rehospitalization is possibly avoidable include "congestive heart failure (CHF), respiratory infection, urinary tract infection (UTI), sepsis, and electrolyte imbalance" (Donelan-McCall, Eilertsen, Fish, & Kramer, 2006, p. 2). These five conditions accounted for "78% of all 30-day SNF hospitalizations" (Donelan-McCall et al., 2006, p. 3).

Patient Protection and Affordable Care Act

Based on the history of fragmented care and the rising costs for service delivery, it is clear that that the health care system in the United States is fragmented with incentives that are not always congruent with health care needs of consumers (Naylor et al., 2012). The national debate about healthcare will have a significant impact on restorative healthcare in the LTC and home care settings. The Patient Protection and Affordable Care Act (ACA) of 2010 that would provide millions of Americans access to health insurance has met with resistance from several forces. Although no system is perfect, the ACA is a thoughtful response to the crisis in access to healthcare for millions of Americans. Although the U.S. Supreme Court has ruled on the case before it regarding ACA, the debate about health care continues to be a source of national discussion with large constituencies from all political points of view.

The ACA provides increased federal funding to develop services that address the diverse needs of disabled individuals and recognizes the importance of family caregivers (Reinhard, Kassner, & Houser, 2011). However, as with most incremental legislative attempts, the ACA will require ongoing adjustments for it to have the most beneficial affects across the landscape of health needs across the United States. Naylor et al. (2012) analyzed three provisions of the current act and concluded that there may be unintended consequences for individuals falling under three of the provisions of ACA. The three areas of concern are in the Hospital Readmissions Reduction Program, National Pilot Program on Payment Bundling, and the Community Based Care Transition Program (Naylor et al., 2012). Essentially the result of the three provisions may lead to poor outcomes for some individuals.

Naylor et al. (2012) suggest that improvement of ACA provisions would include implementation of evidence-based transitional care procedures, revising strategic and operational plans, developing assets for vulnerable older adults and their family caregivers, and developing performance-based systems that are mindful of appropriate assessment instrumentation and reporting protocols. Applying these principles to restorative health care practice in LTC and home care is difficult because of the wide range of clinical settings and services needed. Patient need is wide ranging, and limited resources raises many questions for how these needs can be met. For example, what are ethical treatment options, who has access to health care, and who bears the cost of health care? Without access to resources for medical, mental health, and social services, a corrective health problem could become a permanent condition. Affordable health care is an important social benefit that is not available to millions of citizens in the United States, and in the LTC setting, this limitation remains prominent. The Patient Protection and Affordable Care Act of 2010 address LTC including SNFs.

Paying for Services: Long-Term Care and Its Alternatives

The new Patient Protection and Affordable Care Act (ACA) (2010) aims to provide at-home alternatives to nursing home care. The Community Living Assistance Services and Support (CLASS) Act provides provisions for at-home care and makes LTC insurance by automatically enrolling all Americans, offering a choice to opt out (Kimball, 2010). Participants will pay a premium for 5 years, and a $50 a day cash benefit will be available for those with functional limitations allowing them to use the $50 to make up for the cost of LTC services. The intent of this provision is to offer flexibility to individuals who receive home services and to prevent nursing home placement (McCarthy as cited in Kimball, 2010). One of the goals of health care reform, according to McCarthy, was to offer more accessible and affordable care for LTC costs, thereby offering the chance to reduce costs.

CLASS also targeted the coverage gap for Medicare Part D with regard to medications (Kimball, 2010). Drug manufacturers will offer a 50% reduction to Part D recipients beginning July 1, 2010, for brand-name medicine and biologics (Kimball, 2010). The Patient Protection and Affordable Care Act of 2010 provisions regarding LTC were preserved by the U.S. Supreme Court in their 2012 hearing (Span, 2012). The ACA supports older adults and individuals with disabilities remaining in their homes rather than going to nursing homes. For instance, the Community First Choice Option provides states with assistance with the cost of in-home services for individuals who may have to be in a LTC facility. In addition, the Balancing Incentive Program will increase the match for Medicaid fund where there is less coverage provided for home and community assistance. When the ACA takes effect in 2014, the court's ruling was that states that refuse to expand their Medicaid coverage cannot be penalized, and as a consequence, it is possible that millions of people may be negatively affected. In the long run, the ACA will improve the overall health of senior citizens in a number of ways.

Planning for Death in Long-Term and Restorative Home Care

Death is an inevitable part of the life cycle, and the thought of death engenders fear and denial among many people (Thompson, Bott, Boyel, Gajewski, & Tilden, 2011; Wasabi, 2012). Many individuals in our society spend most of their time ignoring and avoiding this fact, at least until it affects them indirectly. It is usually at this time that an individual struggles with feelings of loss, separation, guilt, fear, and anger. Many individuals fear the unknown that death will bring and the loss of independence that often comes with a chronic illness. Family members fear making decisions about a loved one, especially regarding continuing or discontinuing one's life. The older adult individual and the family member often turn to science and medicine for the answers. The current approach to death by many health professionals is not experienced by the dying individuals as supportive or compassionate as the end of life approaches (Wasabi, 2012). Often physicians continue to provide treatment for individuals who are dying and to not confirm the short time that patients have to live, and this denial of death by medical professionals robs individuals of the opportunity to process their own thoughts and feelings about their impending death.

Physicians, as representatives of the scientific and healing community and leaders of the interdisciplinary team, are often sought out and expected to have the answers and make sense of decisions. For physicians, the emphasis on preserving life and keeping patient's pain free at all costs can remain strong. As physicians cannot always handle the full responsibility of dealing with the possibility of death, and because they are part of an interdiscipli-nary team that includes social workers, the social worker is often sought after to help the individual or the family cope with death.

Before the health care social worker can successfully help the family or the individual to deal with factors related to death and dying, several areas must be examined. First, the health care social worker must become aware of his or her own feelings regarding death. Many social work practitioners, not unlike their medical counterparts, are uncomfortable with the subject of dying. To assist in understanding the concept of death, it may help for the social worker to become acquainted with how death is viewed in other coun-tries and by certain religions. By becoming aware of the alternative concep-tions of death and the legitimating of the role of death, social workers may become somewhat desensitized to the perception or mysticism surrounding death in this country. Once desensitized, the health care social worker is able to address these alternative concepts to individual patients or their family and friends.

The second concern in helping individuals deal with death is to know the resources or services available in the community that might assist the individual to prepare for death. One such service is the hospice program. Hospice services, which are funded by Medicare, offer services that include both inpatient and in-home services (Bullock, 2011). Social workers in the hospice setting provide holistic assessments using the biopsychosocial–spiritual perspective that supports individuals and their families as they approach death (Bullock, 2011). These programs do not focus on prolonging life beyond its natural end. Often, in these programs, the social worker serves as part of an interdisciplinary team designed to assist the individual and family members in preparation for natural death.

LIVING WILL

The health care social worker must also be familiar with the implementa-tion of a *living will*. For more information on this topic, see Chapter 11 in this book. Most individuals are aware of the need for, and do complete, a will that declares who will receive their money, property, and other worldly goods. However, the concern about advanced directives is a discussion that can be beneficial for patients and their families at the end of life. As patients lose decision-making ability, they are more likely to have their wishes carried out if they have completed a living will so that family members understand their wishes regarding life support (Silveira, Kim, & Langa, 2010). The living will is a document that allows an individual to state, in advance, preferences relating to the use of life-sustaining procedures, in the event of a terminal illness. In completing a living will, many individuals are given the chance to state when they want to avoid unwanted life-sustaining measures. This type of will can be especially helpful to family members who are frequently left with the burden of making this decision when their medically ill relative is mentally incapacitated. Without such a will, family members may avoid making this type of decision because they may believe that initiating such a procedure gives them too much control and responsibility over the medically ill person. A living will is generally created by simply expressing one's wishes while in a state of sound mind and body and having the document legally witnessed.

CHAPTER SUMMARY AND FUTURE DIRECTIONS

More social workers are needed in the area of LTC (NASW, 2008b). There is much speculation on why social workers are not serving in this area, and part of this can be related to the roadblocks and ethical dilemmas that have been identified in this chapter. When these professionals feel frustrated and not valued, a sense of powerlessness to impact change can result in dissatisfaction. This can be further complicated by policy changes and organizational responses that create anxiety, confusion, and dissatisfaction among those providing direct patient care. Some of this response to change is related to the disruption of comfortable patterns of behavior, ethical practice concerns, and the insecurity with the unknown changes. Furthermore, the subsequent demand for greater clinical accountability and the pressure to develop best practices to benchmark effective care may also be causing difficulty (Watt, 2001). Regardless, the exact reason warrants further research on the direct causes of job dissatisfaction, and how satisfaction could be increased, thereby attracting more social workers to this area of practice.

Armed with a wealth of experiences, varying health conditions, and differing attitudes, behaviors, and levels of functional impairment associated with aging, older adult patients are possibly the most diverse group of patients with whom social workers will work with. McLeod and Bywaters (2000) validate the need for social workers in health care and report that there is substantial scope for social work involvement by working toward greater equality of access to existing health and social services. Furthermore, social workers need to be active in securing more information and a better understanding of the balancing of responsibility that needs to occur between the federal government and the states in providing adequate funding and reimbursement for home care services (Caro, Porell, Sullivan, Safran-Norton, & Miltiades, 2002)

Strategies for surviving the changes in the LTC system will include social workers realistically assessing their position. This includes careful appraisal of the sources of support for the social worker within the agency. Equally important is to participate in shaping how social workers are viewed establishing their role as a knowledgeable, positive, and supportive resource to support staff, coworkers, and administration (Neuman, 2000). New and different ideas and contributions to increase patient empowerment in the

LTC setting are needed (McWilliam, Ward-Griffin, Sweetland, Sutherland, & O'Halloran, 2001). Whether in a LTC facility or home care, emphasis and awareness on cross-disciplinary patient case reviews and consultations will continue to ensure that patients receive the benefit of a broad range of expertise they need. For the multiple professions working with the population such as nursing, occupational therapy, physical therapy, and speech therapy, among others, collaboration for the betterment of patient care is paramount.

In-service education programs and ongoing case review with other disciplines give social workers the opportunity to display clinical expertise. Establishing standardized biopsychosocial screening criteria for nurse case managers can be instrumental in incorporating social workers in the plan of care of patients (Moore-Greene, 2000). To ensure increased cost-effectiveness of the LTC services, information should always be gathered on incidence of institutionalization, hospitalization, functional impairment, and mortality (Miller & Weissert, 2001), in addition to resource utilization measures such as the number of visits, length of stay, and total direct care time spent with each patient (Adams & Michel, 2001).

Social workers are uniquely qualified to provide clinical services in this important area of practice. Social workers can instruct staff in the intrapsychic, interpersonal, and psychosocial aspects of patients' lives, demonstrate the efficacy of clinical social work interventions, and support staff who are encountering difficulties in proving patient care. By blending their knowledge of environmental and systems assessment and intervention with psychosocial expertise, social workers will need to shift helping efforts to support patient and system needs. Social workers should take advantage of opportunities in this change process by being proactive and creative as the home care social work profession redefines itself.

For providing the best practices in patient care, conducting a prescreening of patients in LTC is expected, taking into account as relevant the unique needs of nontraditional patients such as children, adolescents, and persons with disabilities. Knowledge of chronic health conditions can help to avoid unnecessary admissions and proper placement in home care maximizing an individual's independence and own support systems. Furthermore, if all the emphasis is placed on the medical needs of the patient, what will happen when the mental health needs require increased attention? In the long-term setting, we still have not fully recognized the importance of the mind–body connection, and how addressing only the medical condition will always continue to fall short.

Analyzing the role of the social worker in a LTC setting presents many challenges. Social workers are aware of the importance of asserting autonomy while recognizing the limitations of the policies that govern the facility and work to reduce the power imbalance between residents and staff. Finally, an important function of the social work is to allow for patient independence and maximizing the patient's own voice in decision making.

Glossary

Caregivers   Individuals who assist their family members to stay in the least restrictive environment possible.

Case management   A method of providing services whereby a professional social worker assesses the needs of the patient and the patient's family, when appropriate, and arranges, coordinates, monitors, evaluates, and advocates for a package of multiple services to meet the specific patient's complex needs.

Coordinated care   Patient care strategies that follow a management philosophy designed to improve patient care outcomes.

Home health care social work   Providing services to the patient in the home or the least restrictive living environment possible.

Restorative home care services   This term is used interchangeably with home health care services.

Social work in long-term care settings   Provision of services in the area of assessment, treatment, rehabilitation, supportive care, and prevention of an increased disability of people with chronic physical, emotional, or developmental impairments. These practice settings are generally multidisciplinary and can include general hospitals, chronic disease hospitals, nursing homes (skilled nursing facilities and intermediate care facilities), rehabilitation centers, hospices, residential centers for the developmentally disabled, day care programs, home health care programs, and so on.

Home care services   This type of service refers to social services that are provided to individuals and families in their home or in community and other home-like settings. Home care includes a wide array of services including nursing, rehabilitation, social work, home health aides, and other services.

Home health resource groups (HHRGs)   Based on the responses to items on the OASIS assessment, an HHRG, which consists of a weighted score that is intended to result in a payment that reflects the intensity of care required.

Interim payment system   This is a system in which home health agencies received payment from Medicare under a cost-based reimbursement system where a per-visit cost is implemented, and as many visits as deemed necessary for patient recovery by skilled nurses, therapists, and social workers are allowed.

Outcome and assessment information set (OASIS)   This is a core standard assessment data set to be used in home care developed by the Health Care Financing Administration (HCFA). The OASIS is a federally mandated assessment tool that must be completed every 60 days.

Personal support services   Services that include assistance with mobility, personal hygiene and care, and providing emotional support and physical satisfaction.

Professional support workers   Trained providers that assist with increasing quality of life for the patients served by providing supportive care needs such as assistance with mobility, personal hygiene and care, and emotional support.

Prospective payment system (PPS)   On October 1, 2000, home care entered a new era of reimbursement where payments under the PPS are based on a 60-day "episode" of care, instead of the "per-visit" reimbursement that Medicare had formerly paid. This episodic reimbursement system is based on a national payment rate that is adjusted to reflect the severity of the patient's condition.

Re-enablement   This is a practice perspective where the patient is viewed as a person with abilities that is empowered to regain abilities lost as a result of illness or injury.

Questions for Further Study

1. Do you believe that the role of the restorative home care social worker will continue to change? If so, what future changes do you anticipate happening?

2. In the case example in this chapter with Mr. and Mrs. Delgado, if you were the social worker in this case, what services would you offer?

3. Do you believe the health care social work in the long-term setting will continue to change? If so, what future changes do you anticipate happening?

4. Would you like to be a home care social worker? Why or why not?

ACTIVITY

Find a social worker working in the home care field and ask him or her the following questions:

- What would you identify as the biggest roadblock in performing your job to your satisfaction?
- Are you satisfied or dissatisfied with your job in long-term or homecare?

Websites

Institute for Health, Health Care & Aging Research
Local, state, and national health care and policy issues
www.ihhcpar.rutgers.edu

HIV/AIDS
The Detroit Community AIDS Library offers some of the most useful information on this topic.
www.lib.wayne.edu/sites/dcal

Alzheimer's Association
Information about chapters, caregiver resources, medical and public policy information, and links
www.alz.org

DeathNET
Specializes in information concerning euthanasia, suicide, living wills, and terminal illnesses. Dying with dignity theme, houses archives of Dr. Jack Kevorkian.
www.choicesandchallenges.sts.vt.edu/modules/end-of-life_websites.htm

Family Caregiver Alliance
Information about statistics and research, public policy, publications, and more
www.caregiver.org/caregiver/jsp/home.jsp

The Center for Independent Living (CIL)
CIL is a national leader in helping people with disabilities who live independently and productively.
www.cilberkeley.org/

American Public Health Association (APHA)
APHA is an association with members from over 50 occupations in the public health field. A unique, multidisciplinary environment of professional exchange and study.
www.apha.org/

Today's Health Care Social Worker

Name: Holly Bailey, LBSW
List State of Practice: Alabama
Professional Job Title: Director of Social Services, Long-Term Care Facility

Duties in a Typical Day
To ensure that the resident's needs are met, my weekly duties include facilitation of care planning meetings, which consist of input regarding a patient's progress toward individual care objectives. I work as part of an interdisciplinary team that consists of nurses, nurse's aides, a dietitian, and an activity director. I am also responsible for quarterly assessments, which are submitted to the state on the care provided. I am also responsible for making phone calls and coordinating the needs of our patients with families and their support systems. I work closely with the nurses on developing and implementing any behavioral management objectives that are needed.

1. **What do you like most about your position?**
   I work in a close-knit agency where staff and patients and family all work together to support the patients we serve. We are a Christian-affiliated facility, and many of the patients and their families share a common bond with other residents and their families. I also love helping patients to become more independent or secure the services they need to meet their own needs.

2. **What do you like least about your position?**
   One negative aspect of my position is what I refer to as "jackpot justice." Because many attorneys advertise to the community to encourage lawsuits against nursing homes, this advertisement encourages certain individuals to look for problems or magnify problems that might otherwise be easily addressed.

3. **What "words of wisdom" do you have for the new health care social worker who is considering working in a similar position?**
   I find this work very rewarding. I feel like my job has purpose when I can help a patient who has to live in chronic pain everyday to gain more independence and self-respect. No matter how busy you get always, remember to take time to allow for one-to-one interaction with the patients you serve. Just listening and making efforts to help can make a patient feel so much better.

(continued)

Today's Health Care Social Worker (*continued*)

4. **What is your favorite health care social work story?**

My favorite case example happened when I helped a patient who suffered muscular dystrophy. This resident reached the point where he could no longer sit in his own wheelchair. He was forced to spend most of the day in a reclining geriatric chair, and he constantly told everyone how unhappy he was. After consultation with others, I found a special wheelchair that could be purchased, but it was not covered by insurance and it was so expensive that his family could not afford it. After making some phone calls, I was able to find a sponsor. The local Easter Seals Association purchased the chair and helped us to adjust it to the resident's needs. Now the resident can be seen self-propelling by in his new wheelchair. To add to the final touch, our activities director made a license plate for the back of his wheelchair that says "Roll Tide." This is the motto for the University of Alabama football team.

CHAPTER 11

The Roles and Services Provided by the Hospice Social Worker

AnneMarie Jones and
Sophia F. Dziegielewski

In this chapter, the roles of the hospice social worker are identified to help increase understanding of the current tasks and functions relative to these professionals. These roles are varied and require flexibility as well as individualized care. This chapter emphasizes the need for social workers in this setting to be empathetic listeners while providing information to facilitate admissions and continued care. This requires close collaborations with the nurse case managers and other members of collaborative teams. In addition, the role of the social worker remains essential in providing concrete services to facilitate an improved quality of life for both the patient/client/consumer (hereafter referred to as patient) and his or her family. Therefore, the focus of the hospice social worker is to focus all supportive services toward the patient and his or her family, suggesting ways to help with coping strategies as well as grief work.

Services in the forefront include assessment of the patient and family needs, coordination of services such as spiritual, transportation, and education concerning advanced directives and death and dying. In hospice, there is often a misconception that hospice hastens death and that the patient will become addicted to morphine or other drugs; therefore, information in this area is essential. This chapter emphasizes the role of the social worker as a team member who strongly supports helping all individuals and their families cope with problems and stressors that allow patients to die with dignity.

Table 11.1 Hospice: Patient Age Category for Receiving Services in 2010

• Less than 24 years	0.4%
• 25–34 years	0.9%
• 35–64 years	16.1%
• 65–74 years	15.9%
• 75–84 years	27.9%
• 85 years plus	38.9%

Source: Information from *National Hospice and Palliative Care Organization, Facts and Figures: Hospice Care in America.* (2012).

HEALTH CARE SOCIAL WORK AND HOSPICE CARE

Hospice care according to Bullock (2011) involves end-of-life care that utilizes "… multidimensional assessment and interventions provided to assist individuals and their families as they approach death" (p. 88). Basically, the goal of hospice care is to support the patient and the family, with open acknowledgment that no cure is expected for the patient's illness. Hospice care includes physical, emotional, social, and spiritual care provided by a public or private agency that may or not be Medicare approved. According to the National Hospice and Palliative Care Organization (NHPCO), facts and figures in 2010, 82.7% of the hospice patients were 65 years of age or older—and more than one-third of all hospice patients were 85 years of age or older (National Hospice and Palliative Care Organization, 2012). The pediatric and young adult population accounted for less than 1% of hospice admissions (Table 11.1).

The basis for hospice programs is the belief that care can be given in a familiar setting such as a hospice instead of a clinical setting such as a hospital. The hospice is expected to create a supportive environment in which a person who has a life-threatening illness will be treated with respect and allowed to end his or her life with dignity and with palliative care. So, the individual will be prepared for a dignified death that is satisfactory not only to the person, but also to those who participate in the person's care (McSkimming, Myrick, & Wasinger, 2000).

HOSPICE AND PALLIATIVE CARE

Many people are confused about the differences between *hospice* and *palliative care* as these terms are sometimes used interchangeably. The primary difference is that anyone with a serious illness can receive palliative care regardless of the time he or she is expected to live. In hospice, a physician must certify the terminal nature of the condition and the life expectancy; this is not required in palliative care. In hospice care, the physician must determine that the patient is in the final stages of a terminal illness and will no longer benefit from traditional medical treatment, whereas in palliative care this is not required. What these two types of care share in common is the focus on managing the patient's illness and keeping the patient as comfortable as possible (Icanberry, 2012).

The goal of hospice is to provide care and address the needs of the terminally ill patients. To address this care, both in-patient and in-home services can be furnished. In order for a patient to be considered eligible for hospice, a physician must examine the patient and write an order for the patient to receive hospice care, either at home, in a hospital, or in a skilled nursing facility (SNF). Patients usually do not receive services that are deemed rehabilitative, such as physical therapy, occupational therapy, or speech therapy, unless there is another illness not related to the hospice diagnosis. A patient can receive the same services at home, at the hospital, or at a facility.

At the onset of care, there may be some patients or their family members who have chosen not to sign a DNR (do not resuscitate) order. At the point where death is rapidly approaching, families can choose to allow their loved one to be placed in a hospital or facility where there are medical professionals available around the clock. The doctor, patient, and the family makes the decision as to where the terminally ill patient will go. If the patient lives alone and is eligible to go to a SNF, then the social worker will make those arrangements. If there is sufficient family able to help the patient around the clock, then home may be the preference. There are some hospitals that actually have dedicated rooms or an entire wing for hospice patients.

In palliative care, the focus is on providing care and managing pain with those who have chronic and life-threatening illness. In the past, after the onset of a serious illness, death often came quickly (Lynn, Schuster, & Kabcenell, 2000). This made palliative care and the compassionate supportive care; it provided an essential ingredient for end-of-life transitions. As technology continues to progress, this difference may be recognized somewhat differently. In current practice, one major difference between palliative and hospice care is that in palliative care the emphasis can also focus on disease prevention therapies that are designed to prolong life (Altilio, Otis-Green, Hedlund, & Fineberg, 2012). For example, it might be used in the oncology setting to assist a patient to be as comfortable as possible while treatments are in progress. Regardless of the setting, however, the emphasis in either hospice or palliative care is strong on maintaining the quality of life. This will generally involve taking into account the whole person as well as his or her family, helping networks, and support systems. According to Altilio et al. (2012), "Palliative interventions affirm life and treat dying as a natural process" (p. 591). As the population ages, and living with chronic illness is becoming more common, it is no surprise that interest in palliative care strategies is also growing.

In 2009, the National Consensus Project for Quality Care, focusing primarily on nursing care, identified eight domains essential for providing quality palliative care. These eight domains address the comprehensive needs of the patient afflicted with a chronic life-threatening illness. In the first domain, the structure and process of the care are outlined with the use of a collaborative team approach employing well-trained professionals and volunteers. It utilizes a system of care model, often used in conjunction with a hospice that supports ongoing outcome-driven performance measures that focus on treatment outcomes and measure success. A second guideline addresses the need for managing the physical aspects of the care provided. Pain management is the focus using state-of-art management strategies shown to be effective allowing the patient to have the maximum level of comfort available.

The next five domains provide the guidelines for the psychiatric, psychosocial, cultural, and spiritual aspects of the patient, and how these need to be included in the treatment strategy. According to these guidelines, the psychological and psychiatric aspects of the care needed are identified. From this perspective, the psychosocial and mental health needs of the patient are addressed with particular emphasis on helping the patient and families deal with grief and address bereavement. In addition to supporting the patient during the process of care additional support is always built into the care model to also assist the family after the individual has died. A postdeath bereavement plan is outlined taking into account the cultural and spiritual needs of the family. In the last domain identified, ethical and legal aspects of care are identified. From this perspective, all who support the care of the patient and his or her family need to be knowledgeable of any legal or regulatory aspects. End-of-life supportive strategy and the legal documentation that prepares for it are stressed that outline the needs and desires of the patient who is now deceased.

THE FUNCTION AND ROLES OF THE HOSPICE SOCIAL WORKER

The role of the hospice social worker is to provide comprehensive assessments with the use of the biopsychosocial and spiritual assessments. This approach allows for taking into account not only the medical aspects of the patient but also the person-in-environment or person-in-situation who has long been the stance for social work practice. Many of the patients in hospice care suffer from chronic pain and this may require heavy pain sedation that can cloud their individual judgments. When a loved one is in chronic pain, it can also complicate the responses of the caregivers and other family members who are not sure how to approach certain subjects or address his or her own feelings of guilt. To provide a comprehensive assessment information related to: "... previous experiences with pain and illness, remote and immediate loss experiences, and pain and illness related behaviors as well as information about functioning, communication and conflicts, social supports and resources, and cultural and spiritual values and networks, "will all need to be taken into account (Altilio et al., 2012; p. 597).

In completing a comprehensive assessment, one of the most important roles for the hospice social worker involves whether or not he or she is culturally competent. This component of social work is essential in hospice mainly because people's culture, race, ethnicity, religion, and family values are being dealt with as they face end-of-life issues. Without cultural competency, hospice social workers run the risk of alienating patients and their support system. The hospice social worker has to be aware of what actually influences the belief system and the perception about end-of-life issues to help the patient and the family (Bullock, 2011). Since often having difficult conversations are based on knowledge and trust awareness of these biopsychosocial cultural and spiritual aspects becomes critical to ensuring quality social work services based in competence and integrity.

The role of the social worker is critical to the family planning process, and efforts are made to help family members deal with the patient's illness and impending death in the most effective way possible. To foster an atmosphere of support and caring, the social worker tries to facilitate open communication between patient and family. It is believed that successful transition and eventual acceptance of the diagnosis and prognosis will allow the grief work to begin. The hospice social worker will be expected to assess levels of stress—especially the ones that affect coping and prognosis. In addition, special attention needs to be given in assessing the spiritual needs of the patient and his or her family and helping them continue to adjust and accept.

The hospice setting has a strong interdisciplinary focus with a team approach that will continually assess environmental safety concerns. For many health care social workers in this setting, the services provided can vary but often include: education in the area of death and dying, teaching and patient and family education, referrals to outside community resources to assist with basic human needs, education, and assistance in regard to advanced directives and end-of-life decision making.

Other factors essential to supportive care can include concrete services such as: assistance with transportation arrangements, nursing home placement, and monitoring financial status to secure additional care for the patient as well as referrals within the agency and the community for spiritual interventions, volunteer support, and services to the children. The Center for Workforce Studies & Social Work Practice (2010) provides a comprehensive overview and outlines the functions that social workers in hospice and palliative care can complete (see Table 11.2).

When supportive counseling is provided, it can be direct counseling to the patient or others in his or her support system. Caregivers need this supportive counseling as often they feel exhausted when assuming the role of a full-time caregiver, making the role of the social worker essential to just help the caregiver, feel more at ease. Therefore, one of the first tasks of the social worker is to review what is realistic for the family member to do. Once this is complete, it is time to address grieving and complete an initial *bereavement risk assessment* for the caregiver. This assessment assists the patient and family to identify strengths that help cope with loss. Families are supported and time is always allowed for the patient and family to progress through the stages of grieving. Related to the end-of-care other duties of the hospice social worker involve updating the bereavement care plan after the death and assessing the type of bereavement program to be initiated upon death of the patient. Also, referrals are provided for bereavement support services. The goal of the service is to provide superior quality, competitive value, and outstanding service in collaboration with the interdisciplinary team. Long-term goals are

Table 11.2 Hospice and Palliative Care Overview of Functions

Providing supportive counseling and psychotherapy for individuals, couples, and families.
Providing psychosocial education on an individual and group basis to patients and their support systems related to coping skills, the hospice and palliative care philosophy, and nonpharmacological symptom relief.
Providing in-services to other service providers and organizations and leading community education workshops.
Planning for discharge, identifying, and linking patients with resources while also coordinating care and care planning as well as helping patients to navigate the systems related to their care and end-of-life decisions.
Facilitate advanced care planning and life care planning and mediate conflicts within families, and between professional caregivers and the organizations responsible for such care.
Participate in interdisciplinary team care planning conferences and ethics consultations.
Document all professional activities performed for the patient and his family during and after transition and end-of-life activities decisions have been reached.
All information modified from NASW Center for Workforce Studies & Social Work Practice (2010).

to provide the medical community and community-at-large with education and outreach. The delivery of services to the patient and family is the one of the most important aspects of the hospice's responsibilities (Johnson, 1998).

Working with the Family and the Support System

In addition to in-home and in-patient care, efforts to address the needs of the support system are also addressed. To provide this additional support, educational and supportive counseling services are available to the patient, the families involved and the interested community members. Supporting the family is important and most hospice programs provide direct education helping family and friends to learn how to be better caregivers. It does not matter if the patient is in a skilled facility or at home; the family is seen as central to the patient's care. Most of the education requires helping the family to support the patient and assumes the stance familiar to social work, "start where the patient is."

Education and Supportive Counseling

The role of the hospice social worker when working with the family can be varied; however, most agree it is to assume a supportive role for the family and the patient's support system. The social worker may need to provide education about death and dying and to support the patient and his or her family. The social worker will need to address the needs of the patient and family and provide short-term intervention as well as immediate crisis counseling to address the above-mentioned problems. From this perspective, the patient and the family are treated as a unit; each person is as important as the other. Services provided generally involve linking the patient and family to appropriate community resources, so family members do not have to worry about juggling caregivers to care for the patient at home, picking up prescriptions, taking time off from work, and so on.

Knowing what is available is essential in assisting significant others and other family members to understand the purpose of hospice care and to prepare for the inevitable. The family will need to be supported and be given education about advanced directives and helping patients through a life review where they can look at what has happened and what is to come with a plan that relies on teaching and developing coping skills for both the patient and family. For family members making the decision to have a loved one die at home will take adjustment and this will require knowing the resources available as well as planning how to utilize them. Family members who serve as caregivers will often need homemaking services, additional respite, and arranging for shift work involved in offering continuous care for imminent death.

Families may need homemaking services and additional respite time but may not know how to verbalize this need. Most families are quick to admit when they feel medically naïve and have had no past caregiving experience and that they are unfamiliar and afraid of assuming this new type of role. Families are often apprehensive because they just did not know how to cope with people, especially a loved one who is now that ill. End-of-life care can be frightening and many family members may fear they or others would not take adequate care of their loved one. They may be concerned about the negative side effects related to intensive pain management, although they do not want their loved one to be in pain.

Education and supportive discussions with members of the treatment team are especially important if they felt guilty about possibly doing something improperly as the new caregiver (e.g., gave wrong dosage of medicine). Assuming the responsibility for caregiving for their loved one is a big responsibility and the caregiver can feel overwhelmed with the basics of what to do next. The patient's family will need a great deal of support and this support needs to come from family, friends, hospice, the community, and the church. Nolen-Hoeksema, Larson, and Bishop (2000) feel strongly that the most common benefit from hospice that participants mention is receiving emotional support.

The role of the hospice social worker is a supportive one providing compassionate, palliative care, and counseling for all that will be involved in the dying process. The social worker can help with psychosocial problems, and with this extra support the caregiver is freed to focus only on the patient and grieving process. Therefore, in terms of supportive counseling for dealing with the family member on hospice, it is central to help the family to realize that all helping efforts will need to start where the patient is and what he or she needs. In this role, the family member is taught not to take an adversarial role and never argue with their loved one but rather to recognize and remain supportive to his or her concerns.

Energy is placed on validating the patient's feelings and creating an environment where the educator, whether a social worker, nurse, or other team member, encourages the family or friend to support the patient and listen while not arguing. For example, say the social worker is talking with the patient and he or she becomes very angry because he or she believes a deceased lovef one has said something that he or she could not possibly have said. The best thing for the family member to do in this situation is support the loved one and neither confirm nor deny what the person believes but rather normalize the emotion being experienced as opposed to the behavior. For example, the social worker might say, "I can see this is bothering you. Let us take some time to talk about it." Rather than be confrontive, it is always best to respond to the emotion being displayed. Once the agitation has been addressed, the patient can be redirected with a statement that may relate to an immediate activity or event. To further assist the caregivers with the provision of emotional support, all caregivers involved with the patient's care should participate in the treatment process and subsequent treatment planning. This will assist the family to be involved in either the direct or indirect care and feel a part of the process.

Many families feel strongly that they want their loved one to go "somewhere" with a home-like setting when the time comes to pass on. Families want to be assured that their loved one will be cared for compassionately until he or she dies. Some hospice organizations utilize what is termed a *Hospice House.* The Hospice House can provide palliative 24-hour care by professionals, where it can be explained to the family that they would still be very involved in the care of their loved ones. The essential feature of the Hospice House is that families can stay involved but will not be the actual full-time caregivers.

Lastly, taking on this type of responsibility for the family will indeed impact all areas of their life. Many caregivers may express concerns about employment and cannot afford to give up their income while trying to take care of their loved one in the home. For family members, this fear is so pronounced that family members are forced to face the intense emotional burden of losing a loved one as well as the fear of incurring the expense of end-of-life care. Costs of medications, personal assistance, institutional care, and lost wages can be quite substantial, and generally are not covered by insurance. The reality is that shift work, home health aides, and other services are costly. This needs to be explained and availability for problem solving is essential. For the hospice patient, the good news is the benefits generally cover most medications and some personal assistance. When limitations do exist, the patients and family members also need to be made aware by explaining the Medicare and other insurance benefits and limitations, as well as any limitations within the system of care being offered.

Bereavement and Preparing the Family

Patients under hospice care are generally given 6 months or less to live. This means that death is inevitable and preparing for death is an important component of hospice care. This requires that the hospice social worker be available to discuss issues related to death and dying, and many times this type of discussion will begin to take shape at the initial session. In the bereavement process, feelings and emotions run high and the patient and his or her family can easily become confused with what is said. There may also be an element of denial where the person may not want to hear or face what is considered inevitable. Therefore, the social worker will need to take his or her time to be sure that the information is clearly stated and there is ample time for discussion of feelings.

In the initial interview, the social worker can also help to provide written material that outlines what is being discussed. This way the patient and the family can once again review what was said at a convenient time after the information has been shared. It is not uncommon for the patient or family members who participate in this initial interview to say they were not told certain information and did not feel prepared as to what to expect. The nice part of providing supplemental written information is that it allows the family to review what was written and process it further. The grieving and adjustments process will need to start long before the patient's death.

In hospice, the team works closely with the patient and family before, during, and after the death of the patient. There needs to be time for the patient and family, but mostly for the family to ask questions about the dying process before it happens. Discussing what to expect is important as it starts the healing process. Phrases commonly used in death and dying should be outlined. For example, many hospice workers use the term "death rattle." The death rattle is where the patient produces a labored breathing sound that seems to gurgle or rattle with each labored breath. In this case, the role of the social worker is essential in explaining to the family members that their loved one's voice may rattle but he or she is not trying to speak, as this labored breathing is part of the dying process. When meeting with the family, it might be helpful to listen with them, so the sounds can be explained as they occur. Also, the family members may think the person is choking but they need to be assured that this is not the case. It can be explained that the actual reason for the rattling sound may not be clear as it could relate to the diminished ability to swallow or a problem with secretions. However, the sound is often associated with the dying process and when this is heard death is generally not far behind.

Another item that must be discussed carefully with the family is the fact that the patient may die within minutes of a family member leaving the room. This information is extremely relevant and knowing this can be beneficial to the family members in alleviating a lot of guilty feelings. It will also help family members to leave the patient and get rest. The social worker can assist by helping the family to say their goodbyes without viewing it as being morbid. That way, if the patient does pass away within minutes of one's departure, it is not as hard to accept and the family won't feel that they could have prevented the death.

Prior to the death of the individual, the work of planning for the funeral needs to be started. The hospice team will work with the family in determining which funeral home will come to pick up the loved one's body, and if the person is to die at home, which process will be followed. Planning the funeral will take time and should not be rushed, so starting early is important. Also, the cultural and religious preferences of the patient and the family should always be identified to ensure the person has the type of funeral service preferred. Since hospice provides a comprehensive approach to care, it is not uncommon for the hospice team members to attend the funeral. For family members, this attendance can help make the grieving process a little easier as they see the social worker, RN, or CNA who worked with the patient as a real part of the family in participating in the ceremony to honor the patient's life.

After the patient dies, hospice organizations keep the family on a bereavement list for up to 1 year. While the family's names are on this list, the hospice workers are available for calls and visits (though not as often as before the death) to help with the adjustment. Having this support is central to the grieving process.

The following are some of Medicare's guidelines for bereavement services through hospice:

Medicare Hospice CoP: §418.64(d) Standard: Counseling services—Bereavement counseling.

1. Bereavement counseling. The hospice must:
    i. Have an organized program for the provision of bereavement services furnished under the supervision of a qualified professional with experience or education in grief or loss counseling
    ii. Make bereavement services available to the family and other individuals in the bereavement plan of care up to 1 year following the death of the patient. Bereavement counseling also extends to residents of a SNF/NF or ICF/MR when appropriate and identified in the bereavement plan of care
    iii. Ensure that bereavement services reflect the needs of the bereaved.
    iv. Develop a bereavement plan of care that notes the kind of bereavement services to be offered and the frequency of service delivery (NHPCO, N.D.).

Spirituality and Pain Management

According to *Merriam-Webster's Dictionary* (2012), spirituality is "the quality or state of being spiritual" and is concerned with religious values. According to the National Hospice and Palliative Care Organization (n.d.), pain can keep you from eating and sleeping. In addition, physical pain can cause you to lose peace of mind and hope. Managing pain is one of the goals of hospice care. Hope is a major part of spirituality and if hope is lost because of bad pain management, then the patient's physical pain can actually decrease the quality of life.

Pain management and spirituality vary from person to person and from religion to religion. In order for a patient to have a dignified death, the social worker must be culturally sensitive to a patient's needs. Many times a patient's pain can be managed easier if the caregiver, whether a professional or a family member, is aware of the patient's spiritual or religious beliefs.

In 2002, the World Health Organization (WHO) stated that "Spiritual care is an integral part of the palliative care approach" (Abbas & Dein, 2011, p. 341). Scholars assert that since humans are "spiritual beings," there must be a connection between spirituality and healing (Narayanasamy, 2007). Social work students are taught very early in their educational career to put their religious beliefs aside when working with patients. In other words, they need to be aware of the patient's religious or spiritual beliefs to help the patient to put the death in perspective based on those beliefs. One of the reasons that social workers need to ask about religious beliefs is to help to determine what is a religious experience or belief as opposed to pathological behavior or beliefs that are induced by medications, abnormal grief, or the disease process (National Hospice and Palliative Care Organization, 2011). In hospice care, patients are usually concerned about the "afterlife," which includes where they will spend it, what it means to them, or the fact that they can't go there until they have said good-bye and made peace with a family member.

Keeping Patients Pain Free

A basic premise that underlies hospice care is striving to keep patients comfortable, and in many cases that means as "pain-free" as possible. A prevalent concern of almost all hospice patients, caregivers, and family is related to pain management, especially what is needed and how much is too much? Patients and families can walk a fine line between trying to keep their loved one pain-free and the fear that they will be overmedicated. Families and patients often want more supportive information about the medications that are being used for pain management, especially the misconceptions that surround morphine addiction and what may happen if given too much pain medication. Patients and families will need to have concrete strategies that they can use with their loved ones to help them know there is hope for dealing with their chronic pain (Ellner & Woods, 2012).

Patients may also request help with learning how to deal with their condition, as well as the need for outside and family support. In a study done with an Australian palliative home care service, the most compelling predictors of family satisfaction and outcome were family care perceptions (ranked number one), family members' ages, family functioning, and the length of time that patients received the care service (Medigovich, Porock, Kristjanson, & Smith, 1999).

Pain management is an issue that the patient and family have to deal with. However, there are nuances that most hospice patients and family don't deal with because it may imply that the end is closer than they think. If the pain is managed to the point of the patient thinking he or she is no longer ill or dying, that is not a good "side effect." If the patient or family is so afraid of the patient being over-medicated that they withhold medication, this is also not a good "side effect." The best scenario for both the patient and the family is for the hospice team to continue to reiterate the purpose of pain management. They must also continuously encourage the patient and family to be open and honest about pain and how it will affect everyone involved.

Lastly, in traditional pain management, the cost of certain medications may cause patients and families to struggle with what is covered and what is not. Many medicines are expensive and when entering hospice care discussions on what medications to start and discontinue may be in the forefront of the discussion. Or based on the premise related to hospice care, certain medications may not be utilized if they carry preventative assumptions. A careful consultation with the hospice treatment team can help to identify these issues. The social worker's role is essential to answer the questions that come up related to the psychosocial issues associated with pain management and the death and dying process. Giamberardino and Jensen (2012) and the selected chapter authors provide a good resource for addressing the needs of individuals in controlling their pain while taking into account the numerous problems that can occur with symptom interactions.

Beyond Concrete Services and Advocacy

In terms of advocacy, to adequately meet the needs of their patients and families, more funding is needed through an increase in the hospice medicare benefit and/or the use of fundraisers. If not available, "hospice-type houses" would be beneficial.

The term "MediCaring," as used in Lynn (2001), offers one way to learn how to finance and deliver care for the terminally ill by consciously matching payment coverage with the appropriate service group(s). This would target services for patients who are ill enough to die (instead of using the 6-month guideline), build a continuum of care from provider to provider (i.e., home, hospital, or nursing home), and provide flexibility in financial reimbursement to cutting-edge care providers. Yet, there is the ever-present uncertainty of the future of Medicare as a whole and this in a time when the baby boomers are coming of age and people will live longer with more chronic illness. The challenge now becomes finding an assessment tool or measurement outcome that can be utilized to address the needs of the interdisciplinary team, the patient, the caregiver, and the family.

One way to meet these challenges with respect to documenting impact to outside audiences may be to focus less on measuring the most unique aspects of hospice, which includes such difficult concepts to measure as dying with dignity. Merriman (1999) found it might be more useful to use universally accepted measures of aspects of "dying well" that are based in ethical principles or on consumer research. It is generally accepted that, with few exceptions (so few that they would not skew the data in populations), individuals should not die in pain, alone, or while enduring medical treatments they do not want. These measurements may be fairly easily devised, although other challenges remain in their implementation.

Our health care system is more adaptive to dealing with prevention and efforts to save lives rather than allowing nature to take its natural course, and this emphasis on life over death creates a clear gap between acute care and hospice care. Continuity and comprehensiveness of care for all people are main concerns and key factors to the quality of life that a person can expect. Using national guidelines, two breakthrough collaboratives involving 83 provider organizations generated a list of the promises that a good care system should make to patients who face serious, life-threatening, and eventually fatal illnesses (Lynn, 2001):

* Proven medical treatments;
* Treatment that ensures comfort and avoids overwhelming symptoms;
* Continuity, coordination, and comprehensiveness;
* Advance care planning (ACP), so that complications are anticipated and optimum treatment is ready to be implemented, rather than emergency efforts;
* Customized care reflecting patient preferences;
* Thoughtful use of patient and family resources (financial, emotional, and practical); and
* Assistance to make the best of everyday.

Dying and death are universal realities, but these taboo subjects are not often talked about with family members and even less frequently in mixed company. The importance of discussing end-of-life wishes with family or those who may have to make financial and medical decisions for another is imperative. The best time to discuss views about end-of-life care is before a life-threatening illness has been diagnosed or a crisis happens. Special attention should always be given to addressing racial and ethnic differences as certain cultures may be more or less open to developing advanced care planning (ACP) (Carr, 2012).

This attention and cultural awareness helps reduce the stress a family member may experience in making decisions for a loved one's end-of-life care. ACP can involve the living will, a designated health care surrogate, and durable power of attorney. Planning for what is to come and preparing these documents can help both the patient and the loved one to avoid anxiety and doubt. Oftentimes loved ones may not know what the patient would have wanted done with respect to medical treatment and financial responsibilities. Also, when in a very stress-producing situation, not having a clear plan and knowing the wishes of the hospice patient can increase concerns related to preparing for the loved one's death. Having such information can also assist the physician in providing the care the person wants and addressing issues surrounding the choices made by that person.

The Importance of Hospice Care in End-of-Life Decisions

One of the best ways to prepare the individual and family for end-of-life issues is to help empower the patient and the family to make treatment decisions before getting sick. It sounds cliché but it's true. If a person in his or her twenties makes a living will or sets up power of attorney with a family or friend, when that person turns 60 and has to deal with a terminal illness, it can be helpful to have already discussed and made decisions about the end. Most people are aware of the case of Terri Schiavo in Florida, who was on life support for many years and no one was sure of her treatment decisions. Finally, her husband made a decision and it was argued all the way to the U.S. Supreme Court (Schavio case highlights eating disorders, 2005), but his wishes with the uncertainty of hers were finally acknowledged and implemented. It seemed very difficult for her parents to deal with the final decision. Advanced planning and starting these types of discussions can help to avoid this type of agony. And this makes preparing in advance extremely helpful.

Sudore and Fried (2010) state that the problem with planning in advance is that many people believe they will change their attitudes and beliefs about treatments at the time of the illness. Since early preparation usually occurs when the person is healthy, one assumes that at age 60 or 80 one may not want to receive certain treatments, such as life support. However, again with the reminder of Terri Schiavo, she was only 27 when she suffered major brain damage. It stands to reason that early preparation would have saved her and her family years of suffering if they knew what she wanted or didn't want (to be on life support) near the end of her life. Also, filling out a living will does not have to be permanent and it can be updated as the years continue and situations change.

Advanced Directives

Advanced directives is very important for patient care planning and involves a detailed personal conversation with the patient (when possible), family, and loved ones about the issues surrounding the patient's wishes for end-of-life care. Hospice social workers can help the patient and family approach such difficult subjects, allowing for a plan that honors the patient's wishes and desires about end-of-life care.

Advance directives are instructions that can be given in writing or verbally to family and friends about what type of medical care an individual wants if he or she loses the inability to communicate his or her decisions (Advance Directive *vs*. Living Will, n.d.). "A living will is a type of advance directive, which takes effect when a patient is terminally ill" (p. 1). See the sample copy of a living will at the end of this chapter. These documents are important because there is no need to guess what type of treatment the patient would have wanted. It usually eases the minds of the family members. However, a living will can cause problems when family members are guilt-ridden and are unwilling to let the patient go without any heroics, such as wanting CPR performed each time the patient is in distress. In this situation, it is wise to contact an attorney to determine who will have power of attorney over the patient's health care needs. To get the process started, there are forms and instructions available on the Internet.

Ensuring Quality and Evidence-Based Hospice Care

What about quality? In 1998, Hunt et al. outlined that since the final outcome is death, finding specific performance measures to address satisfaction with care is difficult. Furthermore, the lack of standardized measures documenting the quality of hospice care as advanced in the National Committee of Quality Assurance's Health Plan Employer Data and Information Set 3.0, falls short when many hospice providers are expected to seek certification from Medicare and The Joint Commission. The National Hospice Organization suggests that it is important to validate the effectiveness of the program and that every hospice should have a method by which to survey the effectiveness of all services, including social work services (Archer & Boyle, 1999; Kovacs, 2000). In addition, the roles of the social worker in end-of-life care can be varied from helping patients and families to understand the loss to how to prepare and address anticipatory mourning (Colòn, 2012). This requires a comprehensive assessment of the effectiveness of hospice services that includes all participants involved in the giving and receiving of services (Fontaine & Rositani, 2000). The impact of hospice care can potentially be evaluated at several different levels and would be demonstrated in different ways at each level.

In day-to-day practice at the individual hospice level, the important impact of hospice care is in meeting the needs of terminally ill patients and their families by improving clinical status and maintaining or improving quality of life. At this level, the impact of hospice services can be documented through measurement of clinical, psychosocial, needs fulfillment, and quality-of-life outcomes. Outcome measurement remains a relatively new concept in hospice care, but many hospices now add this technique to their quality and performance improvement efforts (Merriman, 1999). The lack of performance and outcome measures is problematic and needs to be addressed in each hospice, so service delivery and patient and family satisfaction are of the highest quality. For the patient being served, measuring evidence-based care has been more successful. For example, Vlaeyen, Morley, Linton, Boersma, and de Jong (2012) outline a fear-avoidance model of practice that takes into account the patient's perspective related to chronic fear and how to identify the obstacles and challenges that need to be faced.

Evidence-based research is limited, however, for assessing the impact of hospice services. Even more disconcerting is the fact that there is very limited information and research available that addresses what additional services are needed to make the hospice experience more effective for the patient and the family. In this area, measuring effective practice, particularly ACP will need to take into account how different racial and ethnic differences can affect the way patients and families embrace care. For example, using logistic regression to examine 2,111 adults from the Knowledge Networks study Carr (2012) found different opinions and subsequent acceptance of ACP among Whites, Blacks, Latinos, and Asians. For example, Carr found that Latinos and Whites with less education were less likely to discuss their preferences when it came to completing the living will, whereas Asians were more likely to have living wills but less likely to participate in discussions related to its creation. Recognizing these potential differences is important information for social workers as well as others on the team seeking to provide evidence-based practice. It also points to the importance of moving beyond individual care and advocating for patients' rights that ensure public policy is created taking into account such awareness.

To ensure evidence-based practice, a comprehensive assessment of care is needed. This means that in addition to measuring patient and family satisfaction through various measurement tools and surveys, the service delivery concerns of the patient, family, or hospice worker need to be evaluated as well. Perhaps limited evidence-based preventive and wellness care is what differentiates it from traditional acute medical care. Most of the scales and instruments often suggested for use in hospice care can be attributed to measuring the aspects of medical care which were developed primarily to measure a person's quality of life and follow the assumption of traditional medicine (Archer & Boyle, 1999). This may complicate measuring the care delivery of hospice services from a traditional medicine perspective.

One way to measure service delivery and satisfaction in this area is to look directly at the opinions of social workers working in this coordinated care environment. These social workers have first-hand knowledge from the patient and family, and their own experiences with service delivery, to be an effective voice in how and what services are needed to better serve this patient population in the health care setting. It is imperative to identify and address all factors and issues involved concerning end-of-life care to best achieve quality of life for the patient and his or her family, and who better to ask than the people receiving and delivering hospice social services? This makes the role of the hospice social worker important as she or he needs to ask the receivers of care and their families how they feel about the individualized services being delivered. Therefore, perhaps the most logical solution would be to ask the people responsible for service delivery and the people receiving services what are the outcomes related to hospice care, and how different are these outcomes from traditional medical services?

Archer and Boyle (1999) conducted an evaluation of caregiver satisfaction with social services in a large hospice in Atlanta, Georgia. The purpose was to obtain information from the primary caregivers regarding their degree of satisfaction with the services provided by the social work staff. The last question on the survey asked how the social worker could have made the hospice services more beneficial to the family. The majority (84%) of the responses was extremely positive. The other respondents in which 9%

stated that they would have wanted hospice services sooner and 7% stated that they had experienced some difficulty with coordination and delivery of hospice services.

A large long-term study of families served by hospice found that nearly 95% said that hospice had been helpful (Nolen-Hoeksema et al., 2000). Still, about 30% of family members said there was something they wish hospice had done differently. Again, the participants in this study were "overwhelmingly" positive in their views of the hospices. People with some complaints had stated they needed:

1. More daily or constant care.
2. More "good" information about preparing for the patient's condition and death.
3. More or less information and support from the hospice staff.

Other respondents had a conflict with an individual hospice staff member. Many felt that any deficits in hospice's terms of care were due to lack of adequate funding or resources. Although this study looked at the characteristics of the family members who are associated with their satisfaction and not the actual satisfaction with services provided, it does support my findings of what are the perceived service needs of the family.

Teno (1999), in her article regarding care for the dying, provides the reader with a brief overview of current problems with measuring satisfaction. Again, the author does not address what the problems with service delivery are as viewed by the patient, family, or caregiver; but she does support the assertion that the patient, caregiver, and family are key factors in improving services for the terminally ill. She believed that individuals who were dying are not the only patients being served, and the importance of the family in the treatment process cannot be underestimated.

Self-Care for the Social Worker

For social workers, this area of care can be very stressful. Working with patients and families approaching a loved one facing end-of-life care decisions can lead to stress and burnout (O'Donnell et al., 2008). In this setting, social workers, as well as other team members, are exposed to heavy emotional situations where they may feel the treatments provided are not necessary and prolong the suffering of the patient (Altilio et al., 2012). The constant exposure to stressful situations and the requirement for professional empathetic listening can also affect the therapeutic services offered. For social workers, self-care will require the balancing the professional and the personal roles that are to be performed and making sure that will allow them to continue their practice over time.

Social workers often feel the need to help everyone else through difficult times, but when they are stressed, they usually ignore the feelings or any symptoms leading to mental or physical ailments. Social workers who work with the terminally ill, whether in hospice, AIDS, or oncology, for example, need to make sure they have great support. This can be in the form of social support from a good friend, family member, spouse, and so on. Or the support can be professional in the form of a pastor, counselor, or psychiatrist. Pomeroy (2011) tells of a story of her working in an AIDS clinic, where patients died weekly. She states that:

> As a way of coping with this situation, the executive director hired a psychiatrist to conduct weekly group sessions that were required for all practitioners at the agency. Attending to our own grief and loss experiences is of paramount importance if we are to be effective and present for our patients. (Pomeroy, 2011, p. 102)

Social workers need to recognize that they are human beings with emotions just like everyone else and work toward keeping boundaries intact to focus on helping the patient. The stress-provoking services provided to patients in these types of settings should not be underestimated (Pulido, 2012). Having a specific outlet is important. For example, the social worker can play sports, work out at a gym, find a favorite humorous movie or situation comedy that requires no major thinking, known as "mindless" laughter. This is needed to relieve stress. Burnout can come easily for many professionals. But for social workers who are dealing with death and dying on a daily basis, it seems to happen more often. But if there is adequate support within the agency as well as in his or her personal life, many social workers can serve their patients well, take care of their personal needs and have an enjoyable career in hospice.

CHAPTER SUMMARY AND FUTURE RECOMMENDATIONS

This chapter outlined the role of the hospice social worker which generally involves helping patients and families cope with the dying process. The services provided include psychosocial assessment and intervention, information about community resources, as well as education about death and dying and advanced directives. Taking into account the racial and ethnic differences of the patient served should always be at the forefront of ACP decisions (Carr, 2012), as well as recognizing and addressing the spiritual needs of the patient and his or her family. Therefore, it is clear that supportive services need to go beyond concrete service provision as the roles for the patient and family will change dramatically.

The needs for more respite, night sitting, shift work, and perceptions of other family members not involved in the care will also need to be addressed. Concerns about anticipatory grief and loss, the dread of losing the loved one, and how they will get along without him or her will become more pronounced. Expressing concerns about the sense of loss that occurs and when they have to say good-bye to those they love is a difficult and often daunting task.

Lynn (2001) reminds us of the fact that one-third of families of seriously ill, hospitalized, well-insured patients report a major financial change such as loss of most income or having to move because of the costs of illness. When the caregiver burden becomes too great, the need for a Hospice House is evident as well as more home health aides and/or homemaking services to assist the patient and caregiver.

In general, satisfaction surveys regarding hospice care have been found to have a high number of positive responses. To assess the needs of families more effectively, one must be aware of the possible caregiver bias and significant factors that may contribute to that bias (Archer & Boyle, 1999). A factor that may bias the information is the possibility that the person who responded to the survey was caring for a patient who was not as incapacitated, had fewer nursing issues, and died at home.

In closing, it is clear that social workers in the hospice setting provide a valuable service to the patient, caregiver, and family, allowing them to better attain quality of life and service. The main areas for continued advocacy appear to be related to respite services provided in the home. When a patient stays at home to die, the family can be encumbered with a terrible burden if the family members do not feel supported; therefore, the entire situation must be addressed immediately. This difficulty is linked directly to the amount and intensity of care needed by the patient, the ability of the caregiver to care for the patient, the support system of the patient and caregiver, and the services available to the patient and caregiver. There are other mitigating factors such as physical and mental health of the patient and caregiver, the ability of the caregiver to take time off work, and the financial concerns of the patient, caregiver, and family that add to the challenge of caring for the dying patient at home. This is one the most intense and trying circumstances, and it can leave the patient, caregiver, and family very vulnerable.

Glossary

Bereavement risk assessment   This is an assessment that the hospice social worker completes with the caregiver of the loved one who is receiving the hospice service. The assessment is designed to identify strengths that help cope with loss. Once the risk assessment is completed, it is used to identify where families need the greatest support while progressing through the stages of grieving.

Hospice   Hospice care is a special way of caring for people who are terminally ill and their families. The goal of hospice services is to care for the patient and the family, with open acknowledgment that no cure is expected for the patient's illness.

Hospice care Hospice care includes physical, emotional, social, and spiritual care provided by either a public agency or private company that may or not be Medicare approved.

Hospice House This is where end-of-life palliative 24-hour care is provided by professionals where the family can stay involved but will not be responsible for the actual full-time care as the primary caregiver.

Questions for Further Study

1. What is the role of the hospice social worker?

2. What services does the hospice social worker provide?

3. What services or additional services can hospice social workers provide that would be of benefit to the families served?

4. What services or additional services could be provided to better assist caregivers in the bereaving process?

5. What are some of the most important concerns that you believe might be expressed by patients/families?

6. What is the best way to address concerns expressed by the family and what is the role of the social worker as part of the treatment team?

Sample of a Living Will

LIVING WILL DECLARATION OF _____

To my family, doctors, hospitals, surgeons, medical care providers, and all others concerned with my care:

I,_____, being of sound mind and rational thought, willfully and voluntarily make this declaration to be followed if I become incompetent or incapacitated to the extent that I am unable to communicate my wishes, desires, and preferences on my own.

This declaration reflects my firm, informed, and settled commitment to refuse life-sustaining medical care and treatment under the circumstances that are indicated below.

This declaration and the following directions are an expression of my legal right to refuse medical care and treatment. I expect and trust the above-mentioned parties to regard themselves as legally and morally bound to act in accordance with my wishes, desires, and preferences. The above-mentioned parties should, therefore, be free from any legal liabilities for having followed this declaration and the directions that it contains.

DIRECTIONS

1. I direct my attending physician or primary care physician to withhold or withdraw life-sustaining medical care and treatment that is serving only to prolong the process of my dying if I should be in an incurable or irreversible mental or physical condition with no reasonable medical expectation of recovery.

2. I direct that treatment be limited to measures which are designed to keep me comfortable and to relieve pain, including any pain that might occur from the withholding or withdrawing of life-sustaining medical care or treatment.

3. I direct that if I am in the condition described in item 1, above, it be remembered that I specifically **do not** want the following forms of medical care and treatment:

   A. _____
   B. _____
   C. _____
   D. _____
   E. _____
   F. _____
   G. _____
   H. _____
   I. _____
   J. _____
   K. _____

4. I direct that if I am in the condition described in item 1, above, it be remembered that I specifically **do** want the following forms of medical care and treatment:

   A. _____
   B. _____
   C. _____
   D. _____
   E. _____
   F. _____
   G. _____
   H. _____
   I. _____
   J. _____
   K. _____

(*continued*)

Sample of a Living Will *(continued)*

LIVING WILL DECLARATION OF _____

5. I direct that if I am in the condition described in item 1, above, and if I also have the condition or conditions of _____, that I receive the following medical care and treatment:

_____

_____

_____

_____

_____

_____

This Living Will Declaration expresses my firm wishes, desires, and preferences and the fact that I may have executed a form specified by the law of the State of _____, may not be used a limiting or contradicting this Living Will Declaration, which is an expression of both my common law and constitutional rights.

I make this Living Will Declaration the _____ day of _____, 20____.

_____

Declarant's Signature

_____

_____

Declarant's Address

WITNESS STATEMENTS

I declare that the person who signed or acknowledged this document is personally known to me, that he/she signed or acknowledged this Living Will Declaration in my presence, and that he/she appears to be of sound mind and under no duress, fraud, or undue influence.

_____

Witnesses' Signature

_____

Witnesses' Printed Name

_____

Witnesses' Address

I declare that the person who signed or acknowledged this document is personally known to me, that he/she signed or acknowledged this Living Will Declaration in my presence, and that he/she appears to be of sound mind and under no duress, fraud, or undue influence.

_____

Witnesses' Signature

_____

Witnesses' Printed Name

_____

_____

Witnesses' Address

NOTARIZATION

STATE OF _____, COUNTY OF _____

Subscribed and sworn to before me his _____ day of _____, 20_____.

_____

Signature of Notary Public

My commission expires: _____

Source: Sample Living Will Form. Retrieved August 13, 2012 from estate.findlaw.com/living-will/sample-living-will-form.html

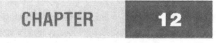

CHAPTER 12

Case Management and Discharge Planning

*Diane C. Holliman
and Sophia F. Dziegielewski*

The purpose of this chapter is to explore and identify issues related to professionals working in case management and the practice of *discharge planning*. In this chapter, case management and discharge planning are defined and described, and a case exemplar is presented to show the tasks and complexities of case management and discharge planning when assisting patients/clients/consumers (hereafter referred to as patients). In case management and discharge planning, the person's medical needs are important, but assessing the person's social environment and support system is essential for successful continuity of care. If a person's health cannot be maintained outside the care setting, the person is at risk for readmission and further health and psychosocial difficulties. In case management and discharge planning, it is not uncommon for both social work and nurse case managers to perform this function. Because these two professionals often share the same roles and responsibilities, learning more about how these jobs are perceived is critical. Topics explored include the role and tasks of the case manager and discharge planner, and how social workers can collaborate with nurses and other professionals in these roles. Recommendations are made for steps toward evidence-based case management and discharge planning in social work.

HISTORY OF CASE MANAGEMENT AND DISCHARGE PLANNING

The Settlement Houses (1890–1910) in New York and Chicago provided a foundation for social workers, allowing these early professionals to guide families through private and public services while helping to mobilize their communities for empowerment, education, and improved quality of life. This practice of developing relationships, assisting, negotiating, educating, referring, and providing follow-up are important aspects of case management that have always been a part of social work practice. Since 1975, case management has been recognized as a method of service delivery with the primary purpose of improving quality of care to vulnerable population and controlling costs (Frankel & Gelman, 2012). Case management approaches have been utilized in health and mental health settings and are defined as a collaboration process that assesses, plans, implements, coordinates, monitors, and evaluates the options and services required to meet an individual's health needs, using communication and available resources to promote quality, and cost-effective outcomes (Frankel & Gelman, 2012).

Case managers seek to ensure that all patients receive the services that they need in a system that sometimes appears fragmented and difficult to navigate (Golden, 2011; Rothman, 2002). The tasks in case management can vary; however, for the most part it includes the completion of psychosocial assessments, initiation and implementation of advanced directives, assisting in connecting to resources and insurance verification for hospital stays, provision of community resources, and completing referrals for services and durable medical equipment. It also includes more supportive services such as crisis intervention support services and assisting patients with medication understanding and compliance (Beaulieu, 2012; Frankel & Gelman, 2012).

If case management is seen as an umbrella, discharge planning would be beneath it. Simply stated, discharge planning is a function of case management that creates a bridge to the next level of care. For example, in the mental health setting, when a person is released from one level of psychiatric care to another level, the plan that fosters this connection is called the *discharge plan*. In case management, discharge planning is an essential function that facilitates continuity of care. In the hospital setting, discharge planning would involve preparing for a patient to go from an inpatient medical bed to another less intensive facility such as a skilled-care nursing home. In this setting, discharge home from the hospital would start with a referral from the medical team for this level of care. Once the referral is received, the social worker would communicate with the patient and family, locating a nursing home for the patient and applying for admission. Once the patient is ready for admission and a nursing home bed is secured, completing paperwork and information for discharge is necessary. Again, the social worker would communicate with the patient and family to make sure they are aware of these final arrangements.

Another aspect of discharge planning can occur in the emergency department when an individual presents with symptoms of depression and anxiety although there is no medical or psychiatric reason that the person should be admitted to the hospital. In this situation, the social worker would meet with the patients to discuss their current situation and work with the patients to create a discharge plan reflective of any outpatient care needs. The major concerns of the patient are noted and often times it can be something as simple as the individuals are reluctant to discuss what is wrong with them because of the fear that families, friends, employers, and other members of their support system will label them as "crazy." In creating a comprehensive management plan, the available care options are explored and questions regarding protected confidential and private information are outlined. Also, the discharge planner and the patient can discuss what information needs to be shared and what does not. In creating a comprehensive care plan, the social work discharge planner may set up appointments to get the patient stabilized.

Helping patients obtain the services they need can be time intensive as case managers and discharge planners are presented with problems complex and multifaceted (Sargent, Pickard, Sheaff, & Boaden, 2007). Ideally, the roles of the case manager and the tasks that are to be performed should reflect the transdisciplinary nature of the team providing the care.

When providing these services physicians, nurses, social workers, patients, family members, and other identified systems will be expected to work together sharing expertise to provide seamless quality care. To provide comprehensive care, it is expected that the patients and their identified families and support systems always should be included in the case planning (Sargent et al., 2007). In case management and discharge planning, plans need to be mutually negotiated and always include the patient as part of the process; listening carefully and gathering their input in the planning (Cawthorn, 2005). In advocacy for the rights of persons with disabilities, it is often echoed "Nothing about us, without us!" (T. Shakespeare, personal communication, July 9, 2012).

In coordinated care, family practice physicians (Parsons et al., 2012), nurses (Cawthorn, 2005; Tahan, 1998), and social workers (Ferguson & Schriver, 2012; Xie, Hughes, Sutcliffe, Chester, & Challis, 2012) all participate in discharge planning and case management with evidence to support the effectiveness of their services. There is a growing body of evidence that supports how important case management and discharge planning services are for increased patient satisfaction, reduced length of stay and recidivism, and better health and mental health outcomes (Fabbre, Buffington, Altfeld, Shier, & Golden, 2011; Fontanella, Pottick, Warner, & Compo, 2010; Maus, 2010; Parsons et al., 2012; Saleh et al., 2012; Wilson, 2012; Xie, Hughes, Sutcliffe, Chester, & Challis, 2012). Yet, more research is needed that focuses on transdisciplinary and patient-centered care and research.

Schuetze's (2006) article, "Shining the light on the '800 lb gorilla' of professional rivalry in case management," described the rivalry between the different professions performing case management services. To address this rivalry, social work case managers and other professionals in the field need to acknowledge the existence of the rivalry. Once acknowledged, open discussions are needed to identify the causes and possible solutions enticing social workers, nurses, and other related professionals to work together. Schuetze goes on to state that case management is still developing and that there are multiple professionals from different disciplines and each professional brings their own strengths to the table. There are some differences among the disciplines, however; conversations based on mutual respect and collaboration need to occur.

Ferguson and Schriver (2012) contend, however, that because of power and pay differentials between social workers, nurses, and other health care professionals is so great. Bringing these different disciplines together will not be a simple task. Ferguson and Schriver's recommendations for social workers in these competitive and multidisciplinary (not transdisciplinary) settings is for social workers to advocate for themselves. This will require making connections with their professional organizations, peer-reviewed literature, as well as educational settings. These disciplines need to come together and define more clearly what the social work role is in case management and discharge planning.

In addition, social workers need to formulate these definitions and share them with state and federal regulating bodies starting an impetus toward change. Whether it be at a hospice, hospital, nursing home, and other discharge planning and case management settings advocacy is essential. Social work leadership in communities is critical for influencing policies and procedures at the state and federal boards and offices. Another area for attention is to add to the growing body of evidence-based outcomes studies on social work's participation, expertise, and success in case management and discharge planning. These macro interventions can lead to greater influence and power for social work that can translate into more jobs for social workers and higher salaries.

Other opportunities for social workers in private practice can include serving as health care advocates, long distance caregivers and geriatric case managers. In these roles, social workers are paid by patients and families to help navigate the system and provide case management and discharge planning in a complex and fragmented health care system. An example of when one of these professionals could be used would be when a person is diagnosed with early Alzheimer's disease. Alzheimer's is a devastating and frightening diagnosis for patients and families. In the early stages of the disease, this private practitioner could assist the patient in writing advanced directives, listening to the patient and family members individually or as a group as they express their concerns, helping the patient and family wade through the medical information and options they are given, and assisting them with individual and longer-term problem solving.

MODELS OF CASE MANAGEMENT

Several theories and perspectives from social work are useful in describing case management. *Systems theory* originates from sociology and biology, and in social work and case management it is used to describe how human behavior is a result of interactions between people and their social systems (Rogers, 2006). In the case study in this chapter, the nursing home, the volunteer who speaks Spanish, community resources that the social worker connected Mr. Marco with such as Medicare, Medicaid and his other insurance, his local pharmacy, and transportation, as well as his family, neighbors and community are part of his social system, and all of these entities in his social system have roles, boundaries, and subsystems, and they interact together. Systems continually strive to maintain their status quo and resist change. For example, for Mr. Marco leaving the nursing home, even though it is seen as a positive change for him, will be a change and there will be new roles for him and systems and subsystems that he must interact with. By seeing his situation through the lens of systems theory, the social worker can understand the stress and possible discomfort of this change for Mr. Marco.

Ecological theory takes the importance of making connections further by describing people as being actively involved in their own development and takes into account that environments and systems are actively changing too. A principle of ecological theory is that the way people understand their environments and experiences significantly affects their perceptions and quality of life (Rogers, 2006). For Mr. Marco, the interaction with the volunteer enabled him to complete the paperwork and provided a positive social outlet for him while he was in the nursing home. In exchange by helping Mr. Marco, the volunteer realized what needed to be done for her own mother. Ecological theory provides an explanation for how the social worker shaped this situation.

Ecosystems approach combines systems and ecological theory. Both systems and ecological theory provide similar, but slightly different explanations of how systems interact with each other. Systems theory (role, boundaries, homeostasis, differentiation, and subsystem) and ecological theory (adaptation, energy, interdependence, and transactions) have distinct terminology, but both can be used together to describe how interactional processes and systems affect the behavior of individuals and systems (Rogers, 2006).

In effective case management, social workers must address the *micro* (facets of personality and individual functioning including the biological, psychological, developmental, emotional, spiritual, and financial), *mezzo* (elements of a person's immediate environment, in the case of Mr. Marco the volunteer was part of his mezzo system), and *macro* (larger social systems that affect a person such as Medicare, health insurance, language barriers, and cultural issues) (Rogers, 2006). Especially in Mr. Marco's case, the *strengths perspective* enabled the social worker to see that there was a way to reach Mr. Marco's capacity for growth, change, and adaptation (Rogers, 2006). All of these (systems theory, ecological theory, ecosystems approach, micro, mezzo, and macro levels, and the strengths perspective) provide frameworks for understanding the complexities of case management.

CASE EXEMPLAR

Recently, Mr. Marco, a 60-year-old Hispanic male, suffered a stroke that left him in need of rehabilitation. He was discharged from the hospital to a skilled nursing facility where he received the care he needed to prepare himself to once again return home. Mr. Marco was informally labeled as being difficult as often he said, "Yes," but the physician and other health care team members were not sure how much he really understood. In preparing for discharge from the facility, it was clear that Mr. Marco could perform most of his activities of daily living independently. He could bath himself, although at times he was somewhat unsteady on his feet. He could walk and get himself to the dining facility. He did become very frustrated when he was faced with his personal situation and often just threw up his hands when some of the team members tried to talk with him about his continued care.

Although he was no longer in need of a restrictive level of care, the physician in charge of his care asked the social worker to assist Mr. Marco to return home. As a case manager, the first role is to help connect Mr. Marco with the community resources he needs to return home. After leaving the skilled facility, he would need updated information related to Medicaid, Medicare, and his other insurance policies. He would also need to apply for Social Security disability. When the social worker asked Mr. Marco about working with him on this, he immediately looked at the forms she had and said, "Just leave them, I do not need any help." The social worker asked if he was sure and he said, "Yes, I am very sure, please leave." The social worker left the room as requested but said she would be back later after lunch to check on him. When she got back, the papers had been moved around but nothing was completed. The social worker noted that he was very friendly to one of the volunteers who spoke fluent Spanish. They often chatted and seemed to have good rapport. The social worker asked her if she minded going with her on the next visit with Mr. Marco. She agreed. When they both walked into the room, Mr. Marco began to speak with the volunteer in Spanish. The two joked about the weather and what he had eaten for lunch and his "gringo salad."

The social worker asked the volunteer to leave the room for a minute and asked Mr. Marco if he would let Ms. Vasquez, the volunteer, help with filling out the paperwork. He agreed. When she came into the room, it became obvious that Mr. Marco did not read English and the three of them worked together to get the paperwork completed. Although Mr. Marco could speak English, his health literacy was a real issue and he did not trust the social worker to make sure the paperwork was filled out correctly.

For Mr. Marco, he felt overwhelmed by the amount of information he was getting and he was not sure how to communicate with social worker nor did he trust the social worker to make sure he had filled out the paperwork correctly. The social worker in this situation quickly learned how important it is to listen to what the patient was and was not saying. Once rapport had been established, Mr. Marco did not hesitate to ask for a bilingual worker to help clarify what he was requesting.

When the social work case manager became aware of the language difficulties, she asked the patient if he wanted another case manager who spoke Spanish. He said no, he was fine with her as long as she continued to get "a little help from her friends." The social work case manager took the time to listen to her patient and his needs. In addition, the bilingual helper told the case manager she enjoyed assisting as now she might be able to use what she was learning to help her own mother navigate the system of care.

To help Mr. Marco, the social worker also spent hours on the phone with local agencies, funding sources, community advocates, and whomever she could think of to help get her patient the services he needed to maintain his desire to stay in his own home. When Mr. Marco was discharged from the facility, she made one final check to make sure he had all of his medications and supplies that he needed to get him settled at home. She also wanted to make sure he knew the procedure for renewal of his prescriptions at the local pharmacy and transportation arrangements for his next physician's visit.

THE ROLES AND FUNCTIONS OF THE CASE MANAGER

There are numerous functions the case manager performs; several important roles are *assessor, advocator, negotiator, educator and teacher, broker and facilitator, record keeper, evaluator, tracker and manager of follow-up*, as well as recognizing crisis and providing *crisis intervention* when needed. Additional duties include determining eligibility for concrete services, developing resources, and providing direct assistance and treatment.

When serving as an *assessor*, the case manager systematically reviews the patient records to look for problems or issues of concern that may present and interfere with the discharge plan. Once identified, the social worker works as a team member and shares her observations of the patient and the patient's situation. Skilled in assessment and treatment, the social worker is in the ideal position to help the team to explore and identify specific needs for the patients and their families. Support networks are identified and availability is assured. The information is synthesized and a comprehensive assessment is completed and the information gathered is used to start the process for coordinated care delivery reflective of a biopsychosocial–spiritual assessment to practice. In assessing the needs of the patient, case managers have guidelines or questions that they must ask for this purpose. Professional interviewers use basic counseling skills and provide direct personal support to those they are interviewing.

As an *advocator*, the case manager is expected to assess the situation and speak out to advocate and make recommendations that are in the best interest of a patient's safety, medical condition, self-interest, and biopsychosocial–spiritual needs. The biopsychosocial–spiritual needs include the family and social support system in each identified problem and the advocacy to address it. The patient's economic and financial concerns as well as perceived mental health and assessing overall quality of life are given top priorities. Patient advocacy is required in case management when the patients or their support systems cannot speak or act for their own protection and safety. In its most simplistic form, advocacy can consist of making recommendations to the patient, treatment team, family and support system, referral agencies, the community, policy makers, and other mezzo and macro systems.

As a *negotiator*, the case managers often assist individuals, programs, organizations, and communities in making compromises that benefit the patient and those in their support system. Negotiation also can help to increase relations with a referral source. There are numerous instances when negotiation is needed, but specific examples include getting the patients' families to take them home for a visit during the holidays when they may have been initially reluctant to do so. Or working directly with a community agency and assisting them to secure the services, they need to better assist the patient placed in their care.

The case manager may need to serve as *educator and teacher* and help the patients apply this problem-solving information to their situation. This type of intervention can involve working with individuals, small groups, or larger groups through teaching. Topics commonly covered by case managers are stress management, navigating the health or mental health system, wellness, substance abuse, living with chronic illness, budgeting, and employment resources. In this role, teaching and educating rests with empowerment where self-sustaining behaviors can be developed where patients and their support systems feel empowered and are able to generalize this information to other situations.

In the role of *broker and facilitator*, the case manager works closely with the team as well as the patients and their family and support systems. As a broker and facilitator, the case manager makes referrals or links the patients and their support systems with health care services, social service organizations, government programs, and other appropriate resources. To be most effective, the broker and facilitator must know how these outside organizations function and have clear and consistent communication with them.

Oftentimes, assuming the role of *record keeper* and *evaluator* is a task in case management that is necessary for meeting organizational standards and the requirements for payment of services (insurance companies, Medicare, and Medicaid) as well as to measure practice effectiveness. Record keepers must keep patient data in a format that is organized, available for the agency, and secure (confidential). Today, most record keeping is done on computers and in a format that meets the organization's standards. It is not uncommon for social workers to serve as service coordinators especially when most patients will require two or more services. Organizing when the patient receives the services, transportation (if necessary), payment of services, and assuring that there is not duplication of services or gaps in services are parts of service coordination. The goal of service coordination is to provide seamless continuity of care and quality of care. As an evaluator, the case managers evaluate their patients, their own practice, and the practice of their programs to ascertain whether they are meeting their goals or outcomes. Evaluation is done in the service of helping others and improving services and includes looking at efficiency (the ratio of costs (time/effort/financial costs) to outcome) as well as effectiveness. Oftentimes, this goes hand-in-hand with record keeping.

As a *tracker and manager of follow-up*, the case manager focuses on patient resiliency and self-sustainment. These activities can occur during the service provision or after the patient leaves the facility, agency, or practice. Follow-up calls, home visits, surveys, and annual appointments are ways to determine whether the patients are still meeting their goals, improving, or if they need additional services.

It is also not uncommon for the patients and their families to be faced with changes and subsequent decision making that can predicate an extreme reaction to a crisis situation. This sudden state of instability or danger and upheaval makes the role of the case manager essential, providing *crisis intervention* services for helping the patients to explore the situation realistically and develop their own support systems. The experience can bring about physical, biological, mental, emotional, or social upheavals that require immediate attention. A crisis requires immediate action, and in crisis intervention, the case manager quickly assesses the situation, provides support and empathy to those involved, and makes a decision about the level of care or intervention necessary to resolve or stabilize the situation. Case managers commonly intervene in crises such as suicidal gestures, sudden death or loss, drug overdoses, hospitalizations, and loss of financial benefits or other needed services.

In case management and discharge planning, other duties performed often involve determining eligibility and connecting patients to the services they need. Determining eligibility often involves assessing the patients and their support systems for service eligibility using agency or program criteria for initiation or referral for services. Determining eligibility requires knowledge of the referral agency or program and their assessment processes, and how the person being referred fits the criteria.

The case manager is also a developer of resources where an awareness of concrete skills is supplemented by helping to maximize the use of resources through macro intervention skills such as community organization, advocacy, and grant writing. Case managers link patients to the services they need and while performing these duties can become aware of the need for additional organizational or community resources. Providing services establishes fertile ground for systematic observation of gaps in delivery. Once these gaps are identified, conclusions can be drawn from patient-related data and feedback. Community assessments can also be conducted to identify the need for additional services.

Finally, social work case managers cannot only provide the services identified earlier as practitioners, but also can provide direct personal support and treatment. Patients need to state their needs and their needs should be taken seriously. The social worker can provide direct personal support and treatment such as basic counseling skills and helping the patients to problem solve their situation. Social workers are trained and know the importance of showing empathy, actively listening, and reflecting content and feelings, while helping to develop mutually negotiated goals and objectives. The case manager is more than a listening ear, although a case manager can actively listen to the patient's needs. Professionally summarizing the needs of the patient and helping them to develop a plan of action is central to successful and comprehensive coordinated care planning. Other elements of direct personal support and treatment are encouraging and even being able to accept anger and criticism from the patient while maintaining and role modeling professional boundaries.

In summary, the roles and the tasks of the case manager can vary, but to provide comprehensive care at a minimum, they should include taking into account the patients, their families, and their support systems and making sure a complete biopsychosocial–spiritual and cultural assessment is completed. A clear plan for developing a plan to address patient concerns needs to continue to assess the patients and their support systems for unexpected problems, changes, and successes, and troubleshoot or respond to changes in a timely and systematic way. Relative to the case example, efforts need to be used to minimize conflict between subsystems. In the case of Mr. Marco, the social worker would be sure to take the time to establish and maintain credibility (honest, ethical practice) and good public relations with him as well as all systems involved.

STEPS TOWARD EVIDENCE-BASED CASE MANAGEMENT

Bertsche and Horejsi's (1980) time-tested model for case management remains one of the most comprehensive models of case management available (Frankel & Gelman, 2012), but an evaluation strategy and measurement related directly to its efficiency and effectiveness is missing. A push toward evidence-based practice (EBP) in medicine, psychology, social work, nursing, and many other disciplines became prevalent after 1992 (Hjorland, 2011), and evidence and published peer reviewed research to show the effectiveness of case management, discharge planning and social work are still lacking (Ferguson & Schriver, 2012).

Steps toward evidence-based case management will be illustrated by describing micro, mezzo, and macro interventions (see "Interventions" Box) to build a stronger body of evidence-based studies on the effectiveness of case management. Because case management and discharge planning are complex processes including assessing the patient's physical and mental condition and social support, communicating with the multidisciplinary team, referrals to community, government, and financial programs *and* these tasks are done at times when the patient's condition or statuses may be changing

Interventions

Interventions at the micro level (the individual level for social workers): Consistent and thorough documentation that meets organizational requirements and addresses patient problems in measurable terms. Rapid assessment instruments may be used. Interventions are detailed specifically, and follow-up measures are done and results are recorded. Data are kept in a secure place and analyzed over time. From the data, recommendations are made and adjustments are made to practice for more successful interventions.

Interventions at the mezzo level (social worker and elements of their immediate environment): Social worker communicates the importance of EBP to employer and professional organization. Social workers can come together through the National Association of Social Workers (NASW) to discuss evidence-based strategies and practice evaluation, and how they can be done in settings throughout their community. Social worker also networks with Council on Social Work Education (CSWE) accredited BSW and MSW programs for assistance with evaluation and utilizes BSW and MSW students in placements for practice evaluation. At the mezzo level, BSW and MSW programs offer assistance to field instructors and practitioners to practice evaluation and reporting evidence-based results through presentations and publications. Social workers can also collaborate with other practitioners in their settings (nurses, medical doctors, counselors, and physical therapists) who do practice evaluation and show evidence of effectiveness of their practice.

Interventions at the macro level (state NASW, national NASW, universities, CSWE, and health care professional organizations): At the macro levels, direct practice social workers who support EBP can interface with their state chapter of the NASW, national NASW, universities, CSWE, and other health care and professional organizations. Also, of great importance, social work leadership (professional organizations, academic and professional social work programs, and executive directors) must take a look at the case management and discharge planning practice done in all organizations, and not only make recommendations for EBP, but assist them in taking these steps to further support what case managers and discharge planners do and how they can evaluate their practice. The Affordable Care Act (ACA), Hartford Partnership Program for Aging Education, Gero-Rich initiative, and the push for the Dorothy I. Height and Whitney M. Young, Jr. Reinvestment Act at the federal levels are mechanisms to support EBP in social work and discharge planning. Social workers and the leadership of the profession can utilize these to further advanced EBP. Only with this comprehensive effort at the micro, mezzo and macro levels can we move toward showing the effectiveness of case management and discharge planning. This is how we can continue to improve these important services that benefit so many.

and at a time in history where our community, government, and financial programs are declining, measuring the effectiveness of the intervention can be difficulty, and fraught with problems. Measuring the effectiveness of discharge planning may not be as simple as measuring the effectiveness of a blood pressure medication or a surgical procedure. That is why these steps are presented at the micro, mezzo, and macro levels and the interaction of these are needed to move toward evidence-based case management.

NURSES AND SOCIAL WORKERS AS CASE MANAGERS

Nurses continue to take a more assertive role in what used to be the domain of social work. Generally, nurses working in case management perform tasks similar to social work; however, more emphasis is placed on performing medical case management tasks such as patient/family education, infection control, quality management, pharmacy inventory, and teaching professional responsibilities, budgeting, and facilitating patient discharges (Bower, 1992; Hawkins, Veeder, & Pearce, 1998; Parsons et al., 2012; Snow, 2001). In general, nurse case managers focus on the medical condition of the patient, the patients insurance, and ensuring that hospital admissions and lengths of stay remain reasonable (Noetscher & Morreale, 2001). According to Holliman et al. (2003), the duties that are shared are attending meetings, documentation, outpatient responsibilities, budgeting, and facilitating patient discharges (see Tables 12.1 and 12.2). Nurses have a longer history of adapting and managing within the hospital structure (Holliman, 1998).

Table 12.1 Tasks of Hospital Discharge Planners: Social Workers and Nurses

Tasks of All Discharge Planners	
Ten tasks that 85% of the discharge planners performed frequently or almost always	
Task	Percent (%) that performed the task frequently or almost always
Coordinate services and patient discharge	96.0
Interview caregivers for assessment	95.0
Make contacts for referrals	92.2
Review record prior to contact	91.6
Reassure, support, and reduce anxiety	91.5
Establish rapport	90.4
Documentation	89.9
Review workload to set priorities	86.0

(continued)

Table 12.1 (*continued*)

Treatment team responsibilities	
Discuss discharge/treatment options with patients/caregivers	85.4

Tasks exclusive to social work and nursing	

Tasks performed frequently or almost always by 60% of discharge planners	

Task	Percent (%) that performed the task frequently or almost always
Performed by social workers	
Review records to ensure standards are met	75.4
Assess treatment plans and quality of care and service effectiveness	64.1
Performed by nurses	
Provide support to unpaid caregivers	63.3
Assess to see if mental health services are needed	63.3
Know current rules/policies	62.3
Gather, enter, and compile data for reports	62.2
Verify eligibility and insurance status	60.4
Educate patients about medical symptoms	60.3

Table 12.2 Comparison of Responsibilities in Addition to Discharge Planning Performed by Social Workers and Nurses

Social Workers	Nurses
Psychosocial assessments	
Initiate and implement advanced directives	Patient/family education
Child/elder-abuse screening	Insurance verification
High-risk screening	Infection Control
Substance abuse intervention	Employee health
Crisis intervention	Quality management
Individual/family therapy	Pharmacy inventory
Group therapy	Critical pathways

(*continued*)

Table 12.2 Comparison of Responsibilities in Addition to Discharge Planning
Performed by Social Workers and Nurses (*continued*)

Grief therapy	Teaching professionals
Employee assistance programs	Research
Conduct home visits	

Performed by both social workers and nurses
Attend meetings
Documentation
Treatment team responsibilities
Conduct in-service training for staff
Supervision
Outpatient responsibilities
Fundraising
Preparation for audits
Organ donation coordinator
Budgeting

Adapted from Holliman et al. (2003).

Although there are similarities in the roles of both the nurse case manager and the social worker, there are also differences. One basic difference is in philosophy where nurses are trained in the medical model and tend to perceive consumers as patients with a focus on concrete services; whereas, social workers are trained in the biopsychosocial model and often assume a more empowering stance and stress self-determination advocating on behalf of the patient as empowerment and self-determination are standards of the social work profession (NASW, 2008a).

With this different focus, it is not uncommon for conflicts to arise between these two disciplines. Some social workers feel that nurses focus too much on the medical needs of the patient, often ignoring the social needs, and some nurses may feel social workers spend too much time on social needs and do not have enough expertise in a patient's medical condition to make informed decisions (J. Jones, MSW, personal communication, July 16, 2012). Therefore, oftentimes when the nurse case manager determines a patient is medically ready to leave the hospital plans to initiate this process begin. Some social workers would argue; however, before this process can begin, "person-in-situation" and biopsychosocial issues need to be explored. For example, what type of support system does the patient have and are the members of the support system able to care for the patient? This must be evaluated before concrete plans can be made. For social workers, it is not uncommon for the social worker to expect to assess the patient's environment or situation prior to discharge. When this assessment is not done and limited supports are available, discharges can become complicated.

It is a delicate issue when a patient is to be discharged yet refuses to go to a nursing home when they are unable to handle their own activities of daily living (ADL) or their own affairs. The pressure remains great, however, for the case manager to push the patient out the door because there is a lack of coverage or a lack of cooperation from a payer source (Beaulieu, 2012). Every day that the patient stays in the hospital under these circumstances costs the hospital money and pressure for discharge will mount.

Is There a Difference?

In the broadest sense, a case manager is the person who makes the health care system work, influencing both the quality of the outcome and the cost (Frankel & Gelman, 2012). Roles are diverse but perhaps the case manager can facilitate an earlier more supported and stable discharge, negotiate a better fee from a medical equipment supplier, or encourage the family to assume responsibility for assistance with the day-to-day care of the patient. She can be a catalyst for change by seeking solutions that promote improvement or stabilization rather than simply monitoring patient status (Frankel & Gelman, 2012).

Most professionals agree that for the case manager to be best utilized in a medical setting well rounded, broad-based knowledge of all aspects of the hospital is expected (Easterling, Avie, Wesley, & Chimmer, 1995; Frankel & Gelman, 2012). Overall, it appears that social work case managers have contact with patients throughout their admission, and this is different from nurse case managers. Social workers see patients when they are admitted to the hospital to assess the patient's initial biopsychosocial needs. The social worker documents the needs of the patients and follows the patients throughout their entire hospital stay making sure that those needs are being met. The social worker may have to arrange for home health care for the patient, nursing home placement, medical equipment, hospice, transplants, or simply transportation for the patient (Holliman et al., 2003; Nelson & Powers, 2001). The social workers are often able to assess all of the previously stated needs in the short time they meet with the patient. The social worker takes into account the patients' desires, the patients' family's desires, the needs of the patient, the history of the patient, and the potential future of the patient.

The nurse case manager reviews the patients' charts, reviews the social workers, notes, and assesses the patients and their medical needs. The nurse's primary focus is business rather than health care (Noetscher & Morreal, 2001).

If the patient is medically ready to leave the hospital, the nurse advocates for the hospital making sure that the patient's length of stay is financially acceptable for the hospital (Taylor, 2002). The nurse can overlook the social and environmental needs of the patient; however, the social and environmental needs are what the social worker is trained to assess.

The social work case manager has a broader knowledge of the patient's needs and the nurse case manager has a broader knowledge of the hospital needs. At times, instead of working together to facilitate an efficient system, the social worker and nurse are pushing in opposite directions actually extending the stay of the patient and increasing the cost to the hospital (Ferguson & Schriver, 2012; Holliman et al., 2003; Hou, Hollenburg, & Charlson, 2001; Schuetze, 2006).

Income for social work and nurse case managers varies in different settings and across regions. However, in most settings, nurses doing case management make at least $10,000 more per year than social work case managers (H. Faisal, personal communication, August 14, 2012; Ferguson & Schriver, 2012; Hawkins et al., 1998; Holliman et al., 2003). Both social workers and nurses make contributions to case management and discharge planning. Social workers input and services is an effective means of shorting a patient's length of stay, and as a result, decreasing the cost to the hospital (Keefler, Duder, & Lechman, 2001). Nurse case managers also lessen the hospitals cost by facilitating a faster move of a patient out of the hospital when medically ready. Again, social workers and nurses may be doing the same type of work, but nurses are often compensated at a higher rate.In the future, more research is needed in trying to establish how to join social work and nursing and help them to work closer as a team. Enhanced teamwork would allow nurse case managers and social work case managers to use the resources and skills, inherent in each profession, toward the best interest of the patient. Allowing the nurse and the social worker to collaborate on each patient and each patient's needs will allow the team to facilitate an accurate, efficient, and useful discharge plan.

In closing, probably one of the biggest areas of contention with this group was in the area of salaries. This salary differential alone has created a rift between those working in the same role. More research is needed to see whether this is considered the norm and whether social workers should advocate for at a minimum "equal pay for equal work."

CHAPTER SUMMARY AND FUTURE DIRECTIONS

Case management in the behaviorally based managed care setting is an evolving art. Many new nurses and social workers are coming into case management and are surprised by the differences in job rules and responsibilities. Case management in the medical setting involves discharge planning from the hospital, placement in nursing homes, placement for rehabilitation, placement in a transitional care facility, or placement in a facility that the patient was in previously. Case management in a medical setting also involves providing patients with medical equipment, verifying insurance claims, and linking patients to community resources for support groups, educational groups, individual family or group therapy, and community resources to help a patient pay for hospital bills and/or medication (Beaulieu, 2012; Nelson & Powers, 2001).

What seems most unfortunate is that social workers are performing nurse components of the case management job; however, nurses are not performing social work components. This means that many times social workers are given the more difficult and time-consuming cases that require counseling or additional supports. These social workers were well versed in the knowledge of medical terms and procedures and financial information such as Medicare and Medicaid. They also need to be aware of community resources and what is needed to qualify for these services. The social worker needs to have background knowledge in mental health, mental illness, domestic violence, child abuse, drug and alcohol abuse, sexual abuse, and an overall understanding of how people live. All of these components are necessary to be able to help the patients who are served.

Furthermore, for case management teams to function more efficiently in the medical setting, the social worker needs to play a crucial role in getting all medical staff more involved in understanding the needs of the patients served. The social work case manager can also facilitate helping the patients to get their needs met as quickly and as accurately as possible. Medical social work is not for all social workers. Some professionals believe it is less "clinical" than traditional social work. Regardless, the roles and concrete skills provided by these social workers are rich in terms of recognizing what a patient needs and advocating and in many cases directly providing for those services from an individualized perspective. After all, historically, has not that been the clinical core of social work practice?

Glossary

Advocator   In case management and discharge planning, this role involves assessing, identifying and speaking out and completing actions designed to advocate for the patients' needs, and make recommendations that are in the best interest of a patient's safety, medical condition, self-interest, and biopsychosocial needs.

Assessor   In case management, this involves systematically reviewing patients records, talking to team members about their observations of the patients and their situations, interviewing patients, their family and available support networks, and synthesizing and evaluating this information to develop a biopsychosocial assessment for the patients' plan of care.

Broker and facilitator   In this role, the case manager makes referrals or links the patients and their support systems with health care services, social service organizations, government programs, and other appropriate resources.

Continuity of care   The process of continuing a patient's quality of care as they are referred to other levels of care and navigate through the health care system. Continuity of care is necessary today because length of stay in acute care settings is limited and patients are quickly discharged to a less restrictive and less expensive level of care. Continuity of care is a transdisciplinary process that includes the patients, their families, and support systems. Communication, relationship building, coordination, sharing of patient information while following HIPAA and other privacy standards, integration of care, follow-up, and evaluation are components of continuity of care.

Crisis intervention   A method of helping patients to deal with a crisis is a sudden state of instability or danger and upheaval that leads to disequilibrium.

Discharge planning   This is considered a subsection or task within case management that involves facilitating the placement from one level of care to another.

Evaluator   In this role, the case managers examine and measure their therapeutic progress with the patient, their own practice, and the practice of their programs to ascertain whether they are meeting their goals or outcomes. Evaluation is a service provided to measure improvement looking at efficiency (the ratio of costs (time/effort/financial costs) to outcome) as well as effectiveness.

Geriatric care manager   A private practice professional who specializes in helping families who are caring for older relatives. A Geriatric care manager can be a nurse, social worker, gerontologist, or psychologist. See www.caremanager.org/

Handover   Working closely with patients, their families, support systems, and the network of agencies and organizations that provide services to them to improve the efficiency, quality, and productivity of services as patients move through the health care system. The term "handover" is commonly used in European countries to describe this process. See www.handover.eu/

Health care advocates Inc   www.healthcareadvocates.com/ is an example of a private nationwide company that can connect people with physical and mental health–related issues with the appropriate and necessary services. Health care advocates often locate specialists for people and negotiate with insurance companies to access health and mental health services and payment for them.

Negotiator   As a negotiator, the case manager assists individuals, programs, organizations, and communities in making compromises that benefit the patient and those in their support system or a referral source.

Nurse case managers   Generally, nurse case managers review charts and assess for medical needs. The primary tasks include patient/family education, insurance verification, infection control, employee health, quality management, pharmacy inventory, critical pathways, teaching professionals, and research.

Recidivism   Readmission or relapse. In case management and discharge planning, recidivism refers to when a person has been treated in a hospital or other level of care and then returns there with the same diagnosis or problem. Recidivism can indicate that the person was not adequately treated the first time, and recidivism is usually much more costly than primary and secondary prevention.

Record keeper   In case management, record keeping involves documenting what is necessary for meeting organizational standards and the requirements of payers of services (e.g., insurance companies, Medicare, and Medicaid), while also documenting patient care and service delivery. Record keepers must keep patient data in a format that is organized, available for the agency, and secure (confidential). Today most record keeping is done on computers and in a format that meets the organization's standards.

Social work case managers   Generally, social work case managers complete psychosocial assessments, patient/family education, initiate and implement advanced directives, child/elder abuse screening, high-risk screening, substance abuse intervention, crisis intervention, individual/family therapy, group therapy, grief therapy, employee assistance programs, and conduct home visits.

Tracker, managing follow-up and self-sustainment   In case management tracking, managing follow-up and patient self-sustainment involves activities such as follow-up calls, home visits, surveys, or annual appointments to determine whether the patients are still meeting their goals, improving, or whether they need additional services.

Transdisciplinary team   A health or mental health care team composed of members of different professions who cooperate across disciplines to improve patient care.

Questions for Further Study

1. Define social work case management and the social work role in discharge planning. What tasks in case management and discharge planning are uniquely provided by the social worker as opposed to the nurse? How does social work's role differ from that of nursing in terms of the functions performed? What is the physician's role? Develop your definitions clearly and concisely, then meet in small groups in class to discuss your definitions,

and work to come to a consensus on definitions for case management and discharge planning.

2. Conduct a literature review from a social work or a nursing database (or both) and find a study that shows the effectiveness of case management or discharge planning in health care. What are the research questions in this study? What population is studied? What is the intervention? What are the outcomes?

3. Brainstorm with classmates to come up with a study to show the cost effectiveness of discharge planning or case management social work. How would you go about implementing this study in an agency? What do you think the obstacles would be in implementing this study? What would be the opportunities from this study?

CHAPTER 13

Prevention, Wellness Counseling, and Complementary and Alternative Medicine

Sophia F. Dziegielewski
and George A. Jacinto

Health and wellness counseling involves strategies that health care professionals can offer individuals to assist them in maintaining good health while also improving unhealthy conditions in order to prevent illness or disease. The inclusion of complementary and alternative medicine (CAM) with an emphasis on wellness and health is often associated with the medical model in a number of health care settings (Freeman, 2009; Lake & Spiegel, 2007), and fits well with both the strengths based and holistic approaches of social work.

In health care settings throughout history, health and wellness interventions have remained a popular counseling methodology. This type of service was often viewed as an adjunct to other methods of intervention, but with the influence of coordinated care and the paradigm shifts that have occurred in social work and medicine, interest in providing and receiving this type of counseling has become an expected part of practice.

As the population lives longer and medical technologies improve, living with chronic pain has increasingly become a reality for many people. At the same time, there has been an increasing awareness that traditional Western medicine alone may not be able to address patients' needs, and combination approaches can supplement treatment needed because patients often develop a trust with the provider. Suggestibility rankings with the use of placebos and positive interactions with patients can encourage relief and healing. This can be seen at the forefront of developing a relations strategy that welcomes interaction and teamwork. Ellner and Woods (2012) emphasize the importance of building hope while empowering Patients to manage their own flight-or-fight responses. In a supportive role, whether this service is provided directly to patients/clients/consumers (hereafter referred to as patients) or to fellow members of the interdisciplinary team, social workers are making vital contributions in this expanding role for health care practitioners.

The discussion that follows will be concerned with prevention, followed by wellness counseling, and then the various CAM approaches currently used in health care. Each aspect of wellness counseling will be discussed from the perspective of the social work practitioner. The last section of the chapter will include aspects of CAM and its relevance to social work practice.

PREVENTION

Health awareness programs seek to promote wellness as well as prevent health problems from becoming worse. Therefore, prevention is an essential part of wellness counseling. For example, in planning prevention approaches, practitioners study the research that predicts the approximate number of preventable or avoidable deaths that will occur each year. The leading factors attributed to the causes of death in the United States in 2000 were heart disease, neoplasm, cerebrovascular disease, respiratory tract disease, injuries, diabetes mellitus, influenza and pneumonia, Alzheimer's disease, nephritis, and septicemia (JAMA, 2004). These conditions lead to increased health care expenses, thus disease prevention is clearly an overall health care cost-reduction strategy. The actual causes for all deaths in the United States in 1990 and 2000 included tobacco, poor diet, physical inactivity, alcohol consumption, microbial agents, toxic agents, motor vehicle accidents, firearms, sexual behavior, and illicit drug use (JAMA, 2004).

According to the Centers for Disease Control and Prevention, preventable chronic diseases accounted for approximately "75 percent of two trillion dollars spent on health care in 2005" (Prevention and Wellness, 2007, p. 1). Prevention has been divided into three areas that are based on the degree of involvement that is needed for effective intervention. The first type of prevention is referred to as *primary prevention*. This direct form of intervention reduces the susceptibility of individuals to disease (Burger & Youkeles, 2000). It is here that most directed health education strategies fall. The emphasis is on educating individuals so that they will be less likely to engage in health-defeating behaviors. Examples of primary prevention programs are those designed to achieve better community sanitation or warn the population of the danger of cigarette smoking. Other examples can include sex education in the schools or any other programs designed to prevent conditions from occurring.

The second type of prevention is referred to as *secondary prevention*. These approaches are designed and employed for early detection before irreversible damage has occurred (Burger & Youkeles, 2000). In secondary prevention, a problem is identified, and later a strategy is employed to keep it from spreading. Secondary prevention requires active case finding on the part of the health care social worker. This ensures that the effects of the condition are minimized and the spread to other individuals, families, or communities is minimal. The duty of the social worker to initiate early intervention practices is considered essential. For example, when working with HIV-infected patients, secondary prevention strategies are crucial in helping the patient learn how to address, identify, and educate the patient to factors that will reduce the spread.

The third type of prevention is referred to as *tertiary prevention*. In tertiary prevention, the goal is to manage disease to minimize disability (Burger & Youkeles, 2000). This type of prevention is often addressed in rehabilitative/restorative inpatient and outpatient settings. In this form of prevention, the health care social worker helps a patient who has already experienced the problem to recuperate or recover from it. In addition to direct clinical intervention of the problem, the social worker must also focus on building strengths in the patient to assist him or her if the problem is exacerbated. Although prevention is a constitutive aspect of health and wellness counseling, there are also other elements that are associated with this form of counseling.

WELLNESS COUNSELING

Generally, when most professionals think of wellness counseling, they think of providing it to individual patients; however, this type of counseling can be more inclusive and involve an individual, family, group, or community. In today's environment, the need for wellness counseling is expanding. In the past, wellness counseling was usually thought of as the domain of the public health social worker, however, it has expanded to include other social work settings such as community-based agencies. Although a number of approaches have been suggested, most incorporate the "whole" person in the context of the individual's environment as the focus of intervention. The goal of the wellness counseling approach is to assist individuals in planning to live more fully by integrating body, mind, and spirit in a meaningful manner (Smith et al., 2002).

Many health care professionals are now being called on to provide one-to-one counseling in this area and to provide workshops and other forms of health maintenance and awareness services. Community-focused health promotion programming involves group as well as individual strategies. Many times social workers are challenged to provide educational information as part of the counseling dimensions of wellness programming. For instance, one may provide a seminar on wellness and then meet with small groups or individuals to assist individuals in applying the newly learned information to their life routines.

Areas for this holistic type of specialized education and counseling vary from assisting with weight reduction programs and smoking cessation programs to providing information and techniques that address stress management. Wellness counseling offers social workers another area for expansion that will help many social workers do what they really like—provide counseling. A holistic approach to wellness counseling requires one to perceive the patient in the environment paying attention to factors, which include interpersonal exchanges and environmental conditions that impinge on the individual's functioning. The environment comprises one's family, neighborhood, employment setting, and the larger community. The interactions of many people in the community affect the health and well-being of entire population.

Although wellness promotion has been primarily used with middle-class White Patients, a shift toward use in poor ethnic neighborhoods has shown success as well. For instance, The Well, a neighborhood-based health promotion for Black women located in a housing project in central Los Angeles provided an office for a nurse practitioner with a database for scheduling clinic visits with hospitals and health practitioners; an exercise and fitness room; and lounge/library (Brown, Jemmott, Mitchell, & Walton, 1998). The services of The Well included self-help groups, health education, a walking-for-wellness program, facts and feelings workshops, exercise classes, family planning, birthing project, prevention, economic development activities, "sister circles," and health advocacy services. The Well employed the use of social work counseling and empowerment techniques, ownership of the program by neighborhood residents, a convenient neighborhood-based location, a working relationship with a university, and a number of community partnerships.

Social workers can also enter into partnerships with formal health counseling programs and can assist in providing professional services. For example, *employee assistance programs* (EAPs) have gained tremendous popularity. The advantages for health care agencies and providers to support these types of intervention with their workers are apparent. It is beyond the scope of this chapter to explain the historical and current role of social work in EAPs; however, its relevance and applicability is important for establishing further marketability of health care social work.

Whether this service is provided directly to patients or fellow employees, there are three specific benefits that social workers who engage in the provision of wellness counseling can provide. First, social workers have expertise in working and integrating the behavioral biopsychosocial–spiritual factors related to an individual and can use their expertise to demonstrate how these factors can positively affect health and wellness. Maintenance of health and wellness includes is a number of multifaceted tasks such as individual and group counseling, family planning, prevention efforts, economic development activities, community organization, advocacy, empowerment, psychoeducational workshops, marketing, and exercise classes to name a few (Brenner, 2002; Myers, Sweeney, & Witmer, 2000). These tasks are inter-related social work approaches that are well-suited for the trained social work professional who can understand and incorporate these factors into the overall intervention process.

Second, social workers are skilled in counseling and understanding individual and family dynamics. Many times social workers facilitate the instruction of health education when the simple presentation of informa-tion is not enough. Patients may need the additional assistance that only a trained professional can interpret and provide. For example, a patient was recently diagnosed with adult-onset diabetes. He was immediately referred for health and dietary advice because the physician wanted to initiate a trial of dietary control before placing him on medications. After numerous fail-ures for the patient to self-regulate dietary needs, a referral to the health care social worker was made. On interviewing the patient, it became obvious to the social worker that the patient knew exactly what he was supposed to eat and why. The dietary education that was provided appeared adequate. In exploring this further, it appeared as though the patient was angry over his diagnosis and in a misguided way was rebelling against it. In addition, he stated that he did not prepare the meals, his wife did. When asked how he felt about his diet, the patient stated that, "I tell my wife what to cook and she doesn't listen."

In this situation, the social worker was able to help the patient rec-ognize the need to resolve issues regarding acceptance of his own medical limitations and vulnerability. She also invited the patient's wife to attend an intervention session, and together they discussed the implications of his diabetes, and how it was affecting their relationship. At the conclusion of the session, the social worker helped to arrange for the wife and the patient to both meet with the dietitian one more time. After two meetings with the social worker, diet compliance improved significantly and the patient was able to maintain his condition without medication supplementation. This example helps to explicate how the social worker can be a valuable asset in recognizing individual problems and family considerations that could other-wise impede progress.

A third area, which is probably the most important, is that social workers are trained in formal diagnosis, assessment, and intervention. If individuals are experiencing a mental health problem that is beyond their control, the social worker has the capability to address it or refer as appropriate. Schools of social work generally train social workers in the basics of diagnosis, assess-ment, and intervention planning. In practice, these skills are adapted to assist the patient who is intervention noncompliant or in need of attaining more involved health and wellness services. Social workers who are part of the interdisciplinary health team are also trained in this area and can easily adapt to provide this service. Because rapport with patients is seen as essential in social work practice, the development of this process can be further used to allow patients to feel more comfortable and be able to address intervention issues in a quicker or possibly more efficient manner.

Another benefit for inclusion of social work in wellness counseling is a logistic one. Social workers are already part of the health care delivery team. Although agencies may recognize the need for employee assistance, agencies may not have the economic resources to hire someone to provide counseling services. Using clinical social workers who are already familiar with a program and the health care setting can allow health care agencies and service providers to dispense services to their own employees incurring a limited cost.

Finally is the importance the social worker can have in recognizing and initiating self-care strategy for the self and the team. This need for self-awareness and wellness counseling is highlighted with recognition of *vicarious traumatization*. In this phenomena, helping professionals who work with individuals in crisis are repeatedly exposed to trauma through vicarious (i.e., imagining what it is like) means. Many times health care professionals are exposed to individuals who have been *traumatized* and who are repeatedly exposed to the details that surround the trauma. Therefore, the health care provider experiences repeated episodes of trauma through helping the victim (Figley, 1995). In some cases, the helpers themselves may also need assistance with letting the trauma go after helping the victim to deal with it.

Several examples of this include the emergency department team who try to save the life of a child but cannot; the paramedics who must assist in several tragic events in the course of their day to include multiple traffic accidents, drownings, suicides, or homicide attempts; the hospice worker who continually cares for the terminally ill patient; and so forth. Programs for debriefing of health care professionals have been formulated (Pack, 2012); the role of social workers in facilitating this type of "stress-debriefing" or identification of critical incidents in the group setting have been recognized (Pack, 2012).

Awareness in Wellness Counseling

The key task that will increase awareness in wellness counseling is in assisting individuals to become cognizant of what factors are important to maintaining their own health and wellness. The purpose of health promotion counseling programs is to help communicate needed information that will assist individuals in making needed changes; in using this information to develop self-help skills to empower them to address health needs; and to gain access to the techniques or technologies that can help them to meet their needs. This makes health care social work a service that cannot be underestimated. In addition, the social worker can enhance wellness education and skill building by adding therapeutic counseling designed to address barriers that might impede progress.

Implementation of Wellness Counseling

Once health care social workers are made aware of the process of wellness counseling—the theoretical underpinnings and the strategies necessary for patient success—they develop necessary skills and are more prepared to provide formal training, assistance, support, and direct counseling services in numerous health settings. A few of the many areas for health education and maintenance activities in wellness counseling include weight control, cigarette smoking, health and nutrition, sex education, parenthood, preparation for childbirth, family member or significant other illness, terminal illness, and eventually preparation and acceptance of one's own death or the death of others.

The factors that motivate patients to seek and initiate wellness counseling can vary. Many times the symptoms a patient is experiencing may be the reason the individual seeks health care counseling. Kurtz and Chalfant (1991) warn, however, that symptom identification alone may not be enough to initiate help-seeking behavior. In support of this contention, they remind us that only a small proportion of individuals who suffer from health problems actually seek intervention.

In understanding patient help-seeking behavior, it is not only the psychological, anatomical, or biological factors that influence action toward seeking help. It is primarily the psychosocial influences that reflect the patient's daily life as a social human being (Kurtz & Chalfant, 1991). Therefore, social workers need to be mindful that in implementing a health-counseling approach to practice—providing educational information alone is not enough. Interaction between the social worker and the patient, which focuses on the development of specific skills, is highlighted. In health coun seling, the social worker provides psychoeducational intervention in combi nation with the development of concrete skills to address problem behaviors. There are three basic areas that generally constitute the process of health counseling: (a) educational skill building; (b) personal control; and (c) the social environment (Lewis, Sperry, & Carlson, 1993).

Understanding the Dynamics in Wellness Counseling

There are several educational strategies that can assist the health care social worker in providing education as part of wellness counseling. The provision of health education is essential in helping to shape the beliefs of adults while using this knowledge to build motivation for self-change.

To facilitate implementation of the educational process, Chapman (1994) suggests the following strategies. First, when trying to educate someone, use the following three-step strategy: show, discuss, and apply. The goal here is to create an environment where experiential learning can occur. When individuals understand the basics and can see how it is applied, they are able to adjust to the new behavior and incorporate it more quickly (Plescia, Koontz, &

Laurent, 2001). For example, to teach patients to use relaxation training or the technique of deep breathing to relieve stress, there are many stress-reduction tapes available that depict this technique. Yet, none of these marketed tapes is considered the first choice for educating the patient in the technique. In practice, the social worker has the flexibility to customize the experience for the patient, which, in turn, facilitates learning. To educate an individual in the process of deep breathing, whether in an individual or group session, first the process is discussed; second, the benefits of the technique and the uniqueness of these benefits to the patient are emphasized; third, the social worker has the ability to customize the education program to meet the needs of those involved. Simply stated, explaining stress-reduction techniques and the process of deep breathing; demonstrating how it can be completed; and assisting the individual to apply the techniques in a protective and supportive environment can help an individual to understand the process quickly.

A second educational strategy to assist with health and wellness counseling is "repetitive exposure to the information" (Chapman, 1994). This is based on the simple premise that the more times individuals hear something, the more likely they are to remember and apply it. This makes repeating and reemphasizing key points a necessity. The technique of summarization should always be applied. If interested, the reader is advised to read the explanation of this technique as presented in the chapter on time-limited intervention. Basically, in this technique, the patient is asked to summarize at the beginning and the end of the session what occurred. The use of this technique incorporates the principle of repetition in the educational learning format. Furthermore, it also stresses that the patients summarize the session in their own words. The actual self-stating of the goals and objectives covered in a session can help the patient assimilate more quickly. Whether it is a formal therapeutic session or a brief encounter, repeating what was covered or what is expected to be completed can help to clear up misunderstandings or misinterpretations that might otherwise impede change-behavior.

The third technique to facilitate education is to always remember to teach an individual through small increments of change (Chapman, 1994). When physicians are trained to use medications with older adults, the common practice is "dose low and go slow." The same principle applies here. Dose low, by keeping the steps small and go slow, watching the patients and ensuring that they are following the plan developed with the social worker.

The fourth strategy involves emphasis on the benefit to be gained by participating in the program. Clear goals, objectives, and outcomes-based criteria will help. In addition, these goals and objectives must be reviewed periodically to ensure that adequate progress is being made. Individuals are more likely to stick to a program when they believe it can benefit their lives by reducing their susceptibility to disease or illness.

The fifth strategy involves maximizing and directing session time to facilitate education. Oftentimes, reading material or note-taking can reinforce what is learned. In the health-counseling encounter, this is often not possible; therefore, it is not uncommon for the social worker actually to have handouts or notes prepared for the patient. Oftentimes, handouts are used that stress the basic points of what was covered. They can also serve to reinforce the factors presented in the time-limited encounter. It is important to understand the dynamics of health counseling in order to develop more effective interventions for patients. In addition, the holistic paradigm is a model that may accompany dynamic approaches and will further enhance patient success.

A Holistic Model for Wellness Counseling

The person-in-environment (PIE) perspective of social work and the systems perspective are essential elements in the holistic approach to social work practice (Canda & Furman, 2010). In the area of wellness counseling, the person (biopsychosocial-spiritual)-in-environment must be taken into consideration when developing effective interventions with patients.

The use of educational strategies can be found in the work of Myers et al. (2000), who developed what they call *The Wheel of Wellness* which incorporates 16 characteristics of healthy individuals. These characteristics are illustrated graphically on four concentric circles and spokes. The four circles have within them the following five life tasks: (a) spirituality, (b) self-direction, (c) work and leisure, (d) friendship, and (e) love. Myers et al. suggest that a practitioner can use the wheel in counseling through four phases as follows: (a) by using a lifespan focus to introduce the concepts of the Wheel of Wellness model; (b) by conducting an assessment of the individual using the five life tasks; (c) by implementing interventions designed to enhance wellness in selected areas of the wheel; and (d) by providing ongoing evaluation of progress, follow-up, and continuation as needed of phases (b) through (d) mentioned earlier. A number of communities can benefit from this and other models of wellness. Furthermore, the provision of health promotion in poor and ethnic communities may require more nuanced approaches.

Community Intervention for Health Promotion in Poor and Ethnic Communities

Brenner (2002) and Auslander, Haire-Joshu, Houston, Williams, and Krebill (2000) describe several successful wellness-promotion programs within three ethnic communities. Brenner directed the East Harlem Healthy Heart program using a community intervention model that focused on multiple risk factors. The various aspects of the approach included the following: (a) targeting members of the community who reported multiple risk factors such as a high fat and cholesterol diet, hypertension, and smoking; (b) targeting every segment of the community with information about the project that included churches, schools, associations, retail outlets, supermarkets, tenant associations, day care centers, mass media, and elected officials; (c) developing community ownership and involvement in the health promotion programs; (d) volunteer recruitment and training; and (e) social marketing strategies. In addition, the study provides insights into ways in which both lay and professional communities can effectively work together.

Auslander et al. (2000) reported that the use of health promotion that individually targeted the intervention material in combination with community organization techniques demonstrated potential in reducing the risk of diet-related diseases among African American women. The practice of health promotion among poor and ethnic communities offers unique challenges for practitioners to creatively address needs. Another aspect of health counseling is time-limited brief intervention that is effective with a range of populations.

Time-Limited Wellness Counseling

Health counseling as a form of time-limited intervention is different from traditional psychotherapy. Acknowledgment of these differences is the first step in getting health care social workers to become more comfortable in implementing this as a practice strategy. First, wellness counseling, similar to other time-limited interventions, is more action oriented than traditional psychotherapy. Patients are expected to participate actively and engage in motivated self-change behavior to achieve intervention success. If reduction in health risk requires lifestyle changes, participation is essential. To make these lifestyle changes, the social worker must be skilled in how to initiate the patient change process and maintain it.

Second, wellness counseling, similar to the other forms of time-limited intervention, is always brief in duration. Third, and somewhat different from most other forms of social work intervention, is that the primary focus of intervention should always lead to prevention. Last, in traditional psychotherapy, rapport is an ongoing and building process; in health counseling, however, it must be established in the first session. In this method, rapport in itself is only important because it can be used to help facilitate change behavior.

Methods for Time-Limited Wellness Counseling
Lewis et al. (1993) establish the following three criteria for initiating the practice of health counseling: (a) complete a functional assessment; (b) identify personal or change interest; and (c) establish the expected outcome. In establishing a functional assessment, the social worker tries to understand the patient's present health behaviors in terms of the personal and contextual factors. Many times formal assessment procedures, such as a complete social and developmental history, are not practical. When this occurs, a more basic assessment can suffice. From a limited perspective, information about personality style, health beliefs, current level of functioning, and past or current coping behaviors, can assist in formulating a plan. It is also important to assess someone's level of knowledge regarding the

problem and whether the patient is open to change. To start the assessment processes ask the patient the following:

* Does _____ interfere with your daily life? (Name the problem.) If so, how?

Once the problem and/or concerns are identified, assess the patient's interest to initiate change. At this stage of the assessment process, the shift will occur from identifying the problem or concern to what can be done to address it. Focus is placed on clearly identifying the problem or concern along with strategies for addressing it. What is the patient willing to do to change it? Have all possibilities been explored to help make identification of the problem concrete and measurable?

Start with the following question:

* What do you believe is causing the problem or concern? Are there multiple causes or are the patients simply not sure where to begin in defining what they are experiencing?

From an evidence-based perspective, the last questions to be asked in the assessment need to focus on resolution and achieving an expected outcome. Here the individual is assessed to see how willing, realistic, and open the patient is to the change process suggested. Questions to establish this inquiry include the following:

* What specific changes do you expect to make?
* When do you expect to accomplish this?
* What can I (the social worker) do to support you in developing a plan to address your concerns?

COMPLEMENTARY AND ALTERNATIVE MEDICINE

According to the NIH, more than 83 million adult Americans have used some form of CAM in association with medical care (NCCAM, 2012a). In order to more effectively work with individuals, it is important for social workers to become familiar with the types of CAM and its relationship to various physical and mental disorders (Nahin, Barnes, Stussman, & Bloom, 2009). The National Center for Complementary and Alternative Medicine (NCCAM) of the NIH defines CAM as "a group of diverse medical and health care systems, practitioners, and products that are not presently considered to be part of conventional medicine" (NCCAM, 2011). The NCCAM (2012a) divided the many modalities into the following five distinct categories: (a) alternative medical systems, (b) mind–body interventions; (c) biologically based treatments; (d) manipulative and body-based methods, and

(e) energy therapies (see Table 13.1 for details). To find information about current research in this area, refer to the NIH NCCAM website (www.nccam. nih.gov/health) for lists of evidence-based studies and literature reviews related to a range of CAM modalities.

Table 13.1 Complementary and Alternative Medicine

Alternative medical systems

Acupuncture—procedures involving stimulation of anatomical points on the body by a variety of techniques that include penetrating the skin with thin, solid, and metallic needles that are manipulated by the hands or by electrical stimulation.

Ayurveda—uses *pranayama* (alternate nostril breathing), *abhyanga* (rubbing skin with oil, usually sesame), *rasayana* (herbs and mantras during meditation), yoga, *panchakarma* (intense cleansing therapy including diaphoretics, diuretics, cathartics, and emetics), and herbal remedies.

Environmental medicine—focuses on the effect of chemicals, such as pesticides, food preservatives, car exhaust fumes, and formaldehyde, on the immune system. Uses nutritional supplements, immunotherapy, and desensitization.

Homeopathy—uses homeopathic (minute doses of herb, mineral, or animal products) remedies as catalysts to aid body's inherent healing mechanism. Correct remedy treats the physical, emotional, and mental symptoms.

Naturopathy—holistic approach using homeopathy, vitamin and mineral supplements, physiotherapy, TCM, stress management, and herbs.

Traditional Chinese medicine (TCM)—uses herbs, acupuncture, acupressure (shiatsu, *tsabu, jin shin,* and jujitsu), and physical exercise like *t'ai chi chian* or *qigong.*

Traditional healers

    Botanica—store that deals in herbs and charms associated with the Santeria religion.

    Curandero—healer or shaman from Central America who uses herbal medicines.

    Espiritista—Mexican American healer who performs exorcisms and uses the help of kind spirits and removes malicious spirits.

    Hierbero or *Yerbera*—uses knowledge of the medicinal qualities of plants.

    Native Mexican Healer or Medicine Man or Bruja—acts as a mediator between the "spirit world" and the community in order to cure illness or provide spiritual guidance.

    Shaman—acts as a medium between the invisible spiritual world and the physical world, and performs tasks such as divination, influencing natural events, and healing the sick or injured.

    Sobador—treatments include the use of massage and other rubbing techniques.

Mind–body therapies

Biofeedback—relaxation technique to enable people to gain control over autonomic responses, such as heart rate, blood pressure, and voluntary muscle contractions.

Deep breathing exercises—involve slow and deep breathing through the nose, usually to a count of 10, followed by slow and complete exhalation for the count of 10.

Energy healing—practitioner uses hands to channel of healing energy through the hand to the patient's body to restore a normal energy balance.

Guided Imagery—a series of relaxation techniques followed by the visualization of detailed images, usually calm and peaceful in nature. If used for treatment, the individuals will visualize their body free of the specific problem or condition.

Hypnotherapy—technique of focused attention; especially helpful for pain management, addictions, and phobias.

Magnetic fields—the use of electromagnetic fields where the practitioner focuses energy on specific areas of the body.

(continued)

Table 13.1 (*continued*)

Progressive relaxation—involves systematically tensing and relaxing muscle groups from the top of the head to the bottom of the feet. This form of relaxation is used to relieve tension and stress.

Qi gong—Ancient Chinese practice that includes gentle physical manipulation, mental focus, and deep breathing focusing on specific parts of the body. The prescribed exercises are performed two or more times per week.

Reiki—Originating in Japan, this energy medicine method involves the placing of hands on or near the person with the intent to transfer *ki,* believed to be the life force. Distance healing is also included in this practice.

Tai chi—Originated in China as a martial art. The practice involves slow and gentle body movements in combination with deep breathing and meditation.
Therapeutic touch

Yoga—the practice of yoga involves a combination of physical postures, paired with breathing exercises, and meditation to calm the nervous system, and balance body, mind, and spirit.

Relaxation techniques—autogenic training, progressive muscle relaxation, and meditation.

Manipulative and body-based therapies

Chiropractic—diagnoses and treats illnesses that affect the nerves, muscles, bones, and joints by relieving pressure through manipulation.

Massage—lymphatic massage, neuromuscular (deep tissue) massage, and rolfing (facial manipulation)

Osteopathy—uses diagnostic and treatment techniques similar to medical practitioners, but also treats the musculoskeletal system with adjustive maneuvers.

Movement therapies—focuses on the relationship between the musculoskeletal system and body movement.
Alexander technique—corrects muscle and joint coordination, balance, and ease of movement.
Feldenkreis (improves coordination and increases awareness of bodily functions involved with movement), and
Pilates—a movement therapy using physical exercise to strengthen and control muscles, especially those used for posture. Awareness of breathing and control of movements are integral components of pilates.
Trager psychophysical integration—a movement therapy that applies a series of gentle, rhythmic rocking movements to the joints. They also teach physical and mental self-care exercises to reinforce the proper movement of the body.

Biologically based therapies

Botanical medicine—herbs are prescribed for specific symptoms.

Chelation therapy—a chemical process that binds together molecules, such as metals or minerals, in order for them to be removed from the body. Chelation can rid the body of toxic metals.

Diet-based therapies—each of the following dietary labels have specific practices that can be found at the hyperlinks provided below.
Vegetarian diet—www.mayoclinic.com/health/vegetarian-diet/HQ01596
Macrobiotic diet—www.cancer.org/Treatment/TreatmentsandSideEffects/ComplementaryandAlternativeMedicine/DietandNutrition/macrobiotic-diet
Atkins diet—www.atkins.com/Home.aspx
Pritkin diet—www.pritikin.com/
Ornish diet—www.everydiet.org/diet/ornish-diet
Zone diet—www.zonediet.com/
South Beach diet—www.southbeachdiet.com/diet/
Megavitamin—berkeley.edu/news/media/releases/2002/04/04_vitam1.html

(*continued*)

Table 13.1 Complementary and Alternative Medicine (*continued*)

Biologically based therapies

Nutritional supplements—deficiencies are determined through blood, stool, urine, and hair analyses. Adverse reactions between medications and supplements can occur.

Orthomolecular medicine—uses mega doses of supplements; found useful for hypercholesterolemia and AIDS.

Osteopathy—uses diagnostic and treatment techniques similar to medical practitioners, but also treats the musculoskeletal system with adjustive maneuvers.

Information obtained from Dunne & Phillips (2010) Integrative Medicine Communications (1998) Nahin et al. (2009) NCCAM (2012b).

For many mental health care social workers, there has been a pronounced movement toward helping patients to take charge of their own mental and medical health. In accepting this responsibility is the underlining premise that good health needs to involve the promotion of health and maintaining wellness. For many individuals, this involves exploring nontraditional types of treatment and intervention using traditional, alternative, and complementary or integrative approaches to achieving health and wellness. It can also include medications, herbs, vitamins, minerals, and the new so-called functional foods to enhance and support an individual's well-being. Knowledge of these products has become a practice reality as patients use these interventions and preparations as a means to gain greater control over health and well-being.

For health care social workers, creating effective, efficient, and comprehensive helping relationships require that social workers keep abreast of all types of intervention. When conducting assessment, it is important to document all methods and treatments that patients use and to verify that patients have informed their health care providers of the treatments, supplements, and medications they are using. This is necessary because some natural supplements may have a negative impact when taken with prescription medications.

Practice Strategy

Medical treatments in this country remain varied and can range from home remedies shared among family and friends to medications that are prescribed by a physician. Basically, there are two primary approaches to the delivery of medical care as follows: traditional mainstream medicine and CAM. Historically, in this country, the most traditional and widely used form of medicine involves standard drug therapies and surgical interventions. This type of *traditional mainstream medicine* and the practices that reflect this type of intervention strategy clearly require the skill of a trained professional and are generally referred to as mainstream American medical practice.

Today, the majority of physicians in this country share the traditional mainstream medicine philosophical approach and have been trained primarily in this area. But this may pose a problem because patients using CAM may be reluctant to tell their physician about supplements they are taking or alternative therapies they are receiving. Furthermore, they may believe that their physician is not knowledgeable enough about alternative therapies and is not an expert on the patient's individual needs. Heart disease, for example, has been conventionally treated through surgery that entails an extensive risk such as stroke or heart attack that could occur during the operation itself. Many individuals today are electing not to have this invasive procedure at all and choosing to utilize an alternative treatment consisting of a low-fat vegetarian diet, stress management, moderate exercise, and individual and group counseling (McCall, 1998). For some of these patients, it appears that this less-invasive method works effectively and provides a reasonable alternative to the more invasive surgical procedure that was usually performed.

Those professionals who practice medicine, regardless of whether they specialize in traditional approaches or newer, holistic methods, often agree that when traditionally based medical interventions have been proven to work, it is best to use them (Stehlin, 1995). For example, in childhood leukemia, conventional therapies can yield an 80% cure rate; therefore, it would seem unreasonable to switch to something that was not considered to have as reasonable a chance of success. Generally, however, this is not the type of patient who will leave traditional medicine. Rather, it is the person who suffers from a complicated or chronic condition or one for whom allopathic remedies have not been effective enough. In this case, the patient is tired of receiving minimal relief and wants a new and different "get and stay well" approach. For so many individuals whose symptoms cannot be relieved or controlled by conventional medicine, pain-free or symptom-free relief is so seductive that they will quickly drop the more conventional therapies in favor of alternative ones.

A second approach to medical care that has recently gained in popularity is CAM. In this approach, patients generally receive traditional approaches to therapy such as prescription medications, augmented or supplemented by alternative approaches. In this method, a combination approach is explored. According to Stehlin (1995), most alternative approaches are often described as any medical practice or intervention that is utilized instead of conventional treatment that lacks sufficient documentation in regard to its safety and effectiveness against certain diseases and conditions, is generally not taught in United States medical schools, and is generally not reimbursable by health insurance providers (p. 10).

CAM practices and products that are generally not considered part of conventional medicine (NCCAM, 2011) include such techniques as touch therapy, Reiki, massage (e.g., acupressure), chiropractic, magnets, herbals, and naturopathic remedies. Techniques that allow for mind and body control such as herbal preparations and spiritual healing are also used.

See Table 13.1, for a summary and quick reference for some of the different alternative approaches. When patients express interest in this type of therapy, it is important for social workers to encourage their patients to utilize the services of alternative practitioners who are licensed or certified. However, it is important to stress that patients need to keep their physicians informed of herbal or other supplements and treatments they are receiving.

Considerations and Concerns

In 2007, 40% of Americans used CAM during a 12-month period (Barnes, Bloom, & Nahin, 2008). In a study of physicians in the Western United States, Winslow and Shapiro (2002) reported that 76% of physicians reported having patients who reported that they used CAM; 59% reported being asked about CAM treatments by patients; 48% reported suggesting CAM treatments; and 24% reported that they used some form of CAM personally. Winslow and Shapiro reported that 84% of physicians believed they needed more education about CAM treatments, and those who reported using CAM themselves were more likely to recommend CAM to patients. The National Health and Interview Survey in 2007 revealed that 55.11 million adults in the United States had used herbs or supplements (NHIS as cited by Wu, Wang, & Kennedy, 2007). The survey reported that younger adults were less likely to use supplements in 2007 (17.6%) than in 2002 (20.0%). Older adults were more likely to use supplements with an increase in prevalence from 13.2% in 2002 to 19.5% in 2007. In addition, 45.4% of respondents reported that they had shared details of their herb and supplement use with their physician. Wu et al. (2007) caution, however, that the 2002 and 2007 NHIS were not identical and the data sets were not comparable.

More recently, adults in the United States reported that they meet often with CAM providers (600 million) (Eisenberg et al. as cited in Block, 2012). Another study found that 74.6% of adults in the United States reported using at least one CAM treatment (Barnes et al. as cited in Block, 2012). Furthermore, in pediatric care studies, approximately 21% of parents used CAM treatments; however, parents of children with cancer reported a 73% incidence of CAM usage (Noonan as cited in Block, 2012). While the healing models were wide-ranging, the use of at last one CAM therapy was widespread among all ethnic groups, income levels, and age ranges (Hsiao et al. and MacKenzie et al. as cited in Block, 2012).

Using Multiple Herbal and Nutritional Supplements

Polypharmacy and the problems that can occur with the taking of multiple prescriptions and herbal products can have serious consequences. A study of older adults living on both sides of the United States–Mexico border reported that the prevalence rate of polypharmacy was similar; however, the use of poly-herbal and nutritional supplements was reported to be of lower prevalence in Mexico. In the United States, 25% to 50% of adults over the age of 65 take five or more medications daily. Herb use in Mexico had a lower prevalence rate with less than 25% of adults reporting use of herbal products in the previous 12 months (Loya, Gonzalez-Stuart, & Rivera, 2009). The study further suggests that approximately 50% of older adults were at risk for negative affects resulting from drug–drug interactions. At least 33% have the potential of negative interactions between their nutritional supplements and prescriptions medications (Loya et al., 2009).

So much interest has been generated in alternative therapies that the National Institutes of Health established the Office of Alternative Medicine (OAM) in 1992, with a budget of $2 million. In 1998, Congress established the NCCAM as a replacement for OAM to stimulate, develop, and support research on CAM. It now supports both basic and applied research and reported a budget of $127.7 million in FY 2011 (NCCAM, 2012a).

Probably the biggest concern for the health care social worker in accepting and supporting patients who utilize alternative remedies is the assumption that because these remedies are natural, they must be safe (Dziegielewski, 2010b). Unfortunately, this is not necessarily so. What most people do not realize is that many prescription medications are created similarly and utilize many of the same ingredients (Dziegielewski, 2010b). For example, aspirin, a commonly used pain reliever, is derived from the bark of the white willow tree. In addition to this, one cancer treatment medication known as Taxol comes directly from the Pacific Yew tree.

The implications of this "natural is safe" mentality requires further study as patients may be unaware that they are taking preparations that could create problems when combined with prescription drugs or with other natural supplements or herbs. It is important to note, however, that mixing herbal remedies and prescription medicine does not always have a negative outcome. For some mixtures, the results could be quite positive as the herbal remedies may complement the other medications being taken. The worst-case scenario that can result from combining herbal remedies and prescription medicines deserves some attention, though, because it can have serious toxic results that could present severe health risks for patients. For example, drinking the juice of grapefruits seems safe enough, but when a patient is undergoing dialysis, drinking grapefruit juice can inhibit or prevent the absorption of medications used in dialysis (Goeddeke-Merickel, 1998a, 1998b, 1998c). When dealing with any type of medication at all (herbal and natural included), it is essential to remember that any remedy that is powerful enough to affect the body beneficially is also powerful enough to create unwanted side effects (Dziegielewski, 2006, 2010b).

Herbal medications have received an upsurge of interest since the 1990s; they have clearly gotten the attention of the FDA. It may not be long until herbal preparations, similar to their prescription counterparts, are regulated to ensure efficiency and effectiveness for the claims they purport to address. In the United States, the importance of the need for more controlled studies has been recognized and will continue to increase (Bender, 1996). The NCAMM website provides current research in this area (nccam.nih.gov/health/whatiscam).

Today, the herbal industry is thriving with few, if any, requirements placed on it by the government (Marinac et al., 2007). Generally, most of the herbal products are exempt from federal regulation because they are not considered medications. Rather, to get around regulation, many of the herbal remedies are referred to as dietary supplements. In addition, this lack of regulation can lead to lower quality of the product that is supplied. It has been documented in several case studies, and reported by the FDA, that there is little information about the purity, danger, or usefulness of some herbal products (Marinac et al., 2007). Unfortunately, however, this lack of government regulation can lead to confusion and open misinformation. Furthermore, because the DSHEA makes no requirements for product standardization of the active ingredients a product utilizes, it can have sincere effects on a product's bioavailability and efficacy. There is also no required testing in terms of combination issues with OTC and prescription drugs; therefore, it is incumbent upon the user to exercise caution.

Medicinal Herbs

For the most part, *herbal medicines* are derived from plants, leaves, roots, flowers, and fungi, for example, by alcoholic extraction or decoction, used to prevent and treat diseases (Linde et al., 2001). To date, there are well over 600 medicinal herbs available to the consumer (Gruenwald, 2001) without much regulated and standardized testing to clearly establish their effectiveness (see Table 13.2). In the United States, the Dietary Supplement Health and Education Act (DSHEA) of 1994 allows herbs to be sold legally so long as they make no claims for disease treatment on the label (Kroll, 1997). For example, a very popular product used primarily for the treatment of mild depression known as St. John's Wort states in ambiguous terms that it is used "for mental well-being" or "to improve mental health."

Herbal Medicines

The single largest concern for social workers who see patients taking these preparations is the lack of formal regulation. Currently, many herbal products are limited in the testing that has been performed on them, and therefore there is no way to clearly link safety to efficacy. To avoid legal penalties, it is common for these herbal and natural product manufacturers to use vague terminology such as to "support body function" or "safely balances emotions." The lack of regulation can also lead to limited standardization in terms of harvesting, processing, and packaging. Having active ingredients is essential, and ensuring that they stay active is just as important. Without regulation, there is no guarantee that a product is not

Table 13.2 Popular Herbal Medicines

Herb	Clinical applications	Contra-indications	Side effects	Herb–drug interactions
Black Cohosh	PMS, menopause, arthritis, high blood pressure	First two trimesters of pregnancy	G.I. symptoms	May intensify side effects of synthetic estrogen
Chamomile	Peptic ulcers, skin irritations, colic, insomnia, nausea	Ragweed allergy	Highly concentrated tea may be emetic	May interfere with anticoagulant therapy
Echinacea	Viral and bacterial illness, immune system booster	Autoimmune diseases, immunosuppressant therapy	G.I. symptoms	Do not use with immunosuppressant therapy
Evening primrose oil	Bruises, asthma, chronic fatigue syndrome, congestive heart failure, metabolic disorders, PMS, menopause	May trigger latent temporal lobe epilepsy, particularly in people with schizophrenia	G.I. symptoms	Increases risk of temporal lobe epilepsy when used with epileptogenic drugs for schizophrenia
Feverfew	Migraine, allergies, rheumatic diseases	Pregnancy, lactation, children under 2 years	Nervousness G.I. symptoms	May interact with antithrombotic drugs such as aspirin and warfarin
Garlic	Arteriosclerosis, respiratory infections, mouth and pharynx inflammation, cancer preventive	Slow blood clotting pregnancy, lactation	G.I. symptoms, burn-like skin lesions with topical preparation	Increases action of anticoagulant drugs
Ginger	Colic, menstrual symptoms, motion sickness, reduces some chemotherapy side effects	Gallstones, pregnancy	Mild heartburn	In doses exceeding dietary intake, may interfere with cardiac, anticoagulant or antidiabetic medications

(continued)

Table 13.2 Popular Herbal Medicines (*continued*)

Herb	Clinical applications	Contra-indications	Side effects	Herb–drug interactions
Ginkgo	Allergies, dementia, Alzheimer's, cochlear deafness, macular degeneration, depression, stroke	Ingesting the seed can cause severe adverse effects; the fruit should not be handled or ingested	G.I. symptoms	May interfere with MAO inhibitors
Ginseng	Ulcers, edema, cancer, infertility, fatigue, viral illness, red blood cell depletion	Acute illness, cardiovascular disease, diabetes or blood pressure disorders, pregnancy	None known	May increase the effects of phenelzine (Nardil) or other antipsychotics, or blood pressure, antidiabetic, or steroidal medications
Goldenseal	Gastric inflammation, colds, flu, externally for lacerations, skin eruptions	Pregnancy, hypertension; long-term use of large amounts may lower B vitamin absorption and utilization	Large doses may cause convulsions, long-term use may cause elevated white blood cell counts	None known
Green tea	Stomach ailments, chemotherapy, dental caries prevention, cancer, obesity	Sensitive stomach, cardiovascular complications, kidney disorders, overactive thyroid	Large amounts can cause restlessness, tremor, heightened reflex excitability	Tea beverages may delay the reabsorption of alkaline medications
Hawthorn	Coronary artery disease, congestive heart failure, essential hypertension	Pregnancy, lactation; those using drug therapies for blood pressure disorders and other heart failure medications should be closely monitored	G.I. symptoms, headache	May increase effects of digitalis

Kava	Anxiety, stress, insomnia	Pregnancy, lactation, may cause liver damage	Skin rash, G.I. symptoms	May potentiate effects of barbiturates or alcohol
Milk thistle	Chronic hepatitis B, C, D, E, liver disorders, gallstones, skin problems	Alcohol-based extracts are not recommended for severe liver problems	Mild laxative effect	None known
SAMe (S-Adenosyl-Methionine)	Depression, osteoarthritis, alcoholic liver disease	None known	May trigger manic episode	May potentiate antidepressant medication
Saw palmetto	Stage I and II benign prostatic hypertrophy, female androgen excess disorders	Pregnancy, lactation	G.I. symptoms, headache	May interfere with hormonal therapies
St. John's wort	Mild depression, anxiety, anorexia; topically, promotes wound healing	Pregnancy, lactation	G.I. symptoms, photosensitivity	May interact with L-dopa, MAO inhibitors
Valerian	Sleep disorders, anxiety, migraine	None known	May have paradoxical effect	May interfere with anxiolytics, hypnotics, analgesics, and antiepileptics; may enhance effects of kava and other herbs

Information obtained from Integrative Medicine Communications (2000); Lince et al. (2001).

old or that the packaging is sufficient enough to keep the active ingredients active (Kroll, 1997).

This could be a particular problem if substances are brought in bulk or remain in stores for an extended period of time. In addition, this lack of regulation can lead to contamination of the product that is supplied. It has been documented in several case studies (LaPuma, 1999) and reported by the FDA that some imported herbal products in the past have been known to have by-products in them or trace metals that could prove harmful to those that ingest them, for example, lead poisoning or other toxic reactions that might not be easily traced to the herbal product that introduced it. In monitoring this at minimal levels, the FDA has already made harmful links to products such as ephedra, comfrey, chaparral, licorice, pennyroyal, sassafras, and senna.

A particular challenge is determining which herbal remedies may be efficacious. A meta-analysis of systematic reviews of clinical trials of herbal medicines undertaken by Linde et al. (2001) showed that many herbs, including ginkgo, garlic, St. John's wort, echinacea, and saw palmetto were promising, but that methodological problems, including lack of standardization of the tested compounds, compromised the findings. They report that there is no way to know whether "different products, extracts, or even different lots of the same extract are comparable and equivalent" (Linde et al., 2001, p. 4). A recent study (Hypericum Depression Trial Study Group, 2002) showed that St. John's wort was no more effective than placebo for patients with major depression of moderate severity. Interestingly enough, this study also compared Zoloft to placebo and found little difference.

CHAPTER SUMMARY AND FUTURE DIRECTIONS

Wellness counseling has been used in numerous health care settings, in many different forms, and can be traced back to the early beginnings of health care practice. The health care social worker needs to be aware of this growing movement to integrate wellness concepts through alternative and conventional care. In coordinated care strategies, linking a patient to a comprehensive service network is often needed (Bodenheimer, 2008). This integration can serve to help bridge the gap between the two very different approaches to health care. In the meantime, however, it is extremely important that people share with their physicians what they are taking. For health care social workers, however, this method of practice, including wellness counseling and CAM, is increasingly viewed as being both viable and necessary. Approaches to wellness such as the *Wheel of Wellness* (Myers et al., 2000) can provide frameworks with which to conduct practice that holistically conceptualizes the person-in-environment. The use of efficient assessment frameworks will be cost effective and provide services that are needed by patients. Social workers need to assist patients in as timely, cost-containing, and efficient ways of service delivery. This holistic approach allows just that.

The *Wheel of Wellness* provides a holistic approach that includes needs assessment, education counseling, and some aspects of community organization to achieve successful outcomes for patients. Over the years, there has been increased emphasis for the provision and inclusion of education as part of the intervention regime. Education is viewed as an integral service within the holistic approach to wellness promotion. Health and wellness counseling can initiate patient skill building, while emphasizing the importance of prevention and wellness services. Health care social workers are encouraged to approach this type of service delivery seriously. This method can provide a viable, necessary, and marketable way for health care social workers to provide clinical service.

A study of breast cancer patients by Adler and Fosket (1999) showed that only 54% of the patients who were using complementary therapy informed their physician. Combining herbs and other supplements and prescription drugs can have unpleasant and even hazardous consequences. If physicians and other health care providers are not informed about what their patients are taking, they will be unable to use their expertise to help the patients determine whether this is the best remedy for them. For the health care social worker, there is a clear role that requires encouragement of our patients to inform health care providers of all natural remedies they are taking. Therefore, the health care professional can also become familiar with the effects these natural remedies are having on the patients that they serve. This requires a type of *educative counseling* that helps patients learn the benefits and risks of such treatments. It is essential that the social worker perform within the bounds of the National Association of Social Workers' *Code of Ethics* (NASW, 2008a) that addresses practice competence.

Current and future directions for health care social workers will include advocacy with health care agencies to ensure and support the patient's exploration of complementary treatments. Social workers should encourage patients to make informed decisions in terms of what is best for the patient. Patients do not have to accept and automatically commit to a traditional approach to medical care (Seligson, 1998) and, with the current trends toward wellness, if patients are forced to accept these traditional approaches, they most likely will refuse. All health care social workers need to realize during this confluent period of transition in health care that it is necessary to assist patients by encouraging them to seek the information that allows them to make informed choices. If a health care provider seems resistant to a method of intervention, encourage patients to ask them why they believe there is a problem with the proposed alternative approach. By understanding that there may be a reluctance to discuss the use of natural remedies with the mainstream medical community, social workers can help patients to prepare for such discussions. To create effective, efficient, and comprehensive helping relationships social workers need to consider other forms of treatment that could be useful for the patients served. Complementary forms of intervention can also serve as a preventative measure, helping to ensure patient well-being that can be incorporated into conventional therapies. Keeping abreast of all forms of treatment is important for coordinated care.

Future directions in health care will additionally require more congruence between the traditional medical model and CAM. In order to integrate wellness practices, it will be necessary to include research about the complimentarity of both systems to determine the efficacy of a holistic continuum of care that positions the person-in-the-environment. This holistic association among medical, mental health, and alternative practitioners, will take into account all contributing factors affecting wellness. The social worker may function as the organizer of a comprehensive wellness plan that includes active participation of patients, practitioners, and supportive service providers.

Glossary

Alternative medicine   This is often described as any medical practice or intervention that is utilized instead of conventional treatment, lacks sufficient documentation in regard to its safety and effectiveness against certain diseases and conditions, is generally not taught in United States medical schools, and is generally not reimbursable by health insurance providers.

Confidentiality   The information that is obtained about the patient in the conduct of direct practice includes patient identity, content of verbalizations, professional opinions about the patient, and material from records.

Complementary or integrative medicine   In this approach to medical care, a combination approach is utilized whereas patients generally receive traditional approaches to therapy such as prescription medications augmented or supplemented by alternative approaches.

Educative counseling   This is a loosely defined approach to practice that focuses on helping patients to become "educated consumers" and through this information be thereby be better able to address their own needs.

Employee Assistance Program   Services offered by employers to employees to help them address personal, social, or occupational problems that may impede work performance.

Epidemiology   The basic study of the frequency and distribution of a specified phenomenon, such as disease.

Health-belief model   In this model for addressing health and wellness, the core concept of "fear" or recognition of ones "susceptibility" to an adverse health outcome or illness motivates the individual to partake in health change behavior. Oftentimes, the individuals view themselves as in a vulnerable but solvable situation that can be addressed.

Herbal medicines   These are medicines or preparations used for medicinal purposes that are derived from plants, leaves, roots, flowers, and fungi.

Informed consent   This is where patient permission is obtained and secured to participate in the health and wellness counseling being provided.

Modeling   In social learning theory, modeling relates to how individuals learn; they watch which behaviors are rewarded and punished and "vicariously" embrace implications of what they witness.

Primary prevention   This is the first area of direct prevention services where the objective is to reduce the susceptibility of individuals to disease or to prevent social problems from occurring.

Relative or limited confidentiality   Is the form of confidentiality that most social workers ensure. In this form, information is kept confidential that the social worker is not ethically or morally bound to reveal.

Secondary prevention   These prevention strategies evolve around early detection so that methods of behavior change can be employed before irreversible damage has occurred.

Self-control   In the health belief model, this refers to an individual's desire to secure and maintain command of one's state of health or wellness.

Self-reinforcement   Is where the individuals reinforce themselves without an external stimulator, such as in direct reinforcement.

Social learning theory   An intervention model that highlights the importance of social learning through modeling and direct or self-reinforcing of behaviors.

Stress   Any influence that interferes with normal functioning by producing internal stress or strain.

Stressor   A stimulus that causes, evokes, or is otherwise related to the stress response.

Tertiary prevention   In tertiary prevention, the goal is to manage disease so as to minimize disability.

Traditional mainstream medicine   This type of medical practice is most reflective of the application of the general medical model and is generally referred to as mainstream American medical practice.

Trauma   Any event, particularly those outside the realm of usual experience that causes the development of marked distress.

Traumatic stress Intense arousal of feelings related to a particular event or situation.

Vicarious The feelings or emotions that develop from sharing the experience of another person.

Vicarious traumatization In this phenomena, helping professionals who work with individuals in crisis are repeatedly exposed to trauma through vicarious (i.e., imagining what it is like) means and may also begin to feel the effects of the trauma.

Questions for Further Study

1. In what other areas of health care social work practice can health counseling be used?

2. Make a list of several different types of patient problems that can be addressed through health education counseling.

3. What roles for the expansion of health care counseling do you see in the future?

4. What components would you include in developing a health promotion for people with juvenile diabetes?

5. What aspects of health promotion are most appealing to you?

6. What additional skills do you need to provide this kind of holistic counseling?

7. What do you see as the role of the health care social worker in this area?

8. What can health care social workers do to assist patients that utilize these types of treatments?

Websites

Prevention Sites

Agency for Health Care Policy and Research
www.ahcpr.gov

American Health Information Management Association
www.ahima.org

American Journal of Health Promotion
www.healthpromotionjournal.com

American Public Health Association
www.apha.orgwww.apha.org/publications/journal

Association of State and Territorial Directors of Health Promotion and
Public Health Education
www.astphnd.org

How Does the Affordable Care Act Address Prevention?
healthinsurance.about.com/od/reform/f/public-health-reform-and-the-affordable-care-act.htm

National Institute of Mental Health
www.nimh.nih.gov/health/topics/prevention-of-mental-disorders/
prevention-of-mental-disorders.shtml

Prevention
www.prevention.com/homepage

U.S. National Library of Medicine, National Institutes of Health
www.nlm.nih.gov/medlineplus

U.S. Department of Health & Human Services—Health Resources
healthinsurance.about.com/gi/o.htm?zi=1/XJ&zTi=1&sdn=healthinsuran
ce&cdn=health&tm=239&f=00&tt=12&bt=1&bts=1&zu=http%3A//www.
healthfinder.gov

Wellness Counseling Sites

American Journal of Health Promotion
www.healthpromotionjournal.com

Center for Health Education and Wellness
www.jhu.edu/~health

Comprehensive listing of wellness hyperlinks
www.fit.edu/caps/links.php

Complementary and Alternative Medicine Sites

MD Anderson Cancer Center—Complementary/Integrative Medicine Education Resources
www.mdanderson.org/education-and-research/resources-for-professionals/
clinical-tools-and-resources/cimer/index.html

National Center for Complementary and Alternative Medicine
nccam.nih.gov/news/2011/042611.htm

Online Resources—Complementary and Alternative Medicine
www.hopkinsmedicine.org/healthlibrary/conditions/
adult/complementary_and_ alternative_medicine/
online_resources_-_complementary_and_alternative_medicine_85,P00188/

Stanford Prevention Research Center—CAM Medicine Program
camps.stanford.edu/resources.html

What Is Complementary and Alternative Medicine?
nccam.nih.gov/health/whatiscam

CHAPTER 14

Public Health Social Work

Diane C. Holliman

Public health social work is a growing health care specialty that integrates prevention, case management, education, community organization, policy practice, and leadership.

There are several metaphors that compare the development of social work and the development of other professions to the birth of a child. From this perspective, one could say that psychiatry is the father of social work and social justice is the mother of social work, or prevention of disease and social reform were the parents of public health. If we were to follow these metaphors further, we could readily say that health care social work and social work in public health are siblings.

What is clear is that health care social work and public health have a common lineage. Health care social work lends credence to the role of the health care social worker as an integral part of health care service delivery. Throughout history, social work has been at the forefront in providing health care services to patients/clients/consumers (hereafter referred to as patients). Public health, grounded in the biological sciences and epidemiology (the study of the distribution and patterns of disease), has been at the forefront of health promotion, disease prevention, and addressing health disparities. However, as the two grew up together, they had their differences, individuated, and developed into two distinct fields of practice. Each field of practice had its own definitions, goals, and methods of practice. Now both fields of practice have united in partnership each recognized as accomplished professions uniting to address the needs of the population, creating a partnership that would make any professional parent proud.

This chapter will provide an overview of public health and social work's role as these two fields of practice realize there is much in common and together the field is emerging to a new height. The relationship to health care and the role of public health in health promotion, disease prevention, and addressing health disparities will be examined.

HISTORY AND DEVELOPMENT: THE PRACTICE OF PUBLIC HEALTH

In the middle and late 19th century and early 20th century, as professions were developing, the supporting structure of public health was defined. Rich in the profession of social work, Dorothea Dix, Jane Addams, Alice Hamilton, Lillian Wald, Frances Perkins, and many others advocated to assist the mentally ill, bringing awareness to the concerns of this vulnerable population at the community, state, and federal levels. Starting with the settlement houses for immigrants in urban areas, efforts to educate people and communities on germ theory and hygiene were common. Sanitation was also important with basic attempts to educate people about the importance of removing rubbish from their communities, while advocating for clean water and sewage systems. Advocacy efforts included protesting child labor and unfair and unhealthy labor practices for all, as well as supporting women's suffrage and working for peace.

These heroic efforts fell within the realm of public health and social work and led to many of the policies and programs that emerged from the progressive era such as the child labor laws, the Children's Bureau, Women's Suffrage, and "New Deal" reforms (Karger & Stoesz, 2010; Keefe & Evans, 2012; Ruth & Sisco, 2012; Sable et al., 2012). United together in history, both public health and social work walk a similar path and often claim the events in the past as history of their own. Table 14.1 shows the common roots and features of public health and social work, and how the two differ and where social work and public health can come together.

As Sigmund Freud's theories and the general field of psychiatry emerged, social work utilized these discoveries to inform social casework (Pearlman, 1957) and ego psychology (Goldstein, 1995). Social work continued to branch out toward direct practice with individuals and families,

Table 14.1 A comparison of public health and social work.

Public health	Social work
Primary prevention and health promotion	Secondary and tertiary prevention
Targets population	Targets individuals, groups, and families
Courses in epidemiology, health policy, health administration, biostatistics, environmental health, maternal child health, and international health	Foundation courses in practice with individuals, families, groups, communities, and organizations human behavior and the social environment, research and policy

whereas today direct practice (i.e., working with individuals and families) is a prominent part of social work, and the balance of micro and macro practice in social work has remained arguable (Specht & Courtney, 1995).

Public health, on the other hand, is grounded in the biological sciences and epidemiology. And in public health, the unit of analysis is population (Ruth & Sisco, 2012). Examples of a population studied in public health and epidemiology are infants less than 1 year old in the United States, African American males age 65 and over, and females between the ages of 13 and 19 in a city school system. In social work, there is a dearth of studies and interventions focused on primary prevention. Most of the interventions in social work occur after the problems have occurred (Marshall et al., 2011), whereas in public health social work, primary prevention in communities and population is a focal point.

COMMONALITIES OF PUBLIC HEALTH AND SOCIAL WORK

There are many aspects of social work, especially macro practice, that are shared in common with social work in public health. A common backdrop begins with the foundation for practice as both can focus on social reform and both are based on a rich tradition of social justice and ethics. In addition, both focus on eliminating disparities, oppression, and discrimination. The interventions used can include social work macro perspective policy making, policy practice, advocacy, research, and evaluation with all attempts at service delivery assuming a holistic view of problems and solutions. Both support teamwork and that includes the use of multiple teams (as described earlier in this book) such as the transdisciplinary team where all members work together to address and in many cases solve a common problem. Both disciplines take into account the importance of recognizing an awareness and appreciation for how environment, culture, and diversity affect quality of life and need to be addressed at each stage of the intervention throughout the lifespan (beginning to end of life). Both also afford a systematic- and theory-based approach to practice where comprehensive assessments and interventions based on evidence are always at the forefront of any helping activity. These two disciplines and the people who put strategy into action also work hand-in-hand together and are employed in many of the same agencies at the federal, state, city, county, and local levels.

As these two disciplines have emerged, especially from a macro focus, it appears there are more similarities than differences especially when it comes to recognizing the importance of health promotion and primary prevention strategies. From a public health perspective, the focus is often in the group setting as opposed to practice with individuals, which is often the focus of micro level social work practice. Also, when groups are the focus, the services to groups are generally of an educative, problem-solving focus and not necessarily supportive, although this is changing. One major difference, however, is the background where in public health the heritage is rich in epidemiology, biostatistics, as well as social work practice, research policy, and human behavior and the social environment. Public health is similar to social work as it is rich in policy making and advocacy. Social workers in this area are leaders in supporting research activities that are filled with health education. Grant writing is a major function that supports efficient and effective program planning that focuses on wellness and prevention. Participating in encouraging efforts to recognize and assist while providing services in community organization, case management to identify, and decreasing health and social disparities. Specific microlevel interventions including counseling to assist with education and wellness, obesity prevention, promotion of physical activity, and violence prevention are just some of the areas important in public health social work that cannot be ignored (Keefe & Evans, 2012; Sable et al., 2012).

PUBLIC HEALTH, EDUCATION, AND SOCIAL WORK

In the United States, there are many graduate programs that offer a dual MSW/MPH degree, and there are also MSW programs that offer specialty and advanced courses in child welfare, grant writing, health, loss and bereavement, mental health, older adults, and wellness, as well as other courses that would provide a background for public health social work (Keefe & Evans, 2012). Also, foundation and concentration social work content in human behavior and the social environment, community practice, organizational practice, research, social welfare policy and program evaluation provide a background for public health social work.

At this point, there are no certifications or licenses for public health social workers, but there are continuing education opportunities. The American Association of Public Health has a Social Work section that establishes standards for social work in health care settings and contributes to public health social work practice, research, and service (American Public Health Association, 2012).

Today, local (state, county, and parish) health departments deliver the bulk of public health services in the United States (Sable et al., 2012), and the programs generally associated with public health departments are maternal and child health that includes family planning, prenatal care, well child, immunizations, disease surveillance and treatment programs (such as programs to prevent and monitor tuberculosis, HIV/AIDS, West Nile), environmental protection programs (restaurant inspection, water safety, and air quality), and vital statistics (birth and death records). In local health departments, social workers implement and provide direct services such as case management, HIV/AIDS counseling, and family planning. Public health social work is characterized by an emphasis on prevention and health promotion (Ruth & Sisco, 2012), and the multiple and complex interactions between the biological, social, and psychological aspects of the person and their environment.

Field placements and career opportunities for public health social workers are far reaching. Of course, public health social workers can provide case management, leadership, counseling, and education at the local level in public health departments, community clinics, and private agencies. Research universities, medical centers, and state and federal agencies can provide opportunities for public health social workers in research, evaluation, program development, policy making and analysis, grant writing, teaching, supervision, and administration. Public health social workers are also valued internationally in government and nongovernment organizations because of their cultural competency, leadership, and collaborative skills.

HEALTH DISPARITIES AND PUBLIC HEALTH SOCIAL WORK

Understanding the social determinants of health and health disparities is critical for public health and all social workers (Ashcroft, 2010). The social determinants of health are health risk factors that result from the underlying inequalities in society. Social determinants include a person's socioeconomic status, access to health care, neighborhood and employment conditions, and personal behaviors (Fuddy, 2012). The peer-reviewed literature surrounding social determinants of health show that health is essentially a biopsychosocial phenomenon and that increasing employment, raising the minimum wage, improving nutrition, and developing safer and healthier communities is a way to improve health for communities and the entire population (Moniz, 2010).

In the United States, health disparities (or inequalities) have been repeatedly seen among racial and ethnic minorities and people with lower incomes. Rates of heart disease and stroke, cancer, HIV/AIDS, chronic obstructive pulmonary disease, diabetes, and infant mortality are higher among African Americans, Native Americans, and Latinos than White Americans (Keefe, 2010). Miller, Pinet-Peralta, and Elder (2012) analyzed data of nursing home admissions from 2000–2008 and found that Black adults were overrepresented in nursing homes and had higher rates of suffering from chronic conditions such as diabetes, renal failure, chronic obstructive pulmonary disease, asthma, and cardiovascular diseases. Reasons for these disparities are that people from these groups are sometimes more likely to refuse treatment, unable to afford treatment, less likely to stick to their diet and treatment regimens, or they delay seeking appropriate health care. Other reasons may be prior negative interactions with the health care system, incomplete understanding of provider instructions, and a lack of knowledge about how to best access treatment and provider bias.

Healthy People 2020 (2012) is a national public health document. The website www.healthypeople.gov/2020/default.aspx provides a 10-year agenda (2010–2020) for improving health in the United States including looking at health disparities related to access, income, health behaviors, and other social factors. In social work, health disparities are an area we are well equipped to identify and address. Unfortunately, however, evidence of social work interventions in health disparities (similar to some of the other disciplines practicing in this area) is often lacking (Coren et al., 2011).

To address health disparities, social work can be active on both the micro and mezzo levels. Understanding and assessing for health literacy in patients in the context of their support system is one way to do this. Health literacy is a person's ability to read, understand, process, and use health care information to make informed decisions and follow treatment instructions (Liechty, 2011). The case exemplar describes an example of health literacy and access from direct practice and public health social work. Social workers can also address health disparities by advocating for government programs that increase access to health care and reduce poverty. The Affordable Care Act (ACA) with its provisions for access through the individual mandates and emphasis on primary prevention provides great promise for improving care access and reducing health disparities.

ROLES OF SOCIAL WORK IN PUBLIC HEALTH

Public health social workers are involved in many professional activities and roles. These roles span the continuum of direct and indirect practice and require basic to advanced social work skills. The functions include direct personal support and treatment and policy making and leadership assuming common roles such as case manager, facilitator, educator/teacher, advocate, community organizer, grant writing/grant administration, evaluator and auditor, supervision, management, administration, and leadership.

Public health social workers use *direct personal support and treatment* skills throughout the assessment and treatment process. In the first contacts with the patient, the public health social worker develops rapport through active listening, showing empathy, reflecting content and feelings, and summarizing what the patient is saying. The public health social worker continues to use these generalist and basic counseling skills throughout the treatment process. Other direct personal support and treatment skills that may be used as appropriate are encouraging the patient, confrontation, role modeling, and setting boundaries.

Policy making and *leadership* are macro roles that are components of administration. Policy makers could be elected or appointed officials, or they could be administrators, managers, community organizers, advocates, or grant writer/administrators. Examples of policy making in public health social work are introducing a bill in the state legislature for stronger nonsmoking legislation, developing a policy for a well workplace and participating on a national committee to write professional standards for public health social work.

As described in Chapter 12, case management is frequently used in health care social work practice. As a *case manager*, public health social workers assess the patient and their support system, develop a plan of intervention, and link the patient with services and resources. Evaluation of this intervention also is an important part of case management in public health social work.

Public health social workers often engage in the roles of *facilitator* and *educator/teacher* with individuals, small groups, and large groups or classes. Facilitators in public health social work organize and lead therapeutic or psychoeducational groups. Topics for public health social work groups may include support for new mothers, living with HIV/AIDS, and bereavement. Facilitators make sure that the group runs effectively by assuring that the norms and objectives of the group are being followed.

Educator/teacher is a related public health social work role where the educator/teacher provides content and information on topics. An educator/teacher may also provide support, but the focus for the educator/teacher is delivering content rather than support or facilitating group communication.

Serving as an *advocate* is an important role utilized in public health. A public health social worker may act as an advocate with a patient who has been diagnosed with cervical cancer and cannot find a specialist who will treat her because her payor source is not private insurance. As an advocate, the public health social worker can first contact area gynecologists to refer this patient and stress the urgent nature of the patient's diagnosis. The social workers can also inform health care and community leaders that there is a citizen in their district who cannot get needed cancer treatment and point out to policy makers and those within public health agencies that what is happening to one patient is probably a problem for many others, and how to begin the process of assessing the situation. The social worker is in a pivotal position to see what is offered and compare it to the services needed.

Community organizers in public health social work often respond to spe cific community needs such as lack of medical or mental health services or environmental hazards such as unsafe drinking water. Community organizers enable community members to come together to discuss their needs and formulate strategies for advocating for themselves. Community organizers such as Dorothea Dix and Jane Addams are a clear part of the history of public health and social work and offer professional models for community organizers in public health social work today.

As *evaluators* in public health, social workers are expected to assess one's own practice efforts as well as those of outside programs. *Auditors* are evaluators who ensure that organizational standards, policies, and procedures are being followed. Evaluators and auditors can have similar functions and can work together to establish criteria sets or rubrics for evaluation, and audits can be done by someone within the organization (an internal audit) or by an accrediting body or payor source (an external audit). Evaluation and auditors follow systematic steps to assess practice and organizational effectiveness and efficiency.

Grant writing/grant administration is a macro public health social work role that consists of identifying a need, locating a grant that fits the need and the qualities of the organization, writing, editing, and submitting the grant as well as following the grant through the application process. This can include implementing or administering the grant or hiring someone to administer the grant. Examples of grants that public health social workers could write or administer are grants for school-based clinics, funding for medical services for an underserved population, and grants to evaluate programs.

Public health social workers, especially those with the MSW and other graduate training such as the MPH, may find themselves in *administration, supervision, management, policy making,* and *leadership. Administration* is an advanced practice skill that describes the overall *management* of a department, program, or organization. *Administrators* are responsible for the functioning of the organization as well as being visible representatives or the public face of the organization. An example of a top administrator in Public Health Social Work is Loretta Fuddy, MSW, MPH, Director of Department of Health, State of Hawaii.

Management is a clear part of the *administration* which consists of the controlling and structuring of the work of the organization or unit. Management activities are planning, organizing, staffing, supervising, and leading. Examples of management roles in public health social work are serving as a department head in a county public health department and administering a $100,000 grant.

Serving as a *supervisor* is another part of administration and management. Supervision involves monitoring the work of the unit's staff. Supervision can include orienting, training, coaching, mentoring, and evaluating. A supervisor in public health social work could be responsible for the performance of a team of social workers as well as scheduling them and providing them with resources to effectively do their jobs. The supervisor would then report to the manager or administrator as supervision is one part of the overall management and administration of a unit or organization.

Leadership is a quality of influencing others through communication, persuasion, writing, inspiring, and personal and professional example. All public health social workers have the capacity to influence others and their work settings to help patients and improve the quality of services. Specific examples of leadership in public health social work are educator/teacher, community organizing, grant writing/grant administration, policy making, management, and administration.

CASE EXEMPLAR

As the result of a medical examination for his job, Mr. J is told to report to his county health department for further laboratory work. After his medical evaluation at the county health department, he is told that he has HIV. When Mr. J hears "HIV" and his mind goes blank, he becomes numb and feels that his world has come to an end. He knows that he will never be able to tell his wife, his family, or his children. Even though Mr. J. has been speaking English since he came to the United States from Mexico when he was 10 years old, he cannot understand fully what the physician, nurse, and social worker are saying as they give him the diagnosis, explain treatment options, and tell him what he needs to do right now to follow-up, and protect himself and others from the disease.

Despite the advances in HIV medications and treatments since the early 1980s, and the fact that many people have lived with HIV as a chronic illness for decades, HIV remains a devastating diagnosis with clear implications for Mr. J's life and those connected with him, especially his partners in sexual activity and all of the children he has biologically fathered who may also be affected by HIV.

The public social worker is aware that HIV can be a shocking diagnosis and that upon hearing this diagnosis, Mr. J has much to process on a cognitive, emotional, social, and spiritual level. The others on the treatment team remain concerned about the public health issue at hand and are ready to ask questions related to assessing risk for the spread of HIV to others in his immediate sexual network. The team will assess Mr. J to find out his history of sexual and substance-abuse behaviors, and explain the types of medications he should start on immediately and how they should be taken (time of day, amount, with food or not, and possible side effects).

Before this information is gathered, however, the social work will need to assess Mr. J's understanding and health literacy. To start the process, the social worker asks Mr. J what he has heard from the treatment team, what he knows about HIV, and how he is feeling as he hears this information. To start the process, quiet time, silence, and, when needed, just listening, are so important for establishing rapport. As Mr. J describes his situation, the social worker realizes that English is not his first language and there may be a problem with his understanding of the situation. When Mr. J came in he was speaking English very fluently and at that time he spoke without any obvious accent or outward way for the original interviewee to determine there might be a language barrier to his understanding. The anxiety he is experiencing is affecting him in many ways and clearly is influencing his ability to comprehend what he has been told. Spending time with this patient and continuing to assess Mr. J's understanding of all the unsettling and complex information he is given becomes an essential point for ensuring he understands what he has been told. The social worker will also need to carefully access for suicide risk and how he will follow-up through his personal behaviors (sexual activity, drug use, and informing sexual partners and others who may be at risk). Concrete information will also need to be provided, but this information will need to be given to Mr. J in a way he can comprehend so he knows what course of action he will need to take to ensure his own protection and that of others. Mr. J. will need to understand his medication and appointment schedule is all part of improving access to care and health literacy. Public health social workers taking this role can lead to decreasing health disparities.

EVIDENCE-BASED PRACTICE STRATEGY

As leaders in social work and public health, those with an MSW/MPH can influence practice by utilizing, supporting, and advocating for the use of evidence-based practice strategies and program evaluation. Public health social workers can promote evidence-based practice by using interventions that have a track record of working. An example would be a public health social worker who uses weight loss strategies with her patients that have evidence and data behind them from the Substance Abuse and Mental Health Services Administration (SAMHSA) rather than a diet found in a magazine, or a public health social worker who evaluates his weekly groups on smoking cessation to see whether his intervention has an effect on smoking behavior.

At a macro level, public health social work administrators can require that their personnel follow evidence-based practice models and evaluate their work and programs using standard criteria. Grant writers and administrators can insert evidence-based strategies and evaluation into the programs that they are developing. Public health social workers in leadership in professional organizations (National Association of Social Workers, Council on Social Work Education, Joint Commission, and American Public Health Association) can ensure that their organizations support practices that have evidence to show that they are effective and require practice evaluation as part of their standards. This intervention from leadership is needed, and social workers with advanced and specialty training in social work and public health are the ones who can do this effectively and influence not just their own practice, but also the practice of many others.

THE ROLE OF PRIMARY PREVENTION

Prevention is a topic that we hear and read a lot about today. The ACA, even though opinions about it are divided throughout the United States, supports efforts and programs for primary prevention (Coren et al., 2011). Mrs. Obama's *Let's Move* website and Childhood Obesity Taskforce (Let's Move, 2012) are prime examples of a primary prevention programs. Primary prevention programs are interventions to reduce the risk of health, behavioral, or social problems through education, counseling, and individualized or group interventions. Despite social work's efforts in assessment and treatment after a problem has occurred (mental illness, substance abuse, and obesity), the peer-reviewed literature on primary prevention in social work is lacking (Marshall et al., 2011).

Primary prevention is yet another area where social workers have the knowledge and skills to intervene. The following case exemplar is an example of a social worker engaged in primary prevention in a health program in a public school.

CASE EXEMPLAR

LaShay is a BSW who is employed in a grant-supported health program in the public schools in her county. Her county public health department received a grant for this position and her office is located in one of the public high schools. The purpose of her grant is to reduce truancy and improve high school graduation rates by providing counseling and assistance for students where health-related issues may get in their way of meeting these goals. In this county, teen pregnancy rates are much higher than in the other counties in the state, and this is a factor that leads to student absences and dropping out. However, with the grant, the only sex education programs that can be presented are abstinence-only programs, and the administrators at LaShay's schools have cautioned her not to talk about sex with students.

A part of the grant is for LaShay to facilitate two primary prevention groups. One group is for males grades 6 to 8 and the other is for females grades 6 to 8. Students are identified for these groups by teachers who see them as being at risk for truancy and dropping out of school. LaShay is fortunate to have a wealth of educational materials for this age group from the public health resource library and Internet resources from her grant.

In the first meetings of the primary prevention groups, she gives the students a chance to introduce themselves, discusses the topic of primary prevention, and asks the students what topics they would like to cover and what activities they would like to do in the groups. At this first session, she also gathers baseline data from these students from rapid assessment instruments with self-report questions on health behaviors, measures of self-efficacy, and attitudes toward education. From the group discussions, she finds that the males are interested in topics related to strength and athletic performance and that the females are interested in topics related to healthy weight and appearance. From the rapid assessment instrument for health behaviors, she finds that the students report that they regularly eat fast food, do not have family meals, do not have a set-aside time or place for exercise, and that tobacco and alcohol use are common among their family and neighbors. From the scales on self-efficacy and attitudes toward education, she finds that the students generally do not have clear goals for themselves for the next year, next 5 years, or for college and beyond.

LaShay lets these data guide her group sessions. For each group, she opens with a check-in with a directed question such as asking them, "One word to describe their past week" or "One healthy behavior they engaged in during the past week." Then she introduces the topic for the week. For the males, a few of the topics are strength training and body building, healthy living and athletics, and diet for activity. For the females, some of the topics are healthy diet and weight, eating disorders, and eating and clear skin. After LaShay spends 5 to 10 minutes on each topic, she asks the students for questions and ideas surrounding the topic. Then she directs the students toward goal setting for the next week and the upcoming school years. The students set their own goals, some are health related (drinking more water, trying out for basketball); some are related to education (making a "B" or better in math, finishing high school). LaShay teaches the students that the goals must be stated in one sentence, and be measurable and realistic for them to meet.

Each week they talk about the goals, their progress, and whether they need to rethink their goals or their behavior to meet their goals. At the end of the semester, LaShay administers the rapid assessment instruments again and finds that generally the students have increased their self-report of healthy behaviors and that their self-efficacy scores have increased and their attitudes about meeting their educational goals has become more positive.

During both groups, the topics of sex and relationships come up from time to time, and LaShay allows the students to ask questions and make comments in the way that they ask questions and make comments about other things that come up such as athletics and weight loss. However, sex and relationships are never planned group topics and when these topics come up, LaShay redirects the group back to the topic for the session.

From the outcome data and the feedback from the students, LaShay felt good about both groups and thought that she had made some strides in teaching primary prevention and having the students set and meet health behavior and educational goals. She did not know how or whether her groups affected the teen pregnancy rates in her school system, whether the groups would affect their long-term eating, tobacco, or alcohol use, or whether the students would complete high school, but this gave her ideas for a longitudinal study and reminded her that efforts in primary prevention are not always clearly and immediately evident. And, perhaps this is one of the reasons that public health social work is so challenging and exciting?

CHAPTER SUMMARY AND FUTURE DIRECTIONS

In this chapter, the history and integration of public health social work were described as well as educational opportunities and practice roles for public health social work. Health disparities, health literacy, and primary prevention were described and case exemplars were provided to illustrate how social workers can intervene and evaluate their practice in these areas.

Public health social work offers many opportunities for social workers, and with the ACA and today's emphasis on primary prevention, social workers have the skills needed to engage in this specialty. Social workers need to be proactive in defining their roles in this area, shaping their own practice, and practice evaluation. This requires attention to micro, mezzo, and macro practice as well as seeking out opportunities for leadership in health care. Social work has historically been a guest in the health care setting (Dane & Simon, 1991) with medical doctors and nurses being more visible in these settings, but concerted efforts from throughout social work (students, practitioners, educators, researchers, and administrators) is needed to advance public health social work and other specialty areas. We owe it to the population that we typically serve (those without access, with language barriers, and those not connected with resources) to be in these health care settings!

Glossary

Administration In public health social work, administration is an advanced practice skill that can be described as the overall management of an office, unit, program, department, or organization; the administrator is the executive who is responsible for the operations and functioning of the organization. Administration includes leadership, supervision, and making sure that the unit meets governing standards and policies.

Advocacy In public health social work, advocacy can occur at the micro, mezzo, and macro levels. Advocacy is a planned and strategic process to influence policy, resource allocation, and political, economic, and social systems and institutions. Examples of advocacy in public health social work are calling or writing elected officials about proposed legislation and how it will affect public health patients, developing a public service announcement and ad campaign to promote healthy eating in teens, and writing policy at the national level for standards of practice for population such as children, pregnant women, workers, and older adults.

Auditor (internal or external) In public health social work, audits are done to ensure that organizational standards, policies, and procedures are written correctly and being followed. Audits are done using an established criteria, format, or rubric and can be done by someone within the agency (an internal audit) or an accrediting organization (e.g., Council on Social Work Education, The Joint Commission) or payor (e.g., Medicare, Veteran's Affairs) who comes in to the organization for an external audit or evaluation.

Case management Case management is a generalist and direct practice social work role that includes the biopsychosocial assessment of the patient as well as assessment and interviews with their support system, developing a plan of intervention, and intervening often includes linkage to concrete resources, services, and programs. From the evaluation of the intervention, assessment is done to ascertain whether further intervention is needed.

Community organizer In public health social work, community organization is done when a specific public health need in a community is identified (examples are accessible mental health services or clean water), and members of the community come together to express their needs and develop strategies for advocating for themselves. As a community organizer, the public health social worker acts as a facilitator and educator to empower community members.

Direct personal support and treatment   They are direct and generalist social work practice skills that include showing empathy, actively listening, reflecting content and feelings, summarizing, and goal setting. In direct personal support and treatment, encouraging the patient and even being able to accept anger and criticism from the patient while maintaining and role modeling professional boundaries is a necessary skill.

Educator/teacher   Public health social workers may educate or teach patients individually, in small groups, or in larger topics. Topics that public health social workers may teach are models for healthy eating, the elements of good prenatal care, the benefits of breastfeeding and strategies for mothers, HIV/AIDS prevention, and medication and safety for older adults.

Epidemiology   The study of the distribution and pattern of disease, health, wellness, mortality, and life expectancy and their characteristics, causes, and influences in the population.

Evaluator   In public health social work, this could involve evaluating one's own practice or program evaluation. The process of evaluation is following systematic steps to determine the effectiveness of an intervention (could be individual, group, policy, community, or national) and also the efficiency (comparing the costs it takes for the intervention and the benefits of the intervention).

Facilitator   In groups and community organization, public health social workers facilitate or assist in making the groups run most effectively. Strategies for facilitators are making sure everyone in the group gets to speak and that no one dominates, that the group starts and ends on time, and that the norms and objectives of groups are being maintained.

Grant writing/grant administration   In public health social work, grant writing is an advanced indirect practice skill that involves identifying a need, locating a grant that fits the need and the qualities of the organization, writing, editing, and submitting the grant, and following the grant through the application process. If the organization gets the grant, the grant writer may be responsible for hiring personnel for the program or implementing the grant. If the organization does not get the grant, professional grant writers continue to locate grants and projects for community development.

Health disparities   Also known as health inequalities, these disparities are evident in the United States and throughout the world on the basis of income and ethnicity or race. For example, there are health disparities in rates of alcoholism and substance abuse for Native Americans as compared to White Americans. Health disparities are often attributed to social determinants such as income, housing, oppression, racism, and access to health care.

Health literacy   A person's ability to read, understand, process, and use health care information to make informed decisions and follow treatment instructions.

Infant mortality (IM)   Death of an infant prior to its first birthday; one of a nation's leading indicators to measure a country's health and quality of life.

Leadership   An advanced practice skill that involves socially influencing others and gaining the support of others. Leadership is not so much about the day-to-day activities of management, administration, and supervision, but is about influencing and inspiring others. An example of leadership in public health is Mrs. Obama's role in fighting childhood obesity.

Management   Controlling the overall activity of the unit or organization through planning, organizing, staffing, supervising, and leading. Management is a type of administration, but in many cases, managers of units work for or report to the chief executive administrators rather than being the chief executive administrator.

Policy maker   In public health social work, policy makers write, present, advocate, and educate others about policy. Examples of policy making are developing a policy within your agency for workplace wellness, writing a bill for the state legislature for stronger nonsmoking legislation, and participating on a national committee that is writing standards of practice for public health social work.

Primary prevention   Efforts designed to avoid or ward off health and mental health problems before they begin. Examples of primary prevention—educating new college students on recognizing and managing test anxiety; health education programs in middle school on the harmful effects of smoking and drinking alcohol and how to avoid them in settings with peers.

Secondary prevention   Early detection and intervention to keep incipient health and mental health problems from becoming debilitating. Examples of secondary prevention are screening for ADHD in first graders and adults who are 10 to 20 lbs overweight participating in a diet and exercise program.

Social determinants of health   Health risk factors that result from the underlying inequalities in society. Social determinants include a person's socioeconomic status, access to health care, neighborhood, employment conditions, and personal behaviors.

Supervision   Supervision is a management activity that involves regular monitoring of an employee's work. Supervision can include educating staff on the tasks and processes to be done, coaching the staff as they are doing the activity, evaluating the employee's performance, and developing a plan for remediation or termination if the employee does not meet organizational standards.

Tertiary prevention   Limiting the disability associated with a particular disorder after the disorder has run its course typically, tertiary prevention is thought to stabilize, maintain, and when possible rehabilitate. Examples of tertiary prevention are inpatient physical rehabilitation after a person has a traumatic brain injury and a person with chronic obstructive pulmonary disease using portable oxygen.

Transdisciplinary   A team where the members come together to communicate, plan, and work together collaboratively. This is different from a multidisciplinary team where members from different disciplines come together to present their ideas and then come to a solution.

Questions for Further Study

1. Interview your field instructor or another social worker and ask them how they use prevention in their social work practice. Report what you have found in class, and brainstorm with your classmates to explore how social workers can further use prevention in their practice in mental health, acute care hospitals, outpatient clinics, dialysis, and other settings. Differentiate how primary, secondary, and tertiary prevention can be used in these settings.

2. Do a web search of dual MSW/MPH programs. What courses and competencies are needed for this joint degree? As you evaluate the results of this search, develop your own definition of public health social work.

3. What can public health contribute to social work? What can social workers contribute to public health? How do you see these disciplines collaborating and building to reach common goals?

4. Identify and discuss examples of the social determinants of health and health inequalities. Do a literature review of the social determinants of health and health inequalities. Discuss what you think are the most pressing problems today when it comes to the social determinants of health and health inequalities.

Websites

American Public Health Association, Social Work Section
The American Public Health Association (APHA) has 27 sections for members. The mission of the social work section is to establish standards for social work in health care settings and contribute to the development of public health social work in practice, research, and education.
www.apha.org/membergroups/sections/aphasections/socialwork

Centers for Disease Control and Prevention
A federal agency with the purpose of collaborating with agencies and health care providers throughout the United States and world to monitor health, detect and investigate disease, and provide research and leadership in disease control and prevention.
www.cdc.gov/

Healthy People 2020
From the U.S. Department of Health and Human Services; the vision of Healthy People 2020 is a society in which all people live long, healthy lives. This website includes evidence-based national objectives for improving health care for all Americans and identifies national priorities for public health issues.
www.healthypeople.gov/2020/default.aspx

Substance Abuse and Mental Health Services Administration (SAMHSA)
U.S. federal office for behavioral health and substance abuse prevention and treatment. Their platforms include behavioral health is essential to health, prevention works, treatment is effective, and people recover from mental illness and substance abuse. Federal programs and grants are posted on this website.
www.samhsa.gov/index.aspx

The World Fact Book of the U.S. Central Intelligence Agency (CIA)
Up-to-date country-by-country information covering content on government, geography, economics, communication, industry and agriculture, and transnational issues.
www.cia.gov/library/publications/the-world-factbook/index.html

U.S. Department of Health and Human Services (HHS)
The principal agency in the United States for protecting health, especially the health of those who are least able to protect themselves. This federal agency works with state and local governments and health departments.
www.hhs.gov

PART IV

Conclusion

CHAPTER 15

Health Care Social Work: A Product of Political and Cultural Times

Coordinated care, first introduced in the 2000s, continues to require that the role of the health care social worker remain flexible. Adjusting to service delivery needs rich in evidence-based practice principles continues to stress the development of efficient and effective best practices. For the health care social worker, flexibility to accommodate federal, state, and local policy changes, as well as adjusting to the changing roles of other health care professionals has become the state of practice (Browne, 2012b). If social workers do not respond to these demands, then they will be replaced with other professionals who perform similar functions. The purpose of this chapter is to review the factors critical to the understanding and further development of health care social work. Professional issues and challenges will be discussed and suggestions for the future will be highlighted.

AFFORDABLE HEALTH CARE AND COORDINATED CARE

According to the Kaiser Foundation (2007) in 2006, one in every six Americans did not have health insurance and this constituted approximately 47.5 million people. Employer-sponsored insurance was not an option for many of these citizens. With the number of uninsured growing, the pressure for affordable health care has never been greater. The recent passing of the Affordable Care Act (ACA) was just one example (U.S. Department of Health and Human Services, 2012) of efforts to hold insurance companies accountable by setting standards for reform that allow for lower health care costs. This would also guarantee more choices that enhance quality of care. ACA is expected to support health care changes while improving health care access, quality, and service for 32 million Americans who currently do not have health care coverage (Ofosu, 2011).

Coordinated care has a broad-based emphasis, where technology is integrated into the care and efficiency and effectiveness needs go beyond just helping the patient/client/consumer (hereafter referred to as patient). Emphasis needs to be placed on recognizing the need for healthy behaviors and supporting their development (Engstrom, 2012). This type of treatment requires assuring that the greatest concrete and identifiable therapeutic gains are achieved in the quickest amount of time and with the least amount of financial and professional support. This means that the interventions that social workers provide must not only be socially acknowledged as necessary, but also must be therapeutically effective (Franklin, 2002) as well as be specifically individualized to guide all further intervention efforts (Maruish, 2002). For social workers, effectiveness must also reflect our rich history and that all change efforts are firmly based in our ethical and philosophical foundations (Sparks, 2012).

In addition, these services must be not only be individually designed, therapeutically necessary, and effective, but also must be professionally competitive with other disciplines that claim similar treatment strategies and techniques. This has led to the re-birth of all efforts for patient betterment to be outcome-driven and evidence-based to be acknowledged as effective (Donald, 2002). See Figure 15.1.

EVOLUTION OF HEALTH CARE SOCIAL WORK

As outlined in the earlier chapters of this book, the practice of health care social work has changed dramatically over the years. Traditionally, the health care social worker, similar to the entire social work profession, was linked to serving the poor and the disenfranchised. A clearer definition of what the health care social worker does has been further complicated by basic changes in the health care environment which includes scope of practice, the roles served, and the expectations within the patient–practitioner relationship. Furthermore, this definition along with the focus of care is shifting, making the provision of services to patients and their families difficult to anticipate (Ontario Association of Social Workers, 2009). There is now less emphasis on inpatient acute, tertiary, and specialty/subspecialty care, whereas there is more emphasis on ambulatory and community-based care, emphasizing the role of the physician's office, group practice, and health maintenance organizations (Rock, 2002). Services such as case management and discharge planning have increased considerably in importance, highlighting the need for managing the patient relative to his or her immediate situation (Frankel & Gelman, 2012). These changes require social workers to constantly battle

Outcomes-Based Behavioral Health Care

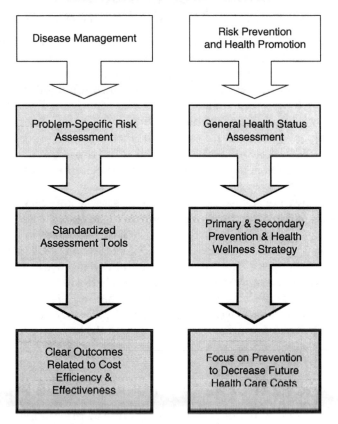

Figure 15.1 Outcomes-based behavioral health care.

"quality-of-care" versus "cost containment" measures for patients, while securing a firm place as a professional provider in a competitive health care environment.

Today, the health care social worker can be viewed as the professional "bridge" who links the patient; the multidisciplinary, interdisciplinary, intradisciplinary, or pandisciplinary team; and the environment. For future marketability and competition, social workers need to move beyond the traditional role of the health care social worker. In the area of clinical practice, new or refined methods of service delivery need to be established and used (Jansson, 2011). Social workers are encouraged to assume positions such as managers, owners of companies, administrators, supervisors, clinical directors, and behavioral care case managers where they can help influence qualifications for services, specific agency policy, services, and procedure.

BEHAVIORAL CARE PRINCIPLES, COORDINATED CARE, AND THE HEALTH CARE ENVIRONMENT

Many events have occurred over the last 25 years that have transformed health care delivery and social work practice. For continued survival in this environment, several steps are suggested for health care social workers: (a) continue to market the services they provide and link them to cost–benefit measurement; (b) present themselves as essential team members on the health care interdisciplinary, multidisciplinary, intradisciplinary, or pandisciplinary teams; (c) never forget the importance of anticipating the environment and the role that political and social influences can have on service delivery; and (d) look beyond the traditional expectations and assumptions historically noted as clinical professional practice in the health care field. New and innovative ideas and methods of service delivery are needed, from rethinking foundations issues in terms of human growth and development (Farley, Smith, Boyle, & Ronnau, 2002) to application of these concepts in an evidence-based framework (Dziegielewski, 2008a; Wodarski & Dziegielewski, 2002). As a field, new and revitalized models to guide practice in social work are needed to compete in today's health care environment. Health care remains a changing environment that requires a resilient social work professional where active attention to health care reform is needed (Zabora, 2011).

ROLES AND STANDARDS FOR HEALTH CARE PRACTICE

All social workers, whether in the role of clinical practitioner, case manager, discharge planner, supervisor, administrator, or community organizer, have been challenged to anticipate our current health care system and the effects it will have on current and future practice. Incremental changes involve compromising and implementing service agreements that are based on the needs/wishes of various political forces. Integrated services and systems that incorporate technological advances must occur under behavioral care principles that make teamwork as well as an awareness of corporate and administrative policies and procedures essential ingredients for success.

Integrated care requires that adequate links be made between the corporate governance structure and the modes and/or agencies that deliver services. Furthermore, coordinated care requires that linkages need be made between coordinated care and other health maintenance organizations, acute care facilities and services, long-term care services and facilities, transitional or home-based services, mental health and substance abuse services, wellness, and prevention services, as well as standard care that may be received in the physician's office (see Figure 15.2). Coordination through referrals, discharge planning, and case management has long been the responsibility of social work; and never before has this role been more important than in today's environment to ensure the continuity of care for each patient served. For each health care social worker engaged in practice, the control of rising health care costs will ultimately be considered his or her responsibility, whether they he or she has the ultimate power to control this trend or not. This leads to accepting responsibility for participation in transformative initiatives that can make the system better for all served (Rosenthal, 2011).

Responsibility for quality service delivery in this cost-containment climate has increased the need for greater emphasis on macropractice. This means that health care social workers must take an active role in ethical

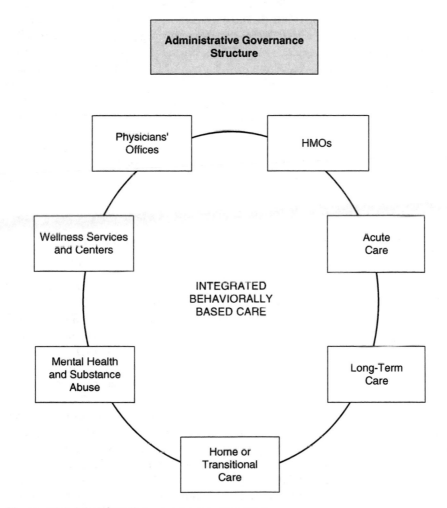

Figure 15.2 Administrative governance structure.

practice while advocating for social action and social change (Sparks, 2012). Social workers must work actively to help society to understand its responsibility to control and regulate the health care industry. Health care social workers, no matter what setting they work in, must help to develop and present a format for approaching problems in the current system and establishing means for addressing them.

FIELDS OF HEALTH CARE SOCIAL WORK PRACTICE

Staff reductions and changes continue to happen throughout the field of health care social work. Yet, health care social workers are not the only profession being targeted for reduction; it is happening across all disciplines as a means of cost reduction. To remain competitive, health care professionals need to be flexible, open, and ready to embrace the future. However, we should never lose sight of our ethical and moral judgment that is needed to steer the profession and ourselves for the betterment of the patients we serve. Corcoran (2012) reminds us of the importance of learning by doing and not being afraid to expand our horizons while utilizing a strengths-based perspective each step of the way. In addition, social workers need to participate in conducting research that can support the work that is being completed on a clinical as well as a research level. Each of the chapters in the special topic sections of this book looks at the issues germane to the field. The biographical sketches of health care social workers throughout the book offer valuable insights into the problems that they confront in everyday practice, and how they believe some of these problems can be overcome.

SHORTAGE OF NURSES: AN OPPORTUNITY FOR SOCIAL WORK GROWTH

Officially, after years of speculation, it has been confirmed that there is a nursing shortage. By all reports, this shortage will reach crisis proportions by 2015 when the United States will experience a 20% shortage of available nurses (HRSA, 2002). In response to this pending crisis, federal and state agencies, legislatures, professional nursing organizations, the health care industry, labor organizations, and private philanthropies have all responded with analysis, recommendations, and in some cases resources (Buerhaus, Needleman, Mattke, & Stewart, 2002). This marshaling of forces has produced a myriad of suggested responses. But the question remains, what does this shortage mean for the role of the nurse as case manager, a role that has always traditionally been filled with social workers. Furthermore, nurses in general report that salary earnings have decreased under managed care principles (Bauer, 2001a, 2001b). Meanwhile, research from the University of Pennsylvania suggests that nursing graduates are leaving the profession in record numbers within the first four years of working (Sochalski, 2002).

In the past, nurse managers would have responded to such a shortage in a fairly typical manner. Retention efforts would be intensified through improved compensation packages and creative scheduling options until aggressive recruitment efforts by educational programs could increase the supply of available nurses (Tanner & Bellack, 2001). However, by all accounts, for nursing professional, this is a shortage unlike any other (Kimball, O'Neil, & Health Workforce Solutions, 2002). Managed care has contributed to a significant increase in the acuity of hospitalized patients (Buerhaus et al., 2002), and the aging population is causing an increased demand for patient care services (Quinless & Elliott, 2000).

This shortage of nurses, who have traditionally been considered essential personnel in the health care field, needs to be openly acknowledged by social workers. Nurses are assuming many of the responsibilities that were traditionally in the domain of social work. For example, this is clearly explicated in Chapter 13, which focuses on discharge planning and case management. As discussed in this book, many nurses continue to assume the roles of the social worker and completing similar if not identical duties at a much higher rate of pay. Therefore, this nursing shortage can be of pivotal importance to health care social workers and serve as a means to take back or increase their role in activities that was previously their domain.

This can only be accomplished, however, by: (1) establishing through evidence-based practice the importance of what they do in helping the patient; (2) responding to social, political, and clinical demands to continue to identify outcomes-based service criteria; and (3) openly advocating and stressing the importance of the service provided in terms of promoting overall health and wellness. Special importance needs to be placed on the increasing numbers of re-admissions and recidivism and how social work services often neglected in today's system can enhance service provision and decrease recidivism.

CONCEPTS ESSENTIAL TO HEALTH CARE PRACTICE

In social work, health care practice needs to continue to incorporate an inclusive biopsychosocial approach that integrates the biomedical and the psychosocial approaches to practice (Browne, 2012b). Important to this approach is understanding the patient's experiences from a perspective that takes into account the interactions among biological, psychological, and societal and cultural processes (Straub, 2012). From this expanded perspective, special attention is always given to inclusion of the spiritual and the cultural aspects of all the patients that social workers serve. It is no surprise that this framework allows the social worker to provide comprehensive assessment of the patient as well as assisting his or her family and community supports. This approach, particularly the focus on the biopsychosocial in its many varied forms, has traditionally been viewed as the basis for social work practice often utilized in the health care area to facilitate transdisciplinary practice and continuity of care (Egan et al., 2011).

Teamwork and collaborative efforts remain strong in health care service delivery and most professionals would agree that good communication is always essential to effective health care (Gehlert, 2012). Yet as a member of the collaborative team, it is not uncommon for blurred definitions and diffuse boundary distinctions to occur between professionals. These problems can result in difficulty defining tasks and obligations. Furthermore, the expectation of blending of roles, tasks, and services can become complicated. Therefore, these blurred and overlapping functions among professionals can complicate the tasks that need to be performed. After all, this tight-knit group of professionals is expected to always act as a team. But this does not have to be viewed as being problematic.

To social work professionals, it can be viewed as a way to expand their role and the services they provide as part of the team. To exemplify this concept, the social worker is encouraged to become a leading professional in the quality review process. It is also recommended that health care social workers highlight the issues related to informed consent. Informed consent requires that the health care provider make the patient aware of the nature of the medical treatments to be given as well as the risks and benefits. To ensure patient confidentiality and privacy, social workers are in a strong position to ensure protecting patient health-related information. Awareness of the Health Insurance Portability and Accountability Act (HIPAA) enacted in 1996, which establishes new rules for the privacy and security of electronic medical records, can help to ensure that *protected health information (PHI)* remains confidential. This privacy rule requires mental health practitioners to develop procedures for controlling the disclosure and use of patient information, whereas the security rule requires the implementation of administrative, technical, and physical safeguards to protect patient information (Bernstein & Hartsell, 2004). Health care social workers can make excellent team leaders and can guide this process, while ensuring that privacy and confidentiality of all health services are provided. They can also expand their roles creating medical–legal partnerships (MLPs) with attorneys. These relationships will allow for a partnership that focuses on identification of legal problems that can have a negative impact on patient health (Colvin, Nelson & Cronin, 2012).

Health care social workers can also serve an active role serving on ethics committees and institutional review boards that protect patients' rights. Health care social workers can be beneficial with their strong ethical code principles to redirect interpersonal considerations (Sparks, 2012).

PRACTICE STRATEGY

Coordinated care that is reflective of outcomes-supported best practices is creating a practice revolution in which the provision of social work services needs to remain an integral component. Interest in time-limited interventions has greatly increased and will most probably continue to increase over the years (Dziegielewski, 2008a). This is especially true in the area of home-based programs or community support services.

Today, practice strategy in the health care environment is often intermittent, whereas each session stands alone and is conducted as if it is the only patient contact that will occur (Dziegielewski, 2008a). Since so many more individuals are living with chronic pain the need to build hope and provide concrete strategies that increase patient empowerment has never been greater (Ellner & Woods, 2012). Coordinated care agencies and employee assistance programs (EAPs) require structured time-limited interventions that are based on outcomes-focused best practice strategy. To take this a step further, it is suggested that social workers continue to learn and use education that utilizes health promotion and other communication strategies that help to create messages that can influence the patient as well as the community at large for improved health promotion and decision making (Edgar & Volkman, 2012). Use of a comprehensive wellness strategy of education and direct intervention, as described in this book, remains a practice reality that cannot be underscored more.

Furthermore, insight-oriented intervention and cure-focused therapy seem to have been replaced by outcomes-based behavioral change, which is considered to be more realistic and practical. Health care social workers (similar to physicians) generally do not cure the problems patients suffer from—nor are they expected to. What is expected, however, is to help patients realize and use their own strengths to diminish or alleviate symptoms or states of being that lead to discomfort. Emphasis on evidence-based practice and outcomes-based behavioral changes are not only expected, but they are also required for "state-of-the-art" practice.

In health care, the use of time-limited and intermittent practice strategies have been clearly established. Models and methods of service delivery, such as those presented in this book, only begin to open the door to what is left to come. Health care social workers are being forced by an environment focused on best practice strategy, fee for reimbursement, capitation, and so on, to continue to demonstrate effectiveness and cost containment in the intervention methods they employ (Gibelman, 2002). Whether social workers like it or not, professional survival dictates change. Behavioral health measurement has introduced a new practice revolution that social workers need to embrace with confidence (Dziegielewski, 2010a).

In general, no matter what setting the health care social worker engages, he or she needs to embrace a more eclectic approach to practice—in which allegiance to one particular model or method is discouraged (Colby & Dziegielewski, 2010). In selecting a clinical practice method in behavioral health, the following considerations are suggested: (a) utilize a time-limited intervention approach; (b) always stress mutually negotiated goals and objectives; (c) use best practices when available and make every effort to include evidence-based objectives that bare behaviorally linked, outcomes-based, and measurable; (d) focus on patient strengths and self-development;

(e) select interventions that are concrete, realistic, and obtainable; and (f) change efforts should be based on the needs and desires of the patient being served—not the preference of the social worker. By adapting this flexible perspective, the social worker will be better prepared to deliver the services expected while maintaining the highest degree of marketability possible.

COST–BENEFIT ANALYSIS

The growth of the over-65 population, the rising costs of health care, and numerous other societal events have stimulated attention and subsequently rocked the delicate balance between cost containment and quality of care. In the resultant health care practice environment, cost reduction is considered the primary maintenance issue. This means that health care social workers must now recognize that at each stage of the intervention encounter, the resultant bottom-line dollar expenditures and savings will be the intended target. To compete successfully, social workers must also show that the services they provide, similar to other professionals in the health care field, can be related to initial dollar savings. An example of this can be viewed in discharge planning from the hospital to home health care services. For example, the social worker must first compute the rate of a general inpatient stay in the medical facility. Generally, most social workers can simply call hospital admissions and ask them for the daily rate for room and board. If a social worker is able to facilitate a discharge home in a timely manner, he or she can simply compute this amount in relation to the cost of an additional in-house stay. With this type of simple calculation, it is easy to see the cost savings that occur with appropriate and timely discharges. This is why discharge planning often receives so much attention.

When patients are discharged with a lack of support services, this can contribute to high recidivism rates. Direct dollar savings have always been difficult for social workers to calculate because little emphasis has been placed on actual prevention of costs. As times change, social workers need to realize the importance of cost–benefit analysis and attach this measurement to every service they provide. Recording and justifying these costs can help social workers to establish the importance of their service from a dollar-driven administrative perspective.

INCLUSION OF PRIVATE PRACTICE: UNITING PHYSICIANS AND SOCIAL WORKERS

For many social workers in health care, the idea of inclusion of private practice might raise a few eyebrows. Yet today, independent private practice or serving in practice within a physician's office remains one of the fastest-growing sectors of social work practice. As social workers become eligible to receive third-party payments for the provision of intervention, and physicians realize the importance of a supportive environment to success in patient care, the area of private practice becomes more inviting. Private practice can serve to develop and expand marketability for health care social workers, particularly those with an interest in providing direct therapeutic intervention to patients.

In the field of social work, the disagreement regarding an increasing market for private practice services continues to rage. Many professionals disagree with the movement toward private practice because they believe it is abandoning social work's original call to serve the poor and underserved. It is further believed that the more social workers enter into private practice, the more spaces will be left open in public sector jobs that were previously filled by social workers. Based on this withdrawal of graduate-level social workers, these positions are now being filled by professionals from other related disciplines. However, in the area of health care social work, this argument is not nearly as relevant. Health care social workers have generally been employed in many areas of social work and continue to serve in the areas of hospital social work, AIDS counseling and education, public health, hospice/counseling and management, home health care, case management, discharge planning, maternal and child health, physical rehabilitation, chemical dependency, and disease prevention and health promotion. Employers of health care social workers continue to be health maintenance organizations, nursing homes, hospitals, clinics, hospice programs, and group homes (NASW, 2005). For future growth, particularly affiliated with physicians' offices or HMOs, entering into private practice arrangements can assist health care social workers to expand their practice arena and, therefore, their marketability. This is particularly true in the area of behavioral health and wellness counseling.

Today, to engage in private practice successfully, the health care social worker must compete for preferred provider status, a position that was virtually unheard of 10 years ago. Membership as providers in coordinated care agencies is essential for health care social workers as it will allow the social worker to accept patients and avoid preauthorization reviews. Mathews (2012) believes that there may be a subtle return to many of the practices of managed care organizations and if this leads to more restrictions that may not always be in the best interest of the patient. All social workers need to be aware and adapt to this type of thinking which is business or corporate focused. Social workers interested in private practice or contracting for services must be aware of the requirements and subsequent limitations relevant to the top tier processes noted in coordination of care. For health care social workers who wish to engage in private practice, partnerships with physicians and other health care providers will remain a critical necessity. Unfortunately, there is no way around them unless the health care social worker is capable of generating only self-pay patients or limits practice to consultation. For more information on managing and creating private practice and whether it is right for you see "Private Practice: When It's Not Right for You (Perk, 2012).

CLINICAL LICENSURE

Generally, in medical social work, a graduate level (MSW) of education is usually required for reimbursement. Almost all states require that social workers be licensed to qualify as providers. The purpose of licensure is to ensure that patients can receive competent, ethical, and moral services. Licensure ensures that social work practitioners have a minimum level of competence necessary to perform professional functions. Health care social workers can benefit from licensure, similar to all social workers. Whether an individual social worker is practicing under the auspices of an agency or not, more emphasis will be placed on licensure and obtaining it to receive third-party reimbursement. Licensure can help health care social workers to maintain current levels of marketability as well as anticipation of future trends. The benefits of the health care social worker being licensed to the patient remain consistent. For health care social workers, licensure at the bachelor of social work (BSW) or the MSW level is highly encouraged.

AWARENESS OF MEDICATIONS AND ALTERNATIVE TREATMENTS

Health care social workers have been forced to examine their intervention methods and modalities with a new vigor. To compete successfully, or more simply stated to survive, in the health care arena, it has become clear that social workers must provide effective and accountable practice. This type of practice must incorporate health care concepts familiar to social work, particularly for those who work in mental health. The techniques medical social workers are expected to know encompass knowledge regarding diagnostic criteria as well as usage and side-effect profiles of the medications so often used in treatment (Dziegielewski, 2010b). Social workers are often called on to give advice for medical treatment or to recommend what medications would best serve as adjunct to the current intervention being provided. And, with the current shortage of nurses, this trend is expected to increase.

Therefore, social workers need to be familiar with current diagnostic guidelines and the medications that are often used. Unfortunately, it was not until fairly recently that social work professionals have addressed the clinical application of psychopharmacology. This has resulted in many of the current resources available being written by non–social work professionals. Yet these other disciplines often do not relate this information directly back to social work treatment principles and strategy. Social workers are, therefore, expected to infuse the field's own practice base and ethical and moral issues into the practice guidelines suggested. Since it is beyond the scope of this text to cover all the basics that are needed in terms of medication knowledge and application, the health care social worker is referred to Dziegielewski's (2006) *Psychopharmacology for the Non-Medically Trained* or Dziegielewski's (2010b) text *Social Work Practice and Psychopharmacology: A Person Environment Approach*.

Although all accredited social work programs generally offer at least one graduate-level course in psychopathology or clinical diagnosis, few offer separate courses in understanding medication or herbal preparation usage. Considering that most social workers may not be required to receive training about medications and herbal preparations in their graduate and undergraduate programs, information reflective of this area is strongly recommended.

Furthermore, knowledge of alternative treatments is also essential. Having knowledge of medications, herbal remedies, and alternative practices are a practice reality for today's health care social worker (Dziegielewski, 2010b). Whether the more radical stance is taken actually to acquire enough education to have limited prescription privileges as suggested by Dziegielewski (1997b), or the more conservative role suggested by Bentley (1997) is adopted, it is clear social workers must have, at a minimum, a general knowledge of medications and their usage. Health care social workers must be familiar with side-effect profiles, dosage routines, and so on, to assist patients to obtain and maintain the most therapeutically productive treatment possible. They must be able to recognize potential problem areas to refer the patient for adequate or revised treatment. Social workers must stay updated with new trends in the field, and how these new medications can affect the patient and the counseling relationship.

LINKING EVIDENCE-BASED PRACTICE WITH BEST PRACTICES

For the health care social worker, the process of recording needs to go beyond the traditional bonds of documentation. Documentation to support and justify evidence-based practice is pivotal. Mixing research and practice yields the type of record keeping employed in the medical setting. This mix must consider the need to achieve both quality of service and cost effectiveness. Although this union may, at times, be an awkward one, the combination is essential to ensure delivery of efficient and effective services.

In health care, a connection between research and practice is critical, and questions to guide the scientific inquiry process include the following: What does the social worker want and need to know about the problem? For example, if there is interest in studying discharge patterns of older adults, is there already a significant amount of information in this area? Is the health care social worker the one that needs to conduct the research? Are other disciplines more suited to completing the study, and if so, what role can the social worker play in this process? For example, if we want to monitor our patients and their responses to medications in the home, we may need some assistance from the interdisciplinary team to accomplish this.

A second important factor is what to do once the information has been gathered in order to determine how it can be used. For example, can the information gathered be used to facilitate the implementation of teen education groups, AIDS prevention programs, and health and wellness education? Unfortunately, identifying the problem may constitute only a small step toward the solution of the problem—particularly, when interest in addressing the problem is not supported in the immediate environment. Many times, the administration may not see the problem as a crucial one to be studied. Administrative nonsupport can leave the health care social worker unaware of the problems and obstacles a nonsupportive environment can create. Administrative interest and investment can be essential in creating a climate open and facilitative of change.

The health care social worker must assess if there are any logistical obstacles present. If so, would measurement be an insurmountable problem? Can the data needed, be obtained? Once the information is gathered, where will the social worker put it? Many times, case records are interdisciplinary in nature and there simply is no room for this type of information. These are just some of the questions that health care social workers must face when they engage in evidence-based practice. Today the pressure to act on this evidence-based means of practice has never been more intense. There is one addition, however, that must be added to this analogy, and that is the concept of cost effectiveness. In today's health care environment, it is openly proclaimed that there must be a balance between quality of care and cost-effectiveness; however, few professionals would argue which one appears to carry the most weight (Dziegielewski, 2010a). In addition to proving that social work practice is efficient and effective, it also must be established that practice can be completed with as little effort and expense as possible.

The health care environment is changing rapidly, and with the tremendous increase in allied health professionals, only the strongest will be able to compete. Not only is this survival important for the profession of health care social work, but it is also essential for the patients who are served. Each day and with every task, the health care social worker completes, the patient's lifestyle and expectations are influenced. Health care social workers help to make their patients better able to relate to their environments. To continue to address the patient-in-environment match in the health care setting adequately, there is no choice—practice and research must be one. When practice and research combine, evidence-based practice results (Wodarski & Dziegielewski, 2002). It is this type of practice strategy that will be best suited to stand the rigor and instability of the coordinated care environment in which the health care social worker must survive.

This book is written to provide a basis for understanding the roles and tasks of the health care social worker when practicing in multiple settings. Regardless of the setting, new technology needs to be linked to evidence-based practice strategy with a direct link to cost containment. To complete this, changes in both research and practice strategy will be required (Rosen & Proctor, 2002). Best practice strategies will need to remain outcome driven to address the scientific vigor needed to facilitate efficient and effective practice. Social work practitioners are urged to learn best practices principles and evaluate the strengths and limitations of these outcomes-driven methods for service delivery.

In evidence-based practice, health care social workers must be aware of emerging technology while mixing practice, research, and cost-containment strategy, and document this accordingly. Intervention plans must show and report success in these areas to justify third-party reimbursement, capitation, and fee for service; yet, this must be done in a limited and often restricted setting. Health care social workers must be able to understand the integration of evidence-based methods and not fear suggesting new and improved methods of documentation that make justification reflective of the professionally therapeutic and economic reality that has been created through the service implemented. If health care social workers engage in evidence-based practice strategy that follows the scientific method, this can also assist to assure that patients are not harmed by practice fallacies that do not involve sound critical thinking (Gibbs, 2002).

DEALING WITH STRESS AND PREVENTING BURNOUT

Any book in the area of health care social work would be deficient if it did not recognize the high-stress environment in which most social workers will be expected to function, and also the importance of dealing with stress and recognizing potential signs and symptoms that could relate to burnout. To help anticipate this problem seminars and training on stress management and prevention of burnout need to be considered (Green & Dziegielewski, 2004). It is believed that participation in these seminars can be effective in increasing understanding and strategies for dealing with stress, thereby allowing professionals to better cope with stressful situations (Deckro et al., 2002).

Health care social workers need to be able to identify: (1) stressful situations; and (2) have an awareness of how to develop and implement strategies to reduce stress. Becoming aware of stress and how to identify it can in itself be preventative. Dziegielewski et al. (2004) encourage the application of psychoeducation regarding stress and using it in a problem-based format. For the most part, the types of work that health care social workers perform are considered very stressful simply because of the types of problems that are encountered. Therefore, teaching strategies to reduce stress and prevent burnout provides fertile ground for future research related to the specific job tasks the health care social worker performs.

Health care social workers will face continued stress throughout their professional careers. Therefore, training health care social workers and other professionals in the health field on how to better cope with stress and burnout and how to apply this information in their academic and professional lives is without a doubt an important area for further exploration.

FUTURE TRENDS: EXPANDING THE ROLE OF THE
HEALTH CARE SOCIAL WORKER

This book presents the basic concepts related to the delivery of social work services in health care. Behavioral health care has been influenced greatly by best practices and outcomes-driven practice strategy. This advent has required the role of health care professionals to change, causing social workers to question the services they provide and ensuring that all service is necessary, comprehensive, effective, and cost containing.

Aronson et al. (2009) remind us that regardless of how hard the times are we must always hang on to what is really important, and that revolves around providing quality patient care. In addition, in today's health care environment, effectiveness must go beyond just helping the patient and must also involve validation that the greatest concrete and identifiable therapeutic gain was achieved with the least amount of financial and professional support (Donald, 2002). This means that not only must the intervention that social workers provide be therapeutically effective—it must also show cost–benefit as well. Health care social workers need to portray themselves as powerful contenders who are professionally competitive with other disciplines that claim similar intervention strategies and techniques. The battle in the health care arena of "more with less" continues to rage. Health care social workers continue to have one strong weapon to bring to the table that should not be underestimated in today's climate of fiscal restraint. Throughout history, social workers have provided similar interventions for less money. In social work, the NASW *Code of Ethics* clearly advises social workers to provide reasonable fees and base service charges on an ability to pay. This makes the fees social work professionals charge competitive when compared with psychiatrists, psychologists, family therapists, psychiatric nurses, and mental health counselors who profess they can provide similar services.

This cost-containment factor can provide enticement to coordinated care agencies to contract with social workers instead of other professionals to provide services of a health and wellness nature. In this era of behavioral health care, this strength is central and with the right marketing, and it can help social workers gain additional ground, adding to their employment desirability.

In general, social workers need to understand the philosophy of the current health care environment; based on this philosophy, they must be willing and able to use evidence-based social work practice strategy with an emphasis on cost containment and outcomes measures to assist individuals, groups, and families (Frager, 2000; Rudolph, 2000). Although medicine and technology have grown tremendously, there are still many uncertainties that persist. It is natural for patients and their families to be confused by the medical options available to them. The health care social worker can help to interpret the medical information as well as take into account the beliefs and expectations of the family allowing for a more comprehensive interpretation that takes into account the families, beliefs, and expectations (Rolland, 2012).

In closing, it is important to remember that the cultural and political environment in which health care delivery finds itself today is changing (Meenaghan, 2001); however, it is not necessarily the downfall of clinical health care social work practice as we have known it. Social workers are not only good practitioners, but they are also skilled activists well aware of the importance of political action and strategy. With this awareness, they can become active in devising and promoting the changes needed for population-level health promotion. It is clear that advocating and achieving policy changes can provide an environment conducive to healthier life styles choices (Delvin-Foltz, Fagen, Reed, Medina, & Neiger, 2012). Social workers need to embrace this challenge and continue to advocate for policy changes designed to support the patients served.

Although crisis can be intimidating—it is also a catalyst to change. Changes impossible before are now possible, but the health care social workers need to acknowledge and accept this challenge swiftly and eagerly. New frontiers that can increase marketability need to be explored and pursued. Empowering patients to link mind–body strategies for intervention and providing them with the skills they need can build hope and resiliency (Ellner & Woods, 2012). Challenge, opportunity, and subsequent risk remain part of the health care social worker's future. In behavioral health care, the provision of social work services with its person-in-environment stance remains an integral component. As health care social workers struggle for survival, they are not alone. The other professional specialties are scared of these practice changes, too. The traditional view of health care social work with its perspective of "treating the total person" and "the person–environment stance" fits beautifully into the current demand for holistic practice intervention that focuses on wellness and prevention. The task for health care social workers remains clear.

The revolution in health care delivery is well underway. Now social workers must decide whether we want to take an active part in this fight or whether we just want to sit at the "gate" and make sure the other medical specialties get through. Realizing the problems within the system and providing a "bridge over troubled waters" will allow the health care social worker to continue to deliver competent, effective, and efficient health care services (Ellis, 2009). If we want it, we will have to fight for it. Engaging in this battle will benefit our patients and us as a profession. If we decide not to advocate for ourselves and assume a position of hesitance and apathy for too long, the importance and strength of the social worker as a crucial member of the health care delivery team will go untold, and the other more assertive professions will be free to claim what once was our turf.

Glossary

Protected health information (PHI)   A term related to protecting private health information and ensuring that this private individual health information is recorded and processed in a way that confidentiality and privacy is maintained. Generally, to release this information, signed consent of the patient (or his or her representative) is required.

Questions for Further Study

1. What do you see as the current role of the health care social worker?

2. What is coordinated care and how will it affect the development of best practices?

3. What are some of the challenges social workers in this field need to be aware of? Once identified, what are some of the ways that these changes can be addressed and later incorporated into the practice environment?

Websites

Health Care and Social Work Jobs
Job openings in the field.
www.quintcareers.com/healthcare_jobs.html

Health and Social Work
Accesses on-line articles.
www.naswpress.org/publications/journals/hsw.html

Home Page
A forum for debate on social work and health care research.
www.scie-socialcareonline.org.uk/

The New Social Worker's Online Career Center
Employment opportunities and job seeking tips.
www.socialworker.com/career.htm

Journal of Social Work Practice
Contents and abstracts of articles in past issues
www.tandf.co.uk/journals/carfax/02650533.html

National Council for Community Behavioral Healthcare
Advocates in Washington to advance the interests of members
and consumers.
www.thenationalcouncil.org/

World Federation of Mental Health
An international nonprofit advocacy organization. Consultant to the UN and of public education programs such as World Mental Health Day. www.wfmh.com

Megasites With Links to Hundreds of Other Sites

World Wide Web Resources for Social Workers
Developed by New York University, this website contains hundreds of links to social work resources in a wide range of topics. www.nyu.edu/socialwork/wwwrsw/

Social Work Search
Providing over 500 different Internet links and related services devoted solely to the social work profession. www.socialworksearch.com/html/about.shtml

Health Finder
Selected online publications, databases, websites, government agencies, and not-for-profit organizations information. www.healthfinder.org/

Today's Health Care Social Worker

Name:	Kendall Basore, MSW, LSW
State of Practice:	Indiana
Professional Job Title:	Social Worker

Duties in a Typical Day:
I am the sole EAP therapist for IU Health Bloomington Hospital as well as IU Health Southern Indiana Physicians. I provide short-term solutions-focused treatment for patients with a variety of mental health needs and make appropriate referrals to outside providers when necessary. I often conduct numerous educational programs for employees in areas such as work–life balance, self-care, stress reduction, and stigma awareness.

As a part of the Crisis Response Team, I also provide hospital-wide and department-specific critical incident debriefing sessions when needed. Finally, I also develop and implement treatment and discharge plans as a therapist for the Inpatient Behavioral Health Unit and assist with crisis management and

(continued)

Today's Health Care Social Worker (*continued*)

suicide prevention as part of the Access Team. However, a typical day usually comprises conducting therapy sessions, documentation, and answering a host of email.

1. **What do you like most about your position?**
   My job has allowed me to get to know many different people from various parts of the IU Health system that I never would have gotten to meet. As the EAP therapist, the role has allowed me to be a part of numerous committees, such as the Self-Care Committee, which actively works to improve work–life balance and reduce stress hospital wide. I am constantly expanding my knowledge of evidence-based practices because I am able to create educational programs around things I am interested in (and that I think will benefit others).

2. **What do you like least about your position?**
   At times, it can be a bit overwhelming trying to balance all the different priorities within my job!

3. **What words of wisdom do you have for the new health care social worker who is considering working in a similar position?**
   Get to know your resources. When I started this position, I was relatively new to the city and did not know what was available both in and out of the hospital system regarding referral options (i.e., other providers, support groups, financial services, etc.). I did a lot of research because it is important to me that I provide my patients with the best services available, as well as numerous options, and it also helps me with networking. As a newer social worker, I have developed a close relationship with my coworkers and use them for support and advice when needed.

4. **What is your favorite social work story?**
   I'm not sure that I have a favorite story. I always feel really touched when I see a former patient and they stop me to tell me how much better they are doing and what a difference it made to come in and talk, especially if they had reservations beforehand due to stigma. I always remind them that it is them, not me, who made the change in their lives, but it does make me feel good to know that I was a part of making an important difference.

Today's Health Care Social Worker

Name: Robin Tripod Patten
State of Practice: Arkansas
Professional Job Title: Director of Social Services

Duties in a Typical Day:
I am the social worker in a small rural, 120-bed hospital. Each day brings different duties. I assist nurse case managers with discharge plans for our patients. That could include nursing home placement, Meals-on-Wheels, lifeline services, and the in-home assistance programs and transportation.

I usually take most of the child abuse and adult abuse hot line calls. I give resources to the domestic violence victims and discuss safety plans if they choose to return to the abusive home. I also assist our patients who are dying and work with their families to help them cope. After the death, I send the families an informational packet about grief. I assist our emergency department in the difficult cases where there has been a tragic death. These cases bring with them a discussion about organ donation. I make referrals for those patients needing drug and alcohol treatments. And finally, I assist with inpatient or outpatient treatment for the patients who have attempted suicide.

1. **What do you like most about your position?**
   I love my job and the different aspects of social work each day brings.

2. **What do you like least about your position?**
   I am the only social worker and sometimes there is not enough time to do all that is required.

3. **What words of wisdom do you have for the new health care social worker who is considering working in a similar position?**
   You will not be able to save the world. However, you can make a huge difference in the world by helping one person at a time.

4. **What is your favorite social work story?**
   On a recent Thanksgiving Eve, a 20-year-old pregnant patient arrived in our emergency department in premature labor. She was 6 weeks premature. She had bruising all over her body, but her face will be etched in my brain forever. Her eyes looked

(continued)

Today's Health Care Social Worker (*continued*)

like a raccoon's facial markings. Really dark around both eyes and even the whites of her eyes were blood shot. Her story was that she had been in a wreck the weekend prior. When pressed about the wreck, there was no police report made because "she had ran off in a ditch and hit her nose on the steering wheel." Supposedly, her uncle came to help her out and her car out of the ditch so there was no need for a police report.

She delivered very quickly. With the baby so premature, she had to stay in the hospital. When the mother came to visit with the baby, I visited with the mother, so did nurses, the obstetrician, and the pediatrician, all trying to get her help for domestic violence. Finally, she confided with a nurse that she was a victim and that is why she came to our hospital because the hospital where she received prenatal care from was already suspicious of domestic abuse and she did not want them to know. I talked with her again and was taught the Duluth Model of the cycle of domestic violence. I tried to get her to allow me to contact her mother. I also tried to get her to go to our local domestic violence shelter but to no avail. She still would not press charges. She still would not give permission to report. She would say the proverbial, "He would never really hurt me" and, "It was me that made him mad...."

As the baby grew and developed, we celebrated when the baby was going to be discharged from the hospital. The pediatrician ordered that the mom come and spend the night at the hospital with the baby to learn how to be comfortable with a sleep apnea machine. The pediatrician ordered that I (social worker) contact the Child Abuse Hotline, which was done. At first, they would not accept the report. The MD called herself and demanded that the home be investigated before she would allow the child to go home in this environment. The birth mom told the DCFS investigator that the baby would not be coming to their home, but to her mother's home. So they closed the case. That Friday night when the baby was to be discharged on Saturday, the mom did not come. On Saturday, when the mom came to visit, she cried and begged the nurses to NOT make her stay all night at the hospital because she could not do that. Finally, she told the nurses she would come back that night. She did not show. Sunday, we received word from local law enforcement that the mom had been murdered—another domestic violence episode and she was choked to death.

(*continued*)

(*continued*)

On Monday, I was finally able to meet the birth mother's mother. It was then that she told me that the final "beating" was the ninth time during this pregnancy she was victimized. The doctor reported that her original facial bruising was due to her being choked—so hard that she passed out. This caused the blood vessels to burst in her face and eyes and caused the labor to start prematurely. The body was trying to deliver the baby before the baby sustained injury as well. The baby was born with a bruise on her chest that was attributed to the domestic violence.

I talked with the mother (grandmother to baby) and she was so frustrated that her daughter would not allow anyone, including her own mother or grandmother, to help get her out of this situation. I explained how our staff tried and tried to provide assistance, but that our hands were tied as well. I did ask for and received written permission to contact our local state senator, Robert Thompson, to tell this story and to ask if he would sponsor a bill to give medical social workers the ability to contact law enforcement in cases such as these. Senator Thompson did draft such a bill, but had opposition from the ACLU and the Arkansas Hospital Association. But in the end, a bill was approved by both houses and signed into law by Governor Mike Beebe allowing medical social workers the ability to contact local law enforcement in instances where a victim of domestic violence is in grave danger. Since that time two other pregnant domestic violence victims have been seen in our hospital and the new law was invoked. Perhaps two lives have been saved.

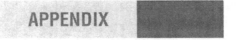
Recognizing Shaken Baby Syndrome

Joshua Kirven and Sophia F. Dziegielewski

UNDERSTANDING AND RECOGNIZING SHAKEN BABY SYNDROME

Health care social workers are competent to deal with a wide array of health crises, but they must be aware of early warning signs indicating shaken baby syndrome (SBS) and its consequences if failure to detect (Coles & Collins, 2007; Molina, Clarkson, Farley, & Farley, 2011). This sometimes brutal and often undetected form of child abuse can be deadly. It was not until 1972 that SBS was first described in the medical literature. Physicians used to think that injuries resulting from SBS were accidental, but as child abuse was studied more diligently, more cases of this syndrome were properly diagnosed (Caffey, 1972, 1974). In fact, neurosurgeons suggest in the United States that the numbers of children being excessively shaken by caretakers are staggering with over 50,000 children in the United States being forcefully shaken by their caretakers every year (Cantu & Gean, 2010). Victims of SBS are infants or children ranging in age from a few days old to 3 years, with some documented cases reaching up to 5 years of age. The majority of the reported cases average being 6 to 8 months old (Kinney & Thach, 2009).

Unfortunately, when the damage is severe, the child may enter into a coma. Those who do survive and recover from the coma often suffer profound mental retardation, spastic quadriplegia, severe motor dysfunction, blindness, varying degrees of paralysis, cerebral palsy, or other grave consequences. SBS is a frequent cause of permanent brain damage and intellectual impairment (Adamsbaum, Grabar, Mejean, & Rey-Salmon, 2010). The damage can be so severe that these babies have lasting effects that leave them as children with special needs. These special needs children often intensify the family dynamic and level of coping strategies of many caretakers. This appendix will examine SBS, overall statistics, problems encountered by health care social workers, and end with suggestions for education and prevention in this area.

The National Institute of Neurological Disorders and Stroke (NINDS) defines SBS as a constellation of injuries to the brain and eye that may occur in young children, with the majority of them being under one year of age, when the child is shaken violently. This violent shaking causes stretching and tearing of the cerebral vessels and brain substance, commonly leading to subdural hematomas and retinal hemorrhages, and these injuries are generally associated with cerebral contusion (an internal bruising of the brain). These injuries may result in paralysis, blindness, and other visual disturbances, convulsions, and death. The anatomy of infants renders them more susceptible to SBS than older children or adults since the head of the infant comprises 10% of his or her body weight compared with just 2% in the adult. Neck muscles have not developed strength compared with later in life, and consequently, the neck cannot absorb the energy generated during a whiplash event such as shaking. Infants at this stage lack head control and muscle mass so they cannot tense their bodies and prepare for sudden force (Kinney & Thach, 2009).

SBS generally occurs when caretakers experience high stress. Fifty years ago, SBS was not recognized as a classification and today it now accounts for more than 20,000 infant deaths per year (Barr et al., 2009). This incidence is growing and is often seen by health care social workers in emergency departments and other placements where they work. Although this focus is very important from a medicolegal perspective, completing a comprehensive evaluation by the social worker could help in educating and helping to remediate the effects of any resultant brain injury (Ashton, 2010).

When this type of abuse is suspected, the law mandates that the health care social worker must report the incident immediately to the State's Department of Children and Families. In order to report effectively, health care social workers need ongoing training on new advances in detection and the renaming of SBS to abusive head trauma (AHT) in much of the new literature, making the terms interchangeable (Findley, Barnes, Moran, & Squier, 2012; Walls, 2006). In further updated literature on inflicted childhood neurotrauma (Fiske & Hall, 2008) or abusive head trauma (Chiesa & Duhaime, 2009), much activity has centered on methods for identifying whether brain injuries are caused by abuse rather than by accidents (Barr & Runyan, 2008).

Unfortunately, the pathophysiology that occurs in SBS starts the moment that the baby is first shaken. Therefore, the severity of cerebral injury will be directly related to the severity of the shaking and the time elapsed during the event. Therefore, the perpetrator must be aware that the vigorous back-and-forth motion causes intense problems within the baby's skull, resulting in serious bruising to the brain as it hits the skull, which in turn causes the subdural bleeding. These factors contribute to cerebral edema and shearing of the blood vessels. As well as causing increased edema, bridging veins can occur in both subdural and subarachnoid compartments, leading to a constriction of the thorax which can also lead to retinal hemorrhages—a classic finding in SBS (Squier, 2011).

Damage also occurs within the eyes of the baby where retinal hemorrhages associated with SBS are attributable to rapid movement of the vitreous body and sudden increased intraocular pressure. This damage is so pronounced because a sudden rise in intracranial pressure is transmitted to the eyes via the optic nerve sheath. This mechanism causes the increased intraocular pressure where the baby could suffer permanent eye damage leading to blindness (Squier, 2011). Based on this finding, it is not uncommon for 30% to 80% of children who have suffered from concomitant intracranial and retinal injury to also have significant visual problems. There appears to be something distinct about abusive head injury with repetitive acceleration–deceleration with or without head impact that results in a pattern of severe retinal hemorrhage (Forbes & Levin, 2010). Therefore, SBS should be looked at closely for consideration in all children under 5 years of age as there may be other causes for retinal hemorrhage other than child abuse (See Box 1).

SBS presents challenges in assessment because on arrival it may not be easily identifiable as it is often obscure and hard to detect (Adamsbaum et al., 2010). The infant who has been a victim of SBS can present in many ways. In less severe cases, some of the symptoms include a history of poor feeding, sucking, or swallowing, vomiting, lethargy or irritability, hypothermia, failure to thrive, increased sleeping and difficulty arousing, and failure to smile or vocalize. Because of the vagueness of the symptoms, SBS may remain unidentified (Ashton, 2010). These types of symptoms can also occur frequently in

---

Box 1 Causes of infant retinal hemorrhage other than child abuse

Hypertension
Bleeding problems/leukemia
Meningitis/sepsis/endocarditis vasculitis
Cerebral aneurysm
Retinal diseases (e.g., infection, hemangioma)
Carbon monoxide poisoning
Anemia
Hypoxia/hypotension
Papilledema/increased intracranial pressure
Glutaric aciduria
Osteogenesis imperfect
Examinations in premature infants with retinopathy of prematurity
Extracorporeal membrane oxygenation
Hypo- or hypernatremia

other infectious processes common to infants and children. Subtle symptoms may occur intermittently for days or weeks preceding the first contact with a health care facility. The caretaker may put the child to bed hoping for natural resolution of symptoms. Instead, the condition of the infant frequently deteriorates (Forbes & Levin, 2010). In more severe cases of SBS, the symptoms are acute and often life threatening. Irreversible damage may already be present. Some of the more severe symptoms include: decreased level of consciousness, seizures, coma, bulging fontanel (indicative of increased intracranial pressure), periods of apnea, bradycardia, and complete cardiovascular collapse. Even when SBS symptoms are life threatening, however, it may go unrecognized. The presentation of such extreme symptoms may lead to misdiagnosis such as traumatic accident, meningitis, sepsis, or unusual neurologic disorders. The characteristic presentation of SBS is the lack of external trauma in the presence of intracranial and intraocular hemorrhage (Walls, 2006). Suspicion of child abuse may not be a consideration because of the absence of surface trauma.

Again, seeing internal injuries is not easy on visual assessment, and to complete the assessment radiological techniques such as computerized tomography (CT) and/or magnetic resonance imaging (MRI) would need to be completed for an accurate diagnostic description (Muni, Kohly, Sohn, & Lee, 2010). A CT scan has become the front line technique in imaging evaluation of the patient with brain injury. CT is generally the method of choice for diagnosing subarachnoid hemorrhage, mass effect, and large extra-axial hemorrhages (Muni et al., 2010). The most common CT finding in the shaken baby is subdural hematoma. It is also the most common cause of death in shaken babies when the death is classified as a homicide. MRI is of great value as an adjunct to CT. It offers better contrast sensitivity and clearer evidence of injury and is useful in determining the age of an injury (Cantu & Gean, 2010). Hand-held spectral domain optical coherence tomography allows high-resolution imaging of the vitreoretinal interface and retina in infants with SBS and has provided insight into the mechanism of various retinal findings (Muni et al., 2010). An ophthalmology exam is one of the simplest and cheapest ways of determining closed injury traumas, especially SBS (D'Lugoff & Baker, 1998). Hand-held spectral domain optical coherence tomography is helpful in the evaluation of patients with SBS (Muni et al., 2010). Retinal hemorrhages occur in about 75% of victims of SBS, indicating that an ophthalmology consultation is paramount on all patients with suspicious histories, including children with unexplained lethargy or seizures (D'Lugoff & Baker, 1998). Except in the first month of age, the presence of retinal hemorrhage in children younger than 4 years of age should serve as a red flag precursor for SBS (Babikian & Asarnow, 2009).

Once the child with a head injury is stable, a skeletal survey may rule out or confirm other injuries. Most abuse is not a single event; therefore, evidence of old injuries may be present. On examination, long bones, skull, spine, and ribs should be x-rayed (Emerson et al., 2007). Old injuries and injuries in various stages of healing are consistent with abuse should be examined.

According to Coles and Collins (2007), the profile of perpetrators is males (80%), with an average age of 23 years (ranging from 14 to 50 years of age) who are related to the victim or to the victim's mother (44% were fathers, 23% were boyfriends of the mother, 2% were stepparents, and 6% were unrelated male babysitters). Furthermore, children who have sustained a brain injury or trauma as a baby will need long-term follow-up with a comprehensive assessment and intervention packages focusing on protective factors and levels of functioning (Ashton, 2010). An astonishing finding in the research that distinguishes SBS from other forms of child abuse is that the mother is the least likely perpetrator (Babikian & Asarnow, 2009; Brennan et al., 2009; Coles & Collins, 2007; Walls, 2006).

SBS is a complex disorder with implications beyond the undeniable need for identification and protection for child victims. Social workers in a hospital setting, office practice, and public health and community practice play a major role in prevention, diagnosis, and treatment of the individual and family affected by SBS.

RISK FACTORS

There are many risk factors associated with SBS. Frequently, new parents are unaware of a child's normal development or an infant's basic needs. This lack of knowledge can create unrealistic expectations of the infant and/or child. Other parents may have a need for nurturing themselves and look, illogically, to the infant or child to fulfill that need. When these expectations are unsatisfied, a parent's stress and frustration increases. Young parents and single parents fall within the parental risk group. Their lack of life experience and immaturity may create unmanageable frustration when faced with an inconsolable infant. A crying infant, combined with poor impulse control in the parent and not knowing how to console their baby, places the child at high risk for SBS.

Another major risk factor contributing to SBS is substance abuse by either parent, and when the family system is under financial distress this could magnify the problem even further (Coles & Collins, 2007). Since most individuals under the influence of mind altering substances lose inhibition and impulse control, the actions that result may be severe and would never have been committed in a non-impaired state.

For example, infants born to substance-abusing mothers are at extreme risk for SBS (Brennan et al., 2009). Addicted themselves, these infants cry for extended periods, and to a mother who serves as the primary caregiver who is also addicted, these infants may seem inconsolable. Her frustration and altered mental status place that infant at high risk for SBS, neglect, and other forms of abuse.

Another factor increasing the risk of SBS is that the overall environment may increase the stress levels of all individuals. Numerous factors, such as financial, social, and physical burdens, which have changed negatively with the birth of a child, contribute to increased levels of stress. Any external factor that places stress on the parent puts an infant at risk for SBS.

Among these factors, lack of financial resources is a major stressor. The infant is at even greater risk if there was a significant effect on the family financial situation with the birth of the baby. Compounding that financial burden is the fact that the presence of a child often decreases the earning potential in a dual-income couple if adequate childcare resources are not available.

In the case of new parents or single parents, the responsibility of an infant often creates social isolation. They no longer have the freedom to pursue individual interests and goals. Things previously taken for granted no longer exist or are difficult to attain. These changes can result in resentment toward the infant. As time goes by, the parent may experience a decreased tolerance for the numerous needs of an infant.

The use of a narrative approach that incorporates an optimal worldview that can help the distressed parent or caretaker struggling with repressed feelings and negative thoughts toward their life being limited (Kirven, 2001). An optimal worldview can be added to the clinical milieu of the social worker in offering an alternative framework that can help parents or caretakers trying to make sense of this new reality and trying to find a more fulfilling life. This approach offers a practical coping strategy in strengthening the parent's/caretaker's protective factors.

In addition, physical elements of the surroundings, parent, or child may be risk factors. A parent with a physical disability may experience increased difficulty caring for an infant, leading to feelings of inadequacy. A child with a physical or mental disability places additional demands on the parent.

Ironically, infants themselves have intrinsic behavior patterns that place them at risk for SBS. The behavior that most often precedes an episode of shaking is crying. Infants spend about 20% of their time crying even in optimal situations with the parents not knowing what is wrong or how to respond (Brennan et al., 2009). Some parents perceive the crying as constant and unrelenting. It becomes even more frustrating when the infant is inconsolable. For example, infants with colic cry even more and often are inconsolable. An inconsolable infant can make the parent feel helpless and increasingly frustrated.

Previously unrecognized as a potential perpetrator of SBS, the family babysitter is an individual that can be considered risky because of immaturity and lack of life experience. When a caretaker from outside of the family is the perpetrator of SBS, there is often a failure to report the onset of symptoms to the parents (Coles & Collins, 2007). This lack of information makes it difficult to determine the time of injury (Christian & Block, 2009). Frequently, caregivers claim that the infant was fine when put to bed and then was unresponsive when later checked (Walls, 2006). A delay in recognizing and seeking early treatment for symptoms associated with SBS increases mortality and morbidity of injuries sustained. Given the number of families who rely on outside childcare, it is essential to target this group for education regarding the danger of SBS.

There have been episodes of SBS that are nonintentional. These "accidents" are linked to lack of understanding of the etiology of SBS. Rough horseplay such as swinging or tossing an infant can cause severe injuries. Or it can be related to cultural practices such as "Calda de Mollera" which is a form of Hispanic folk medicine (Molina et al., 2011). The purpose of the practice is to raise the sunken fontanel in an infant. The practitioner holds

---

From the Field: Social Work

In the emergency department of a local hospital, a 2-month-old baby boy's case was given to the social worker on the unit for assessment. The physician was concerned when the parents were unable to adequately explain what had happened to their baby boy. The baby presented as listless and unresponsive. When the social worker met the family, she recalled having seen them before. The couple had sought medical attention for another child in the past, when the sister had been treated for several broken ribs and a broken arm that were explained by the parents as a result of a fall from the crib. At that time, the social worker reported the case to the Department of Children and Families (DCF). On this occasion, similar to the incident in the past, the social worker should also report the case to DCF. In addition, she should continue to work closely with the family to help better assess what happened to the infant as well as how to best educate the family to be sure they understand the gravity of the situation. This interaction needs to begin with a social worker that is aware of the signs and symptoms of SBS. Once SBS is suspected, reporting the case to DCF is of primary importance as the social worker is a mandatory reporter. The social worker also needs to be available to support the medical team and the family as this is a time of great stress and concern for all involved.

Unfortunately, In the emergency department setting, after reporting the case to DCF and completing the initial documentation and supportive work with the family, the social worker often loses touch with a case. Continuity is limited, and in cases such as this, the reporting social worker is not aware of the disposition or what happens after the referral is made. This disturbs the continuity of care for all, and as much as possible a clear referral process with adequate follow-up can assist with the transitions yet to come.

---

the infant upside down over a pan of hot water. The heels of the infant are then slapped while the infant is simultaneously shaken in an up-and-down motion. The obvious solution to these inadvertent causes of SBS is to educate those who care for infants about the dangers of such practices.

Presentation Case Example

Gill et al. (2009) highlight the difficulties that hospital health care personnel can have in diagnosing SBS, as well as the problems parents can experience when trying to determine if seeking medical consultation is appropriate. They describe the case of a 4-month-old African American boy who was brought into the emergency department by his parents. In the initial assessment, the baby appeared listless and was believed to be in septic shock. The mother stated that for the previous 24 hours her child would not eat, was having trouble breathing, was crossing his eyes, and was having what appeared to be seizures. The parents reported the baby had recently received his immunization shots and the mother noted to the staff that his symptoms resembled what his doctor had warned might occur as a reaction to the shots.

During the health assessment, the mother claimed that the baby had fallen off the bed while his father was caring for him 2 weeks earlier. The mother reported she had contacted her doctor, but was informed by the nurse that since the baby did not lose consciousness he would not need medical attention. On this occasion, the child was observed in the emergency department for three hours without a diagnosis being rendered. No one suspected SBS. Consequently, no referral was made to a health care social worker.

It was not until later when the child was placed in a tertiary care facility that a report of suspected child abuse was filed. Upon further examination, the baby was found to have a fractured skull, internal bleeding, five fractured ribs and both wrists fractured. The child's right eye was bruised and his big toe appeared to be smashed. The father was arrested and charged with child abuse, assault, battery, reckless endangerment, and attempted murder. He was found guilty and sentenced to a minimum of 15 years in prison. The mother was arrested and charged with failure to seek urgent medical treatment for her son and served 6 months.

It was the opinion of Gill and his team that the mother was not guilty of neglect nor did she willfully delay getting the child treatment. Furthermore, in reviewing the dynamics that surrounded this case, it would appear that the child's mother also became a victim. According to Gill et al. (2009), the mother did try to help her child by reporting the child's toe to the pediatrician during a check-up and the doctor gave the child medication. The mother called the pediatrician's office when the child fell from the bed and was informed not to bring the child in. The mother was also informed that after the child was immunized he might have side effects similar to the symptoms he displayed after being shaken by the father. The mother tried to get help for her child but may have been unaware of the extent of his injuries or may have not realized what serious injuries the baby could sustain from shaking. The baby was permanently damaged by his injuries and was placed into a foster home which is a common outcome (Coles & Collins, 2007; Gill et al., 2009).

Working with children and families in a health care setting is the social worker's opportunity to listen to parents and to pick up on cues that may lead to the discovery of families at risk and in need of support before SBS occurs. Without preventative interventions, such families may respond to the pressures in the family dynamics with inappropriate parenting behavior (Patrini, 2002). The end result of such behavior may culminate in a shaken baby.

Parenting can be challenging for even the best of parents at times and not knowing or understanding why a baby is crying can be very frustrating for all involved. For parents, new or additional parental responsibilities often mean juggling with competing priorities to balance work and home life. This juggling is further complicated by simply trying to understand how best to meet children's needs at all stages of their development. Parents themselves require and deserve support. There are some families who are not capable or self-aware enough to be able to recognize their need for help. This is why health care social workers need to be trained to recognize the symptoms of such family pressure and identify needs and provide or assist to access support mechanisms (Patrini, 2002).

Social workers can help parents and caregivers to better understand an infant's behavior. Teaching parenting skills and other concrete skills to help caregivers manage their frustrations could significantly reduce the occurrence of SBS and other types of abuse. Education and support is essential as sometimes parents may shake a child, perceiving it a less violent way than other means to enforce discipline.

The focus of education should focus on anyone who provides support care for the infant. Social workers can assist making sure that new parents can be informed through prenatal care, community education, and their primary care provider. In the hospital setting on the postpartum unit, information about the dangers of shaking an infant should be a part of routine education and supportive care for any new parent. Decreasing mortality and morbidity associated with SBS is achievable through early preventative education. A health care social worker, as a part of preventative management, should assess caretaker stress, discipline practices, substance abuse, and responses to the crying infant. There is increasing recognition nationwide that SBS is not a rare phenomenon, and more and more agencies have begun to distribute printed material describing the problem. The number of public service announcements and billboard ads has also risen. Child care providers, another concerning risk group, need to have mandated child abuse training that includes SBS education before they begin caring for children. Funding and monitoring high-quality childcare is also important so that parents leave their children with safe caregivers. Physicians, social workers, educators, attorneys, families, and others should collaborate to educate the public about preventing SBS. In addition to public education, strategies to reduce the problem should include identifying families at high risk for abuse and providing supports to reduce stress.

All parents need help and support sometimes as caring for children can be very stressful. Parents need to be encouraged that when they feel frustration and about to lose control, they should leave the room and call or contact another adult to watch the child while they calm down. Getting help is important so have the following information readily available:

Child Abuse Support Lines

CHILD HELP (800-4-ACHILD).
National Child Abuse Hot line (800-422-4458).

FACTORS IN ASSESSMENT

SBS is an extremely difficult diagnosis to recognize in the absence of obvious signs of physical abuse. If true for medical personnel, it is at least equally difficult for a layperson. From a health care social worker's point of view, a biopsychosocial assessment could contribute information regarding the health and safety of the home. A review of relevant history of behaviors, values, attitudes, and fears is important to understand what might contribute to parents delaying seeking medical help. Furthermore, community health social workers are apt to be familiar with the barriers that the underprivileged experience through lack of telephones, timely transportation, inaccessible health care, and language and class disparities with caregivers. They are more likely to recognize community-wide illiteracy or compromised educational functioning and can educate and enlighten judges and prosecutors of these problems that are not likely to be present in the life experience of upper-middle class professionals. Likewise, they can share research evidence of the difficulty that families have in identifying drug use in a family member who wishes to conceal it.

Funding for prevention continues to be limited due to the high costs and fear of negligence in many court rulings. Rising costs have caused some decline in prevention funding, although the benefit of prevention can far outweigh the cost of care for a surviving SBS child over his or her lifetime (Ellingson, Leventhal, & Weiss, 2008). It is highly unlikely that these financial and psychological costs can be absorbed by families, and advocacy for preventive services is critical to ensure that the needs of the child and family are met.

In recent years, it has been estimated that just the initial hospitalization for a SBS child is in the hundreds of thousands (Ebbs, 2011). This does not include continuing rehabilitation or medical expenses incurred after the child goes home. Most of these costs are absorbed by society through insurance, government assistance, and increased special education costs (Gutierrez, Clements, & Averill, 2004). Advocacy needs to include prevention, education, and intervention in regards to SBS. The social worker must always be cognizant of signs and symptoms of SBS when working with patients and their families. Workers must be prepared to train and educate parents and caregivers on how a normal infant will develop and grow, what to expect and how to meet a child's needs, and how to handle frustration when stress does occur. Health care social workers must be vigilant for the signs of SBS so that appropriate interventions and protection of the child can take place. Risk factors must also be recognized before the occurrence of injury. Intervention before an episode of shaking may save the life of an infant. There is no greater reward than saving a life.

Important Questions for Health Care Social Workers to Address

* How do we as health care social workers determine the presence and extent of risk factors for a child to become a victim of SBS?
* How can we best be helpful to children and families?
* How do we best teach parents how to teach, guide, and discipline their children?

Specific Recommendations for the Health Care Social Worker

* Become educated about the recognition, assessment and treatment, and potential outcomes of shaken baby injuries in infants and children and utilize this information to assist the patient and his or her family.
* Exercise responsibility by reporting these injuries to appropriate authorities.
* Provide pertinent social and medical information to other members of multidisciplinary teams investigating these injuries.
* Support home visitation programs and any other child abuse prevention efforts that prove effective.
* Provide or have appropriate referrals to resources to educate parents about healthy coping strategies when dealing with their child.

SUMMARY AND FUTURE DIRECTIONS

Parenting is a difficult challenge and under the best of circumstances the stress of a new baby (particularly to young first-time parents) is intense, not only in trying to handle the demands of an infant but also in the changes that take place in the new parent's life—increased responsibility, financial pressure, and decreased independence. Mix in less-than-ideal circumstances, poor or no support from family and friends, substance abuse, or a combination of other stressors, and the temptation to take out these troubles on an unsuspecting, baby is sometimes too great. A baby that cries a lot is another target. Frustration can boil over and picking up a baby and shaking him or her to stop the crying is sometimes an impulsive action. No matter why SBS may occur, the results are devastating (Coles & Collins, 2007). Thousands of serious injuries and deaths occur each year. The best method for the health care social worker to assist with this problem is by taking a proactive approach of education and prevention. Reaching out to caregivers at a young age with more emphasis on SBS in schools; education about SBS as an integral part of prenatal and postpartum care; and diligence among social workers to identify and assess and address potential problems before they occur. A combination of the above could result in many fewer cases of this deadly, brutal, and heartbreaking syndrome.

Glossary

Abusive head trauma   An inflicted traumatic brain injury—also called shaken baby syndrome (or SBS)—is a form of inflicted head trauma that can be caused by direct blows to the head, dropping or throwing a child, or shaking a child violently.

Bradycardia   Slowness of the heartbeat, as evidenced by slowing of the pulse rate to less than 60 per minute.

Cerebral contusion   Contusion of the brain following a head injury.

Cerebral edema   Fluid collecting in the brain, causing tissue to swell.

Failure to thrive   These are infants that appear to develop normally, but then for some reason that is usually unexplained they do not grow and gain weight as would be expected for an infant of similar age and size

Fontanel   One of the membrane-covered spaces remaining at the junction of the sutures in the incompletely ossified skull of the fetus or infant. Although these "soft spots" may appear very vulnerable, they may be touched gently without harm. Care should be exercised that they be protected from strong pressure or direct injury.

Hematoma   A localized accumulation of blood in tissues as a result of hemorrhaging.

Hemorrhage   A condition of bleeding, usually severe.

Intracranial   Within the cranium.

Intraocular   Within the eye

Retinal hemorrhage   Bleeding of the retina, a key structure in vision located at the back of the eyes

Shaken baby syndrome (SBS)   A severe form of head injury that occurs when a baby is shaken forcibly enough to cause the baby's brain to bounce against his or her skull. This jarring can cause bruising, swelling, and bleeding of the brain, resulting in permanent, severe brain damage or even death

Subarachnoid hemorrhage or subdural hematoma   A localized accumulation of blood, sometimes mixed with spinal fluid, in the space of the brain beneath the membrane covering called the dura mater.

Traumatic brain injury (TBI)   An acquired injury to the brain caused by an external physical force, resulting in total or partial functional disability or psychosocial impairment, or both, that adversely affects a child's educational performance.

Questions for Further Study

1. What are the risk factors to be aware of in cases where an infant has been brought to treatment? What factors report mandatory reporting?

2. What are the most important points for health care social workers to identify in order to help educate new parents and baby sitters on the danger of shaking a baby?

3. What types of parents are at greatest risk of SBS and why?

4. What is the impact of marital discord and financial distress on the increase of SBS?

5. What coping strategies work best when a parent is feeling frustrated with the care of an infant?

6. What are potential risk factors that may be related to cultural or religious practices? Once identified, how can these be addressed?

7. What are potential risk factors in detecting SBS with closed-cultural family networks such as Amish, Muslim, and Caribbean minorities (such as Haitian and Jamaican)?

References

Abbas, S. Q., & Dein, S. (2011). The difficulties assessing spiritual distress in palliative care patients: A qualitative study. *Mental Health, Religion & Culture, 14*(4),
341–352.

ABC News. (2006). *Terri Schiavo Timeline*. Retrieved from www.abcnews.go.com/
Health/Schiavo/story?id=531632&page=1#.UB9Cl473Ab0

Abramson, J. S. (2002). Interdisciplinary team practice. In A. R. Roberts & G. J. Greene
(Eds.), *Social workers' desk reference* (pp. 44–51). New York, NY: Oxford University
Press.

Adams, C. E., & Michel, Y. (2001). Correlation between home health resource utilization measures. *Home Health Care Services Quarterly, 20*(3), 45–56.

Adamsbaum, C., Grabar, S., Mejean, N., & Rey Salmon, C. (2010). Abusive head
trauma: Judicial admissions highlight violent and repetitive shaking. *Pediatrics,*
126(3), 546–555.

Adkins, E. A. (1996). Use of the PIE in a medical social work setting. In J. M. Karls &
K. M. Wandrei (Eds.), *Person-in-environment system: The PIE classification system*
for social functioning problems (pp. 67–78). Washington, DC: NASW Press.

Adler, S. R., & Fosket, J. R. (1999). Disclosing complementary and alternative medicine use in the medical encounter: A qualitative study in women with breast
cancer. *Journal of Family Practice, 48*, 453–458.

Advance Directive *vs.* Living Will. (n.d.). Retrieved August 2, 2012, from www
.seniorcarehomes.com/tips-and-resources/advance-directive-vs.-living-will.html

Alperin, R. M. (1994). Managed care versus psychoanalytic psychotherapy: Conflicting ideologies. *Clinical Social Work Journal, 22*, 137–148.

Altilio, T., Otis-Green, S., Hedlund, S., & Fineberg, I. (2012). Pain management
and palliative care. In S. Gehlert & T. Browne (Eds.), *Handbook of health social*
work (2nd ed., pp. 590–626). Hoboken, NJ: John Wiley & Sons.

American Psychiatric Association. (2000). *Diagnostic and statistical manual of mental*
disorders: Text revision (4th ed.). Washington, DC: Author.

American Public Health Association. (2012). American Public Health Association,
Social Work Section. Retrieved from www.apha.org/membergroups/sections/
aphasections/socialwork/

Amoah, A. G., Owusu, S. K., Acheampong, J. W., Agyenim-Boateng, K., Asare, H. R.,
Owusu, A. A., ... Woode, M. K. (2000). A national diabetes care and education
program: The Ghana model. *Diabetes Research and Clinical Practice, 49*(2–3), 149–157.

Anderson, G. F., & Frogner, B. K. (2008). Health spending in OECD countries: Obtaining value per dollar. *Health Affairs, 27*(6), 1718–1727.

Andersson, G. (2009). Using the Internet to provide cognitive behavior therapy. *Behaviour Research and Therapy, 47*(3), 175–180.

Archer, K. C., & Boyle, D. P. (1999). Toward a measure of caregiver satisfaction with hospice social services. *The Hospice Journal, 14*(2), 1–15.

Aronson, J., Sammon, S., & Smith, K. (2009). Managing social services in hard times: Are we doing what really matters. *The Journal of Ontario Association of Social Work, 35*(1). Retrieved from www.newsmagazine.oasw.org/magazine.cfm?magazineid=5&articleid=83

Ashcroft, R. (2010). Health inequities: Evaluation of two paradigms. *Health & Social Work, 35*(4), 249–256.

Ashton, R. (2010). Practitioner review: Beyond shaken baby syndrome: What influences the outcomes for infants following traumatic brain injury? *Journal of Child Psychology and Psychiatry, 51*(9), 967–980.

Atkatz, J. M. (1995). Discharge planning for homeless patients. *DAI, 55*(11), 363A (University Microfilm No. AAC9509698).

Auslander, W., & Freedenthal, S. (2012). Adherence and mental health issues in chronic disease: Diabetes, heart disease, and HIV/AIDS. In S. Gehlert & T. Browne (Eds.), *Handbook of health social work* (2nd ed., pp. 526–556). Hoboken, NJ: John Wiley & Sons.

Auslander, W., Haire-Joshu, D., Houston, C., Williams, J. H., & Krebill, H. (2000, January). The short-term impact of a health promotion program for low-income African American women. *Research on Social Work Practice, 20*(1), 78–97.

Austin, D. M. (2001). Flexner revisited [Special issue]. *Research on Social Work Practice, 11*(1), 1–3.

Axelrod, T. B. (1978). Innovative roles for social workers in home care programs. *Health & Social Work, 3*, 48–66.

Babikian, T., & Asarnow, R. (2009). Neurocognitive outcomes and recovery after pediatric TBI: Meta-analytic review of the literature. *Neuropsychology, 23*, 283–296.

Badger, K., Royse, D., & Craig, C. (2008). Hospital social workers and indirect trauma exposure: An exploratory study of contributing factors. *Health & Social Work, 33*(1), 63–71.

Barber, C. E., & Lyness, K. P. (2001). Ethical issues in family care of older persons with dementia: Implications for family therapists. *Home Health Care Services Quarterly, 20*(3), 1–26.

Barker, A. (2010). Following her lead: A measured approach to providing case management and mental health treatment to homeless adults. In T. Kerson & J. McCoyd's (Eds.), *Social work in health care settings* (3rd ed.).

Barker, R. L. (2003). *The social work dictionary* (5th ed.). Washington, DC: National Association of Social Workers.

Barnes, P. M., Bloom, B., & Nahin, R. L. (2008). *Complementary and alternative medicine use among adults and children: United States, 2007* (National Health Statistics Report No. 12). Hyattsville, MD: Centers for Disease Control and Prevention, National Centers for Health Statistics. Retrieved from http://nccam.nih.gov/sites/nccam.nih.gov/files/news/nhsr12.pdf

Barr, R. G., Rivara, F. P., Barr, M., Cummings, P., Taylor, J., Lengua, L. J., & Meredith-Benitz, M. (2009). Effectiveness of educational materials designed to change knowledge and behaviors regarding crying and shaken-baby syndrome in mothers of newborns: A randomized, controlled trial. *Pediatrics, 123*(3), 972–980.

Barr, R. G., & Runyan, D. K. (2008). Inflicted childhood neurotrauma: The problem set and challenges to measuring incidence [Supplemental]. *American Journal of Preventive Medicine, 34*(4), S106–S111.

Bartlett, H. M. (1940). *Some aspects of social casework in a medical setting*. Chicago, IL: American Association of Medical Social Workers. (Reprinted by the National Association of Social Workers in 1958.)

Bassili, A., Omar, M., & Tognoni, G. (2001). The adequacy of diabetic care for children in a developing country. *Diabetes Research and Clinical Practice, 53*(3), 187–199.

Batalden, P., Mohr, J., Strosberg, M., & Baker, G. R. (1995). A conceptual framework for learning continual improvement in health administration education programs. *Journal of Health Administration Education, 13*, 67–90.

Bauer, J. (2001a). The other half of the picture. *RN, 64*(11), 38–45.

Bauer, J. (2001b). Higher earnings, longer hours: 2001 earnings survey. *RN, 64*(10), 56–63.

Bauer, M., Fitzgerald, L., Haesler, E., & Manfrin, M. (2009). Hospital discharge planning for frail older people and their family. Are we delivering best practice? A review of the evidence. *Journal of Clinical Nursing, 18*(18), 2539–2546.

Beaulieu, E. M. (2012). *A guide for nursing home social workers* (2nd ed.). New York, NY: Springer Publishing Company.

Beck, A. T. (1967). *Depression: Clinical, experimental and theoretical aspects*. New York, NY: Harper & Row.

Beck, A. T., & Freeman, A. (1990). *Cognitive therapy of personality disorders*. New York, NY: Guilford Press.

Beck, A. T., & Weishaar, M. E. (2000). Cognitive therapy. In R. J. Corisini & D. Wedding (Eds.), *Current psychotherapies* (6th ed., pp. 241–272). Itasca, IL: F.E. Peacock.

Bell, S. A., Bern-Klug, M., Kramer, K. O., & Saunders, J. (2010). Most nursing home social service directors lack training in working with lesbian, gay and bisexual residents. *Social Work in Health Care, 49*, 814–831.

Bender, K. J. (1996, October). St. John's wort evaluated as a herbal antidepressant. *Psychiatric Times*. Retrieved July 6, 1999, from www.mhsource.com/edu/psytimes/p964058.html

Benjamin, A. E., & Fennell, M. L. (2007). Putting the consumer first: An introduction and overview [Part II]. *Health Research and Educational Trust, 42*(1), 353–361.

Bennett, C., & Beckerman, N. (1986). The drama of discharge: Worker/supervisor perspectives. *Social Work in Health Care, 11*, 1–12.

Bentley, K. J. (1997). Should clinical social workers seek psychotropic medication prescription privileges? No. In B. A. Thyer (Ed.), *Controversial issues in social work practice* (pp. 152–165). Boston, MA: Allyn & Bacon.

Berkman, B. (1996). The emerging health care world: Implications for social work practice and education. *Social Work, 41*, 541–549.

Berkman, B., Chauncey, S., Holmes, W., Daniels, A., Bonander, E., Sampson, S., & Robinson, M. (1999). Standardized screening of elderly patients' needs for social work assessment in primary care: Use of the SF-36. *Health & Social Work, 24*(1), 9–17.

Bernstein, B. E., & Hartsell, T. L. (2004). *The portable lawyer for the mental health professional: An A–Z guide to protecting your clients, your practice and yourself* (2nd ed.). Hoboken, NJ: John Wiley & Sons.

Bertsche, A., & Horejsi, C. (1980). Coordination of client services. *Social Work, 25*(2), 94–98.

Biancosina, B., Vanna, A., Marmai, L., Zotos, S., Peron, L., Marangoni, C., ... Grassi, L. (2009). Factors related to admission of psychiatric patients to medical wards from the general hospital emergency department: A 3-year study of urgent psychiatric consultations. *The International Journal of Psychiatry in Medicine, 39*(2), 133–146.

Bjork, S. (2001). The cost of diabetes and diabetes care. *Research and Clinical Practice, 54*(1), S13–S18.

Blades, B. (2010). Social work in a for-profit renal dialysis unit. In T. Kerson & J. McCoyd's (Eds.), *Social work in health care settings* (3rd ed.).

Block, P. B. (2012). Developing a shared understanding: When medical patients use complementary and alternative approaches. In S. Gehlert & T. Browne (Eds.), *Handbook of health social work* (2nd ed., pp. 291–317). Hoboken, NJ: John Wiley & Sons.

Bloom, M., Fischer, J., & Orme, J. (2009). *Evaluating practice: Guidelines for the accountable professional* (6th ed.). Boston, MA: Allyn & Bacon.

Blumenfield, S., & Epstein, I. (2001). Introduction: Promoting and maintaining a reflective professional staff in a hospital-based social work department. *Social Work in Health Care, 33*(3–4), 1–13.

Bodenheimer, T. (2008). Coordinating care: A perilous journey through the health care system. *The New England Journal of Medicine, 358*(10), 1064–1071.

Borge, F. M., Hoffart, A., Sexton, H., Markowitz, J. C., & McManus, F. (2008). Residential cognitive therapy versus residential interpersonal therapy for social phobia: A randomized clinical trial. *Journal of Anxiety Disorders, 22,* 991–1010.

Boughtin, A., & Orndoff, R. C. (2011). Future of managed behavioral care. In S. A. Estrine, R. T. Hettenbach, H. Authur, & M. Messina (Eds.), *Service delivery for vulnerable populations* (pp. 431–445). New York, NY: Springer Publishing Company.

Bower, K. (1992). *Case management by nurses.* Washington, DC.: American Nurses Association.

Braun, S. A., & Cox, J. A. (2005). Managed mental health care: Intentional misdiagnosis of mental disorders. *Journal of Counseling and Development, 83,* 425–433.

Brennan, L. K., Rubin, D., Christian, C. W., Duhaime, A. C., Mirchandani, H. G., & Rorke-Adams, L. B. (2009). Neck injuries in young pediatric homicide victims. *Journal of Neurosurgeon Pediatrics, 3,* 232–239.

Brenner, B. (2002). Implementing a community intervention program for health promotion. *Social Work and in Health Care, 35*(1–2), 359–375.

Bristo, D. P., & Herrick, C. A. (2002). Emergency department case management: The dyad team of the nurse case manager and social worker. *Lippincott's Case Management, 7*(3), 121–128.

Brower, A. M., & Nurius, P. S. (1993). *Social cognitions and individual change: Current theory and counseling guidelines.* Newbury Park, CA: Sage.

Brown, K. A. E., Jemmott, F. E., Mitchell, H. J., & Walton, M. L. (1998). The well: A neighborhood-based health promotion model for black women. *Health & Social Work, 23*(2), 146–152.

Browne, T. (2012a). Nephrology social work. In S. Gehlert & T. Browne (Eds.), *Handbook of health social work* (2nd ed.).

Browne, T. (2012b). Social work roles in health-care settings. In S. Gehlert & T. Browne (Eds.), *Handbook of health social work* (2nd ed., pp. 20–40). Hoboken, NJ: John Wiley & Sons.

Bruder, M. B. (1994). Working with members of other disciplines: Collaboration for success. In M. Wolery & J. S. Wilbers (Eds.), *Including children with special needs in early childhood programs* (pp. 45–70). Washington, DC: National Association for the Education of Young Children.

Budman, S., & Gurman, A. (1988). *Theory and practice of brief therapy*. New York, NY: Guilford Press.

Buerhaus, P. I., Needleman, J., Mattke, S., & Stewart, M. (2002). Strengthening hospital nursing. *Health Affairs, 21*(5), 123–132.

Bull, M., Hansen, H., & Gross, C. (2000). Predictors of elder and family caregiver satisfaction with discharge planning. *The Journal of Cardiovascular Nursing, 14*, 76–87.

Bullock, K. (2011). The influence of culture on end-of-life decision making. *Journal of Social Work in End-of-life & Palliative Care, 7*(1), 83–98. doi:10:1080/15524256.2011 .548048

Bunger, A. C. (2010). Defining service coordination: A social work perspective. *Journal of Social Service Research, 36*(5), 485–401.

Buppert, C. (2002). NPs cannot order, certify, or recertify home care, or perform plan oversight. *Green Sheet, 4*(7), 1–3.

Burger, W. R., & Youkeles, M. (2000). *Human services in contemporary America* (5th ed.). Pacific Grove, CA: Brooks/Cole Thomson Learning.

Burgess, E. W. (1928). What social case records should contain to be useful for sociological interpretation. *Social Forces, 6*, 539–544.

Burner, S. T., Waldo, R. R., & McKusick, D. R. (1992). National health expenditures: Projections through 2030. *Health Care Financing Review, 14*, 1–29.

Bywaters, P. (1991). Case finding and screening for social work in acute general hospitals. *British Journal of Social Work, 21*, 19–39.

Cabot, R. C. (1915). *Social service and the art of healing*. New York, NY: Moffat, Yard and Company.

Cabot, R. C. (1919). *Social work: Essays on the meeting ground of doctor and social worker*. New York, NY: Houghton Mifflin.

Caffey, J. (1972). On the theory and practice of shaking infants: Its potential residual effects of permanent brain damage and mental retardation. *American Journal of Disabled Children, 124*, 161–169.

Caffey, J. (1974). The whiplash shaken baby syndrome: Manual shaking by the extremities and whiplash induced intracranial and intraocular bleeding linked with residual permanent brain damage and mental retardation. *Pediatrics, 54*(4), 396–403.

Canda, E. R., & Furman, L. D. (2010). *Spiritual diversity in social work practice: The heart of helping*. New York, NY: Oxford University Press.

Cantu, R. C., & Gean, A. D. (2010). Second-impact syndrome and a small subdural hematoma: An uncommon catastrophic result of repetitive head injury with a characteristic imaging appearance. *Journal of Neurotrauma, 27*(9), 1557–1564.

Caplan, G. (1970). *The theory and practice of mental health consultation*. New York, NY: Basic Books.

Carlton, T. O. (1984). *Clinical social work in health care settings: A guide to professional practice with exemplars*. New York, NY: Springer Publishing Company.

Carlton, T. O. (1989). Discharge planning and other matters. *Health & Social Work, 14*(1), 3–5.

Caro, F. G., Porell, F. W., Sullivan, D. M., Safran-Norton, C. E., & Miltiades, H. (2002). Home health and home care in Massachusetts after the Balanced Budget act of 1997: Implications of cost containment pressures for service authorizations. *Home Health Care Services Quarterly, 21*(1), 47–66.

Carr, D. (2012). Racial and ethnic differences in advance care planning: Identifying subgroup patterns and obstacles. *Journal of Aging and Health, 24*(6), 923–947.

Cawthorn, L. (2005). Discharge planning under the umbrella of advanced nursing practice case manager. *Nursing Leadership, 18*(4), online exclusive.

Centers for Disease Control and Prevention. (Updated October 14, 2009). *Healthy People 2020.* Retrieved July 15, 2012, from www.cdc.gov/nchs/healthy_people/hp2020.htm

Centers for Disease Control and Prevention. (2012a). Department of Health and Human Services: Fiscal Year 2012. Retrieved from www.cdc.gov/fmo/topic/Budget%20Information/appropriations_budget_form_pdf/FY2012_CDC_CJ_Final.pdf

Centers for Disease Control and Prevention. (2012b). Retrieved from www.cdc.gov/hrqol/wellbeing.htm#/four

Centers for Disease Control and Prevention. (2012c). Nursing home care. Retrieved August 25, 2012, from www.cdc.gov/nchs/fastats/nursingh.htm

Chambliss, C. H. (2000). *Psychotherapy and managed care.* New York, NY: Allyn & Bacon.

Chang, D. S., Kang, O. S., Kim, H. H., Kim, H. S., Lee, H., Park, H. J., ... Chae, Y. (2012). Pre-existing beliefs and expectations influence judgments of novel health information. *Journal of Health Psychology, 17*(5), 753–763.

Chapman, L. S. (1994). Awareness strategies. In M. P. O'Donnell & J. S. Harris (Eds.), *Health promotion in the work place* (pp. 163–184). Albany, NY: Delmar.

Chen, S. (1997). *Measurement and analysis in psychosocial research: The falling and saving of theory.* Brookfield, VT: Avebury.

Chiesa, A., & Duhaime, A. C. (2009). Abusive head trauma. *Pediatric Clinics of North America, 56*(2), 317–331.

Christian, C. W., & Block, R. (2009). Abusive head trauma in infants and children. *Pediatrics, 123*(5), 1409–1411.

Colby, I., & Dziegielewski, S. F. (2010). *Introduction to social work: The people's profession.* Chicago, IL: Lyceum.

Coleman, M., Schnapp, W., Hurwitz, D., Hedberg, S., Laszio, A., & Himmelstein, J. (2005). Overview of publicly funded managed behavioral health care. *Administration and Policy in Mental Health, 32*(4), 321–340.

Coles, L., & Collins, L. (2007). Barriers to and facilitators for preventing shaken and head injuries in babies. *Community Practitioner, 80*(10), 20–24.

Colón, Y. (2012). End of life care. In S. Gehlert & T. Browne (Eds.), *Handbook of health social work* (2nd ed., pp. 627–642). Hoboken, NJ: John Wiley & Sons.

Colvin, J. D., Nelson, B., & Cronin, K. (2012). Integrating social workers into medical–legal partnerships: Comprehensive problem solving for patients. *Social Work, 57*(4), 333–341.

Cone, J. D. (1998). Psychometric considerations: Concepts, contents and methods. In A. S. Bellack & M. Hersen (Eds.), *Behavioral assessment: A practical handbook* (4th ed., pp. 22–46). Boston, MA: Allyn & Bacon.

Corcoran, J. (2012). *Helping skills for social work direct practice.* New York, NY: Oxford University Press.

Corcoran, J., & Walsh, J. (2011). *Mental health in social work: A casebook on diagnosis and strengths-based assessment* (2nd ed.). Boston, MA: Pearson. Prentice-Hall

Corcoran, K., & Boyer-Quick, J. (2002). How clinicians can effectively use assessment tools to evidence medical necessity and throughout the treatment process. In A. R. Roberts & G. J. Greene (Eds.), *Social workers' desk reference* (pp. 198–204). New York, NY: Oxford University Press.

Corcoran, K., & Fischer, J. (2007). *Measures for clinical practice and research: A source book* (4th ed., Vols. 1 and 2). New York, NY: Oxford University Press.

Coren, E., Iredale, W., Rutter, D., & Bywaters, P. (2011). The contribution of social work and social interventions across the life course to the reduction of health inequalities: A new agenda for social work education? *Social Work Education: The International Journal, 30*(6), 594–609.

Corey, G. (2001). *Theory and practice of psychotherapy* (6th ed.). Belmont, CA: Brooks/Cole.

Corey, G., Corey, M. S., & Callanan, P. (2003). *Issues and ethics in the helping professions* (6th ed.). Pacific Grove, CA: Brooks/Cole.

Coulton, C. J. (1985). Research and practice: An ongoing relationship. *Health & Social Work, 10,* 282–292.

Cowles, L. A., (2000). *Social work in the health field.* Binghamton, NY: Hawthorne.

Cox, C. B. (1996). Discharge planning for dementia patients: Factors influencing caregiver decisions and satisfaction. *Health & Social Work, 21*(2), 97–104.

Cumming, S., Fitzpatrick, E., McAuliffe, D., McKain, S., Martin, C., & Tonge, A. (2007). Raising the *Titanic:* Rescuing social work documentation from the sea of ethical risk. *Australian Social Work, 60*(2), 239–257.

Dane, B. O., & Simon, B. L. (1991). Resident guests: Social work in host settings. *Social work, 36*(3), 208–213.

Darnell, J. S., & Lawlor, E. F. (2012). Health policy and social work. In S. Gehlert & T. Browne (Eds.), *Handbook of health social work* (2nd ed., pp. 100–122). Hoboken, NJ: John Wiley & Sons.

Davey, M. P., & Watson, M. F. (2008). Engaging African Americans in therapy: Integrating a public policy and family therapy perspective. *Contemporary Family Therapy, 30,* 30–47. doi:10.1007/s10591-007-9503-z

Davidson, K. (1978). Evolving social work roles in health care: The case of discharge planning. *Social Work in Health Care, 4*(1), 43–54.

Davidson, K. W. (1990). Role blurring and the hospital social worker's search for a clear domain. *Health & Social Work, 15,* 228–234.

Davis, S. R., & Meier, S. T. (2001). *The elements of managed care: A guide for helping professionals.* Pacific Grove, CA: Brooks/Cole.

Deckro, G. R., Ballinger, K. M., Hoyt, M., Wilcher, M., Dusek, J., Myers, P., … Benson, H. (2002). The evaluation of a mind/body intervention to reduce psychological distress and perceived stress in college students. *Journal of American College Health, 50*(6), 1–14. Retrieved June 20, 2002, from www.ehostvgwll.epnet .com/ehost.asp

De Jong, P. (2002). Solution-focused therapy. In A. R. Roberts & G. J. Greene (Eds.), *Social workers' desk reference* (pp. 112–116). New York, NY: Oxford University Press.

De Jong, P., & Berg, I. K. (2002). *Interviewing for solutions* (2nd ed.). Pacific Grove, CA: Brooks/Cole.

De Jong, P., & Berg, I. K. (2012). *Interviewing for solutions* (4th ed.). Belmont, CA: Brooks/Cole.

Delvin-Foltz, D., Fagen, M. C., Reed, E., Medina, R., & Neiger, B. L. (2012). Advocacy evaluation: Challenges and emerging trends. *Health Promotion Practice, 13*(5), 581–586.

DeNavas-Walt, C., Proctor, B. D., Smith, J. C., & U.S. Census Bureau. (2011, September). *Income, poverty, and health insurance coverage in the United States: 2010* (Current Population Reports, P60–239). Washington, DC: U.S. Government Printing Office. Retrieved from www.census.gov/prod/2011pubs/p60-239.pdf

Depoy, E., & Gilson, S. F. (2003). *Evaluation practice: Thinking and action principles for social work practice.* Pacific Grove, CA: Brooks/Cole.

De Shazer, S. (1985). *Keys to solution in brief therapy.* New York, NY: W. W. Norton.

Deter, H. (2012). Psychosocial interventions for patients with chronic disease. *Biopsychosocial Medicine, 6*(2), Online publication. doi:10.1186/1751-0759-6-2

Dictionary.com. (2012). *Nurse*. Retrieved May 23, 2012, from www.dictionary .reference.com/browse/nurse?s=t

Diwan, S., Balaswamy, S., & Lee, S. E. (2012). Social work with older adults in health-care settings. In S. Gehlert & T. Browne (Eds.), *Handbook of health social work* (2nd ed., pp. 392–425). Hoboken, NJ: John Wiley & Sons.

D'Lugoff, M. I., & Baker, D. J. (1998). Case study: Shaken baby syndrome—one disorder with two victims. *Public Health Nursing, 15*(4), 243–249.

Dobrof, J., Dolinko, A., Lichtiger, E., Uribarri, J., & Epstein, I. (2001). Dialysis patient characteristics and outcomes: The complexity of social work practice with the end stage renal disease population. *Social Work in Health Care, 33*(3–4), 105–128.

Dolgoff, R., & Skolnik, L. (1996). Ethical decision making in social work with groups: An empirical study. *Social Work with Groups, 19*(2), 49–63.

Donald, A. (2002). Evidenced-based medicine: Key concepts. *Medscape Psychiatry and Mental Health, 7*(2), 1–5. www.medscape.com/viewarticle/430709.

Donelan-McCall, N., Eilertsen, T., Fish, R., Kramer, A. (2006). *Small patient population and low-Frequency event effects on the stability of SNF quality measures*. Medicare Payment Advisory Commission; Aurora, CO: Division of Health Care Policy and Research. Retrieved from www.medpac.gov/documents/Sep06_SNF_ CONTRACTOR.pdf

Dong, X., Simon, M., & Evans, D. (2012). Elder self-neglect and hospitalization: Findings from the Chicago health and aging project. *Journal of the American Geriatrics Society, 60*(2), 202–209.

Draine, J., & Solomon, P. (2001). Threats of incarceration in a psychiatric probation and parole service. *American Journal of Orthopsychiatry, 71*(2), 262–267.

Druss, B. G. (2010). The changing face of US mental health care. *American Journal of Psychiatry, 167*, 1419–1421.

Duffy, F., & Healy, J. (2011). Social work with older people in a hospital setting. *Social Work in Health Care, 50*(2), 109–123.

Duncan, W. J., Ginter, P. M., & Swayne, L. E. (1992). *Strategic management of health care organizations*. Boston, MA: PWS-Kent.

Dunn, A., & Phillips, C. (2010). Complementary and alternative medicine: Representation in popular magazines. *Australian Family Physician, 39*(9), 670.

Dziegielewski, S. F. (1996). Managed care principles: The need for social work in the health care environment. *Crisis Intervention and Time-Limited Treatment, 3*, 97–110.

Dziegielewski, S. F. (1997a). Time limited brief therapy: The state of practice. *Crisis Intervention and Time Limited Treatment, 3*, 217–228.

Dziegielewski, S. F. (1997b). Should clinical social workers seek psychotropic medication prescription privileges? Yes. In B. A. Thyer (Ed.), *Controversial issues in social work practice* (pp. 152–165). Boston. MA: Allyn & Bacon.

Dziegielewski, S. F. (2005). *Substance addictions: Assessment and intervention*. Chicago, IL: Lyceum.

Dziegielewski, S. F. (2006). *Psychopharmacology handbook: For the non-medically trained*. New York, NY: W. W. Norton.

Dziegielewski, S. F. (2008a). Brief and intermittent approaches to practice: The state of practice. *Brief Treatment and Crisis Intervention, 8*(2), 147–163.

Dziegielewski, S. F. (2008b). Problem identification, contracting, and case planning. In W. Rowe & Rapp-Paglicci (Eds.), *Comprehensive handbook of social work and social welfare: Social work practice* (pp. 78–97). Hoboken, NJ: John Wiley & Sons.

Dziegielewski, S. F. (2010a). *DSM-IV-TR™ in action* (2nd ed.). Hoboken, NJ: John Wiley & Sons, Inc.

Dziegielewski, S. F. (2010b). *Social work practice and psychopharmacology: A person and environment approach.* New York, NY: Springer Publishing Company.

Dziegielewski, S. F. (2012). *Clinical, advanced, intermediate: Preparation for the social work licensure exam.* Orlando, FL: Siri Productions.

Dziegielewski, S. F. (in press). *DSM-5™ in action* (3rd ed.). Hoboken, NJ: John Wiley & Sons, Inc.

Dziegielewski, S. F., & Holliman, D. (2001). Managed care and social work: Practice implications in an era of change. *Journal of Sociology and Social Welfare, 28*(2), 125–139.

Dziegielewski, S. F., & Powers, G. T. (2000). Designs and procedures for evaluating crisis intervention. In A. R. Roberts (Ed.), *Crisis intervention handbook: Assessment, treatment, and research* (2nd ed., pp. 487–506). New York, NY: Oxford University Press.

Dziegielewski, S. F., Turnage, B. F., & Roest-Marti, S. (2004). Addressing stress with social work students: A controlled evaluation. *Journal of Social Work Education, 40*(1), 105–119.

Easterling, A., Avie, J., Wesley, M., & Chimmer, H. (1995). *The case manager's guide.* New York, NY: American Hospital Publishing.

Ebbs, J. D. (2011). *Report to the Attorney General: Shaken Baby Death Review.* Toronto, ON: Attorney General.

Edgar, T., & Volkman, J. E. (2012). Using communication theory for health promotion: Practical guidance on message design and strategy. *Health Promotion Practice, 13*(5), 587–590.

Edinburg, G. M., & Cottler, J. M. (1995). Managed care. In R. L. Edwards (Ed.), *Encyclopedia of social work* (19th ed., Vol. 2, pp. 1199–1213). Silver Spring, MD: National Association of Social Workers.

Egan, M., Combs-Orme, T., & Neely-Barnes, S. L. (2011). Integrating neuroscience knowledge into social work education: A case-based approach. *Journal of Social Work Education, 47*(2), 269–282.

Egan, M., & Kadushin, G. (1999). The social worker in the emerging field of home care: Professional activities and ethical concerns. *Health & Social Work, 24*(1), 43–55.

Elder, S. (2012). Institutions are no place for kids. *The Star Phoenix.* Retrieved September 3, 2012, from www2.canada.com/saskatoonstarphoenix/news/forum/story. html? id=abd23cad-7e40-4e4d-a1c9-d22330410f33

Ellingson, K. D., Leventhal, J. V., & Weiss, H. B. (2008). Using hospital discharge data to track inflicted traumatic brain injury. *American Journal of Preventive Medicine, 34*(4), 157–162.

Ellingson, L. L. (2002). Communication, collaboration, and teamwork among health care professionals. *Communication Research Trends, 21*(3), 3–21.

Ellis, A. (1971). *Growth through reason.* Palo Alto, CA: Science and Behavior Books.

Ellis, A. (2008). Cognitive restructuring of the disputing of irrational beliefs. In W. T. O'Donohue & J. E. Fisher (Eds.), *Cognitive behavior therapy: Applying empirically supported techniques in your practice* (pp. 91–95). Hoboken, NJ: John Wiley & Sons.

Ellis, A., & Grieger, R. (Eds.). (1977). *Handbook of rational-emotive therapy.* New York, NY: Springer Publishing Company.

Ellis, J. (2009). A bridge over troubled waters. *OASW News Magazine, 35*(1). Retrieved from www.newsmagazine.oasw.org/magazine.cfm?magazineid=5&articleid=77

Ellner, M., & Woods, K. T. (2012). *Hope is realistic: A physician's guide to helping patients take the suffering out of pain* [Kindle edition]. Retrieved from www.amazon.com/Realistic-Physicians-Patients-Suffering-ebook/dp/B00913ZTCG/ref=sr_1_3?ie=UTF8&qid=1359675107&sr=8-3&keywords=ellner+woods

Emerson, M. V., Jakobs, E., & Green, W. R. (2007). Ocular autopsy and histopathologic features of child abuse. *Opthalmology, 114*, 1384–1394.

Engel, G.L. (1977). The need for a new medical model: A challenge for biomedicine. *Science, 196*(4286), 129–136.

Engstrom, M. (2012). Physical and mental health: Interactions, assessment, and interventions. In S. Gehlert & T. Browne (Eds.), *Handbook of health social work* (2nd ed., pp. 164–218). Hoboken, NJ: John Wiley & Sons.

Epstein, M. W., & Aldredge, P. (2000). *Good but not perfect.* Boston, MA: Allyn & Bacon.

Estrine, E., Hettenbach, R. T., Authur, H., & Messina, M. (Eds.). (2011). *Service delivery for vulnerable populations.* New York, NY: Springer Publishing Company.

Ethics meet managed care. (1997, January). *NASW NEWS, 42*, 7.

Etters, L., Goodall, D., & Harrison, B. E. (2008). Caregiver burden among dementia patient caregivers: A review of the literature. *Journal of the American Academy of Nurse Practitioners, 20*(8), 423–428.

Fabbre, V. D., Buffington, A. S., Altfeld, S. J., Shier, G. E., & Golden, R. L. (2011). Social work and transitions of care: Observations from an intervention for older adults. *Journal of Gerontological Social Work, 54*(6), 615–626.

Fahs, M. C., & Wade, K. (1996). An economic analysis of two models of hospital care for AIDS patients: Implications for hospital discharge planning. *Social Work in Health Care, 22*(4), 21–34.

Falck, H. S. (1990). Maintaining social work standards in for-profit hospitals: Reasons for doubt. *Health & Social Work, 15*, 76–77.

Falck, H. S. (1997). The social work career in health care: Assessments, predictions, and some advice. *The Newsletter of the Society for Social Work Administrators in Health Care, 23*(4), 1–6.

Farley, O. W., Smith, L. L., Boyle, S. W., & Ronnau, J. (2002). A review of foundation MSW human behavior courses. *Journal of Human Behavior and the Social Environment, 6*(2), 1–12.

Feder, J., Komisar, H. L., & Neifeld, M. (2000). Long-term care in the United States: An overview. *Health Affiliates, 19*(3), 40–56.

Feigelman, W., Jordan, J. R., McIntosh, J. L., & Feigelman, B. (2012). *Devastating losses: How parents cope with the death of a child to suicide or drugs.* New York, NY: Springer Publishing Company.

Ferguson, A., & Schriver, J. (2012). The future of gerontological social work: A case for structural lag. *Journal of Gerontological Social Work, 55*, 304–320.

Figley, C. R. (Ed.). (1995). *Compassion fatigue: Coping with secondary traumatic stress in those who treat the traumatized.* Bristol, PA: Brunner/Mazel.

Findley, K., Barnes, P., Moran, D., & Squier, W. (2012). Shaken baby syndrome, abusive head trauma and actual innocence: Getting it right. *Houston Journal of Health Law and Policy, 12*(2), 209–312.

Fiske, E. A., & Hall, J. M. (2008). Inflicted childhood neurotrauma. *Advanced Nursing Science, 31*(2), E1–E8.

Fontaine, K., & Rositani, R. (2000). Cost, quality, and satisfaction with hospice after-hours care. *The Hospice Journal, 15*(1), 1–13.

Fontanella, C., Pottick, K., Warner, L., & Campo, J. (2010). Effects of medication management and discharge planning on early readmission of psychiatrically hospitalized adolescents. *Social Work in Mental Health, 8*(2), 117–133.

Forbes, B. J., & Levin, A. (2010). Abusive head trauma/shaken baby syndrome. *Pediatric Retina, 17*, 409–421.

Forum of ESRD Networks. (2012). *The end stage renal disease network system.* Retrieved from www.esrdnetworks.org/

Fottler, M. D., & Malvey, D. M. (2010). *The retail revolution in health care.* Santa Barbara, CA: Praeger.

Fox, M. A., Hodgson, J. L., & Lamson, A. L. (2012). Integration: Opportunities for family therapists in primary care. *Contemporary Family Therapy, 34*, 228–243.

Frager, S. (2000). *Managing managed care.* New York, NY: John Wiley & Sons.

Frankel, A. J., & Gelman, S. R. (2011). *Case management: An introduction to concepts and skills* (3rd ed.). Chicago, IL: Lyceum.

Franklin, C. (2002). Developing effective practice competencies in managed behavioral health care. In A. R. Roberts & G. J. Greene (Eds.), *Social workers' desk reference* (pp. 3–10). New York, NY: Oxford University Press.

Freeman, L. W. (2009). *Mosby's complementary and alternative medicine.* St. Louis, MO: Mosby Elsevier.

Fruzzetti, A. E., Crook, W., Erikson, K. M., Lee, J. E., & Worrall, J. M. (2008). Emotion regulation. In W. T. O'Donohue & J. E. Fisher (Eds.), *Cognitive behavior therapy: Appling empirically supported techniques in your practice* (pp. 174–186). Hoboken, NJ: John Wiley & Sons.

Fuddy, L. (2012). Advancing public health today and for future generations. *Hawaii Journal of Medicine and Public Health, 71*(3), 79–81.

Gantt, A. B., Cohen, N. L., & Sianz, A. (1999). Impediments to discharge planning effort for psychiatric inpatients. *Social Work in Health Care, 29*(1), 1–14.

Gehlert, S. (2006). The conceptual underpinnings of social work in health care. In S. Gehlert & T. Browne (Eds.), *Handbook of health social work* (pp. 3–22). Hoboken, NJ: John Wiley & Sons.

Gehlert, S. (2012). Communication in health care. In S. Gehlert & T. Browne (Eds.), *Handbook of health social work* (2nd ed., pp. 237–262). Hoboken, NJ: John Wiley & Sons.

Gelman, S. R. (2002). On being an accountable profession: The code of ethics, oversight by board of directors, and whistle-blowers as a last resort. In A. R. Roberts & G. J. Greene (Eds.), *Social workers' desk reference* (pp. 75–80). New York, NY: Oxford University Press.

Gentry, L. R. (1993). The special caretakers program: A hospital solution to the boarder baby problem. *Health & Social Work, 18*(1), 75–77.

Georgetown University Long-Term Care Financing Project. (2007). *Medicare and long-term care: Fact sheet.* Washington, DC: Health Policy Institute. Retrieved September 5, 2012, from ltc.georgetown.edu/pdfs/medicare0207.pdf

Giamberardino, M. A., & Jensen, T. S. (Eds.). (2012). *Pain comorbidities: Understanding and treating the complex patient.* Seattle, WA: International Association for the Study of Pain.

Gibbs, L. (2002). How social workers can do more good than harm: Clinical thinking, evidence-based clinical reasoning, and avoiding fallacies. In A. R. Roberts & G. J. Greene (Eds.), *Social workers' desk reference* (pp. 752–756). New York, NY: Oxford University Press.

Gibelman, M. (2002). Social work in an era of managed care. In A. R. Roberts & G. J. Greene (Eds.), *Social workers' desk reference* (pp. 16–22). New York, NY: Oxford University Press.

Gilbert, P. (2002). Understanding the biopsychosocial approach: Conceptualization. *Clinical Psychology, 14*, 13–17.

Gill, J. R., Goldfeder, L. B., Armbrustmacher, V., Coleman, A., Mena, H., & Hirsch, C. S. (2009). Fatal head injury in children younger than 2 years in New York City and an overview of the shaken baby syndrome. *Archives of Pathology & Laboratory Medicine, 133*(4), 619–627.

Gingerich, W. J. (2002). Computer applications for social work practice. In A. R. Roberts & G. J. Greene (Eds.), *Social workers' desk reference* (pp. 23–28). New York, NY: Oxford University Press.

GlaxoSmithKline. (2012). The impact of chronic diseases on healthcare. *Triple Solution for a Healthier America*. Retrieved from www.forahealthieramerica.com/ds/impact-of-chronic-disease.html

Goeddeke-Merickel, C. M. (1998a, May/June). Alternative medicine and dialysis patients: Part II. *For Patients Only, 19*–20.

Goeddeke-Merickel, C. M. (1998b, July/August). Alternative medicine and dialysis patients: Part III. *For Patients Only, 22*, 30.

Goeddeke-Merickel, C. M. (1998c, March/April). Herbal medicine: Some Do's and Don'ts for dialysis patients. *For Patients Only, 22*–23.

Golden, R. (2011). Coordination, integration, and collaboration: A clear path for social work in health care reform. *Health & Social Work, 36*(3), 227–228.

Goldstein, E. (1995). *Ego psychology and social work practice* (2nd ed.). Glencoe, IL The Free Press.

Goode, R. (2000). *Social work practice in home health care*. Binghamton, NY: Hawthorne.

Gorin, S. H. (2011). Repealing and replacing the affordable care act: Prospects and limitations. *Health & Social Work, 31*(1), 3–5.

Grabowski, D. C., Aschbrenner, K. A., Rome, V. F., & Bartels, S. J. (2010). Quality of mental health care for nursing home residents: A literature review. *Medical Care Research & Review, 67*(6), 627–656.

Green, C. E., & Dziegielewski, S. F. (2004). Three-part series on self support, self-help, and professional development [Part 1: Stress Reduction]. *Faculty Focus, 3*(2), 3–4.

Green, L. S., Oades, L. G., & Grant, A. M. (2006). Cognitive-behavioral, solution-focused life coaching: Enhancing goal striving, well-being, and hope. *The Journal of Positive, 1*(3), 142–149.

Grimaldi, P. (2000). Medicare's new home health prospective payment system explained. *Healthcare Financial Management, 54*(11), 46–56.

Gruenwald, J. (2001). *PDR for herbal medications*. Montvale, NJ: Medical Economics.

Guild, J. P. (2012). The social worker and the depression. *Journal of Progressive Human Services, 23*, 50–54.

Gutierrez, F. L., Clements, P. T., & Averill, J. (2004). Shaken baby syndrome: Assessment, intervention and prevention. *Journal of Psychosocial Nursing and Mental Health Services, 42*(12), 22–29.

Haber, D. (2010). *Health promotion and aging practical applications for the health professions*. New York, NY: Springer Publishing Company.

Hailey, D., Ohinmaa, A., & Roine, R. (2004). Study quality and evidence of benefit in recent assessments of telemedicine. *Journal of Telemedicine and Telecare, 10*(6), 318–324. doi:10.1258/1357633042602053

Hamilton, G. (1936). *Social case recording*. New York, NY: Columbia University Press.

Hamilton, G. (1946). *Principles of social case recording*. New York, NY: Columbia University Press.

Hart, J., Coady, M. M., & Halvorson, G. (1995). The managed care perspective. *Health Administration Education, 13,* 53–66.

Hartsell, T. L., Hartsell, T. L., Jr., & Berstein, B. E. (2008). *The portable ethicist for mental health professionals: A complete guide to responsible practice.* Belmont, CA: John Wiley & Sons.

Hawkins, J., Veeder, N., & Pearce, C. (1998). *Nurse social worker collaboration managed care: A model of community case management.* New York, NY: Springer Publishing Company.

Health Care Financing Administration. (2000, April). Role of physician in the home health perspective payment system. *Program Memorandum Carriers,* 1–4.

Health Care Financing Review. (2010). Statistical Supplement: Figure 6.1, Growth in Medicare skilled nursing facility program payments: Calendar years 1983–2009. Retrieved August 30, 2012, from www.cms.gov/Research-Statistics-Data-and-Systems/Research/MedicareMedicaidStatSupp/2010.html

Health Resources and Services Administration (HRSA), Department of Health and Human Services. (2002, June 4). *HHS Awards $30 Million to Address Emerging Nursing Shortage* [Press release]. Available at http://archive.hhs.gov/news/press/2oo2pres/20020604.html

Heart and Stroke Foundation. (2011). *Statistics.* Retrieved September 1, 2012, from www.heartandstroke.on.ca/site/c.pvI3IeNWJwE/b.3581729/k.359A/Statistics.htm#stroke

Heeschen, S. J. (2000). Making the most of quality indicator information. *Geriatric Nursing, 21*(4), 206–209.

Heller, N. R., & Gitterman, A. (2011). Introduction to social problems and mental/illness. In N. R. Heller & A. Gitterman (Eds.), *Mental health and social problems: A social work perspective* (pp. 1–17). New York, NY: Routledge.

Helzer, J. E., Kraemer, H. C., Krueger, R. F., Wittchen, H. U., Sirovatka, P. J., & Regier, D. A. (Eds.). (2008). *Dimensional approaches in diagnostic calssification: Refining the research agenda for DSM-V.* Washington, DC: American Psychiatric Association.

Hepworth, D. H., Rooney, R. H., Rooney, G. D., Strom-Gottfried, K., & Larsen, J. (2010). *Direct social work practice: Theory and skills* (8th ed.). Belmont, CA: Brooks/Cole.

Herman, J. L. (1992). *Trauma and recovery.* New York, NY: Basic Books.

Hernandez, S. R., Fottler, M. D., & Joiner, C. L. (1994). Integrating strategic management and human resources. In M. Fottler, S. Hernandez, & C. L. Joiner (Eds.), *Strategic management of human resources in health service organizations* (2nd ed., pp. 3–25). Albany, NY: Delmar.

Hinshaw, S. P., & Stier, A. (2008). Stigma in relation to mental disorders. *Annual Review of Clinical Psychology, 4,* 269–293.

Hiratsuka, J. (1990). Managed care: A sea of change in health. *NASW News, 35,* 3.

Hixon, T. (2012). The U.S. does not have a debt problem …. It has a health care problem.*Forbes.* Retrieved May 19, 2012, from www.forbes.com/sites/toddhixon/2012/02/09/the-u-s-does-not-have-a-debt-problem-it-has-a-health-care-cost-problem/

Hjorland, B. (2011). Evidence-based practice: An analysis based on the philosophy of science. *Journal of American Society for Information Science and Technology, 62*(7), 1301–1310.

Hodgson, J., Lamson, A., Mendenhall, T., & Crane, R. (2012). Medical family therapy: Opportunity for workforce development in healthcare. *Contemporary Family Therapy, 34,* 143–146. doi:10.10007/s10591-012-9199-1

Hofschire, D. (2012). Why health care reform is critical for the U.S. economy. Retrieved May 19, 2012, from www.news.fidelity.com/news/article.jhtml? guid=/FidelityNewsPage/pages/viewpoints-healthcare-economy&topic= saving-for-retirement

Holland, T. P., & Kilpatrick, A. C. (1991). Ethical issues in social work: Toward a grounded theory of professional ethics. *Social Work, 36*(2), 138–145.

Holliman, D. (1998). *Discharge planning in Alabama hospitals.* (Unpublished dissertation.) University of Alabama, Tuscaloosa. (UMI DAI-59-09A 3647).

Holliman, D., Dziegielewski, S. F., & Datta, P. (2001). Discharge planning and social work practice. *Journal of Health Care Social Work, 32*(3), 1–19.

Holliman, D., Dziegielewski, S. F., & Teare, R. (2003). Differences and similarities between social work and nurse discharge planners. *Health & Social Work, 28*(3), 224–231.

Hou, J., Hollenburg, J., & Charllson, M. (2001). Can physicians' admission evaluation of patients' status help to identify patients requiring social work interventions? *Social Work in Health Care, 33*(2), 17–28.

Huckfeldt, P. J., Sood, N., Escarce, J. J., Grabowski, D. C., & Newhouse, J. P. (2012). *Effects of medicare payment reform: Evidence from the home health interim and prospective payment system.* Faculty Research Working Paper Series. Cambridge, MA: Harvard University.

Hudson, C. G. (2001). Changing patterns of acute psychiatric hospitalization under a public managed care program. *Journal of Sociology and Social Welfare, 28*(2), 141–176.

Hunt, K. A., Gabel, J. R., & Hurst, K. M. (1998, September). The truth about hospice. *Business & Health, 16*(9), 67–68.

Hypericum Depression Trial Study Group. (2002). Effect of hypericum perforatum (St.John's wort) in major depressive disorder: A randomized, controlled trial. *The Journal of the American Medical Association, 287,* 1807–1814.

Icanberry, A. (2012). What's the difference between hospice and palliative care? Retrieved August 2, 2012, from www.caring.com/articles/whats-the-difference-between-hospice-and-palliative-care

Ingoldsby, A., Kumar, N., Cohen, M. A., & Wallack, S. S. (1994). Medicare home health care: The struggle for definition. *Journal of Long-Term Home Health Care, 13,* 16–31.

Integrative Medicine Communications. (1998). *An integrative medicine primer.* Newton, MA: Author.

Integrative Medicine Communications. (2000). *A physician's reference to botanical medicines.* Newton, MA: Author.

Jackson, R. L. (2001). *The clubhouse model: Empowering applications of theory to generalist practice.* Pacific Grove, CA: Brooks/Cole.

Jacobsen, L. A., Kent, M., Lee, M., & Mather. (2011). America's aging population. *Population Reference Bureau Population Bulletin, 66*(1), 1–15.

JAMA. (2004). Actual causes of death in the United States, 2000. *Journal of the American Medical Association, 10,* 1238–1245. doi:10.1001/jama.291.10.1238

James, R. K., & Gilliland, B. E. (2012). *Crisis intervention strategies* (7th ed.). Belmont, CA: Brooks/Cole.

Jansson, B. S. (2011). *Improving healthcare through advocacy: A guide for health and helping professionals.* Hoboken, NJ: John Wiley & Sons.

Johnson, P. (Ed.). (1998). *Hospice of health first student orientation* [Brochure]. West Melbourne, FL: Hospice of Health First, Inc. (Original work published 1992).

Jongsma, A. E., Jr., Peterson, M., & Bruce, T. J. (2006). *The complete adult psychotherapy treatment planner* (4th ed.). Hoboken, NJ: John Wiley & Sons.

Judd, R. (2010). Hospital social work: Contemporary roles and professional activities. *Social Work in Health Care, 49*(9), 856–871.

Kadushin, A. (1976). *Supervision in social work.* New York, NY: Columbia University Press.

Kadushin, A. (1992). What's wrong, what's right with social work supervision? *Clinical Supervisor, 10,* 3–19.

Kadushin, G., & Egan, M. (2001). Ethical dilemmas in home health care: A social work perspective. *Health & Social Work, 26*(3), 136–161. Retrieved January 4, 2002, from Ehost online database.

Kadushin, G., & Kulys, R. (1994). Patient and family involvement in discharge planning. *Journal of Gerontological Social Work, 22,* 171–199.

Kagle, J. D. (1995). Recording. In *Encyclopedia of social work* (19th ed., Vol. 2, pp. 2027–2033). Washington, DC: NASW Press.

Kagle, J. D. (2002). Record-keeping. In A. R. Roberts & G. J. Greene (Eds.), *Social workers' desk reference* (pp. 28–37). New York, NY: Oxford University Press.

Kagle, J. D., & Kopels, S. (2008). *Social work records* (3rd ed.). Long Grove, IL: Waveland Press.

Kaiser Foundation. (2007). *The uninsured a primer: Key facts about Americans without health insurance.* Retrieved August 12, 2012, from www.kff.org/uninsured/upload/7451-03.pdf

Kanaan, B. K. (2009). The CHF care transition projects: Final progress report and meeting summary. Retrieved September 5, 2012, from http://www.chcf.org/~/media/MEDIA%20LIBRARY%20Files/PDF/C/PDF%20Care TransitionsFinalMeeting.pdf

Karger, H., & Stoesz, D. (2010). *American social welfare policy: A pluralist approach* (6th ed.). Boston, MA: Allyn & Bacon.

Karls, J. M., & O'Keefe, M. E. (2008). *The PIE manual.* Washington, DC: NASW Press.

Karls, J. M., & O'Keefe, M. E. (2009). Person in environment system. In A. R. Roberts (Ed.), *Social workers' desk reference* (2nd ed., pp. 371–376). New York, NY: Oxford University Press.

Karls, J. M., & Wandrei, K. M. (Eds.). (1996a). *Person-in-environment system: The PIE classification system for social functioning problems.* Washington, DC: NASW Press.

Karls, J. M., & Wandrei, K. M. (1996b). *PIE manual: Person-in-environment system: The PIE classification system for social functioning problems.* Washington, DC: NASW Press.

Kayel, H. S., Harrington, C., & LaPlante, M. P. (2010). Long-term care: Who gets it, who provides it, who pays, and how much? *Health Affairs, 29*(1), 11–21.

Keane, T. M., Marshall, A. D., & Taft, C. T. (2006). Posttraumatic stress disorders: Etiology, epidemiology, and treatment outcome. *Annual Review of Clinical Psychology, 2,* 161–197.

Keefe, R. (2010). Health disparities: A primer for public health social workers. *Social Work in Public Health, 25*(3–4), 237–257.

Keefe, R. H., & Evans, T. A. (2013). Introduction to public health social work. In Public Health Social Work Section of the American Public Health Association (Ed.), *Handbook of social work in public health* (pp. 3–20). New York, NY: Springer Publishing Company.

Keefler, J., Duder, S., & Lechman, C. (2001). Predicting length of stay in an acute care hospital: The role of psychosocial problems. *Social Work in Health Care, 33*(2), 1–15.

Kemp, A. (1998). *Abuse in the family: An introduction.* Pacific Grove, CA: Brooks/Cole.

Kielbasa, A. M., Pomerantz, A. M., Krohn, E. J., & Sullivan, B. F. (2004). How does clients' method of payment influence psychologists' diagnostic decisions? *Ethics and Behavior, 14*, 187–195.

Kim, J. S. (2010). Examining the effectiveness of solution-focused brief therapy: A meta-analysis. *Research on Social Work Practice, 41*(20), 260–270.

Kimball, B., O'Neil, E., & Health Workforce Solutions. (2002, April). *Health Care's Human Crisis: The American Nursing Shortage* [For The Robert Wood Johnson Foundation]. Retrieved November 8, 2002, from https://folio.iupui.edu/bitstream/handle/10244/471/NursingReport.pdf

Kimball, M. (2010). Healthcare reform will impact long-term care. *HealthLeaders Media.* Retrieved from www.healthleadersmedia.com/page-2/LED-248406/Healthcare-Reform-Will-Impact-LongTerm-Care

Kinney, H. C., & Thach, B. T. (2009). The sudden infant death syndrome. *New England Journal of Medicine, 361*(8), 795–805.

Kiresuk, T. J., & Sherman, R. E. (1968). Goal attainment scaling: A general method for evaluating comprehensive community mental health programs. *Community Mental Health Journal, 4*, 443–453.

Kirst-Ashman, K. K. (2000). *Human behavior, communities, organizations & groups in the macro social environment.* Pacific Grove, CA: Brooks/Cole.

Kirst-Ashman, K. K., & Hull, G. H., Jr. (2011). *Understanding generalist practice* (6th ed.). Belmont, CA: Brooks/Cole, Cengage Learning.

Kirven, J. (2001). Minority adolescents in therapeutic foster care: Applying narrative interventions with an optimal worldview. *Journal of International & Comparative Social Welfare, 17*(1), 37–44.

Kongstvedt, P. (2012). *Essentials of managed care* (6th ed.). Burlington, MA: Jones & Bartlett Learning.

Kovacs, P. J. (2000). Participatory action research and hospice: A good fit. *The Hospice Journal, 15*(3), 55–62.

Kroll, D. J. (1997, September). St John's wort: An example of the problems with herbal medicine regulation in the United States. *Medical Sciences Bulletin, 240*, 1–5.

Krupnick, J. L., Green, B. L., Stockton, P., Miranda, J., Krause, E., & Mete, M. (2008). Group interpersonal psychotherapy for low-income women with PTSD. *Psychotherapy Research, 18*, 497–507.

Kurtz, R. A., & Chalfant, H. P. (1991). *The sociology of medicine and illness* (2nd ed.). Boston, MA: Allyn & Bacon.

Kutchins, H., & Kirk, S. A. (1986). The reliability of DSM-III: A critical review. *Social Work Research & Abstracts, 22*, 3–12.

Kutchins, H., & Kirk, S. A. (1988). The business of diagnosis. *Social Work, 33*, 215–220.

Kutchins, H., & Kirk, S. A. (1993). DSM-IV and the hunt for gold: A review of the treasure map. *Research on Social Work Practice, 3*(2), 219–235.

Lake, J., & Spiegel, D. (2007). *Complementary and alternative treatments in mental health care.* Arlington, VA: American Psychiatric Publishing.

Lambert, M. J., & Hill, C. E. (1994). Assessing psychotherapy outcomes and process. In S. L. Garfield & A. E. Bergin (Eds.), *Handbook of psychotherapy and behavior change* (4th ed., pp. 72–113). New York, NY: John Wiley & Sons.

LaPuma, J. (1999). Danger of Asian patent medicines. *Alternative medicine alert: A clinician's guide to alternative therapies, 2*(6), 71.

Laube, J. (2002). Crisis groups. In A. R. Roberts & G. J. Greene (Eds.), *Social workers' desk reference* (pp. 428–432). New York, NY: Oxford University Press.

Lawrence, S. A., & Zittel-Palamara, K. (2002). The interplay between biology, genetics, and human behavior. In J. S. Wodarski & S. F. Dziegielewski (Eds.), *Human behavior and the social environment: Integrating theory and evidenced-based practice* (pp. 39–64). New York, NY: Springer Publishing Company.

Lee, N., & Motzaku, J. (2012). The biosocial event: Responding to innovation in life sciences. *Sociology, 46*(3), 426–421.

Lens, V. (2002). Managed care and the judicial system: Another avenue for reform? *Health & Social Work, 27*(1), 27–35.

Let's Move. (2012). Retrieved from www.letsmove.gov/

Letsch, S. W. (1993, Spring). National health care spending in 1991. *Health Affairs, 2*, 94–110.

Levkoff, S. E., Chen, H., Fisher, J., & McIntyre, J. (2006). *Evidence-based behavioral health practices for older adults: A guide to implementation.* New York, NY: Springer Publishing Company.

Lewin, K. (1947). Frontiers in group dynamics. *Human Relations, 1*, 5–41.

Lewis, J. A., Sperry, L., & Carlson, J. (1993). *Health counseling.* Pacific Grove, CA: Brooks/Cole.

Lewis, S. J., & Roberts, A. R. (2002). Crisis assessment tools. In A. R. Roberts & G. J. Greene (Eds.), *Social workers' desk reference* (pp. 208–216). New York, NY: Oxford University Press.

Liechty, J. (2011). Health literacy: Critical opportunities for social work leaderhip in health care and research. *Health & Social Work, 36*(2), 99–107.

Ligon, J. (2002). Fundamentals of brief treatment. In A. R. Roberts & G. J. Greene (Eds.), *Social workers' desk reference* (pp. 96–100). New York, NY: Oxford University Press.

Limpawattana, P., Theeranut, A. J., Sawanyawisuth, K., & Pimporn, J. (2012). Caregivers burden of older adults with chronic illnesses in the community: A cross-sectional study. *Journal of Community Health.* doi:10.1007/s10900-012-9576-6. Retrieved from www.springerlink.com/content/lj466nx9w80l2j70/

Linde, K., Reit, G., Hondras, M., Vickers, A., Saller, R., & Milchart, D. (2001). Systematic reviews of complementary therapies: an annotated bibliography. Part 2: Herbal medicine. *BMC Complement Alternative Medicine, 1*(5). Retrieved February 10, 2002 from www.biomedcentral.com/1472-6882/1/5

Lipsitz, J. D., Gur, M., Forand, N., Vermes, D., & Fyer, A. J. (2006). An open trial of interpersonal psychotherapy for panic disorder. *Journal of Nervous and Mental Disease, 194*, 440–445.

Lipsitz, J. D., Gur, M., Vermes, D., Petkova, E., Cheng, J., Miller, N., ... Fyer, A. (2008). A randomized trial of interpersonal therapy versus supportive therapy for social anxiety disorder. *Depression and Anxiety, 25*, 542–553.

Loewenberg, F. M., Dolgoff, R., & Harrington, D. (2000). *Ethical decisions for social work practice* (6th ed.). Itasca, IL: F.E. Peacock.

Low, L., Yap, H. H. W., & Brodaty, H. (2011). A systematic review of different models of home and community care services for older persons. *BMC Health Services Research, 11*, 93–108. doi:10.1186/1472-6963-11-93

Loya, A. M., Gonzalez-Stuart, A., & Rivera, J. O. (2009, May). Prevalence of polypharmacy, polyherbacy, nutritional supplement use and potential product interactions among older adults living on the United States–Mexico border: A descriptive questionnaire-based study. *Drugs & Aging, 26*(5), 423–436.

Lum, D. (2003). *Culturally competent practice*. Pacific Grove, CA: Brooks/Cole.

Lustig, S. L. *Advocacy strategies for health and mental health professionals: From patients to policies*. New York, NY: Springer Publishing.

Lynn, J. (2001). Serving patients who may die soon and their families: The role of hospice and other services. *Journal of the American Medical Association, 285*(7), 925–932.

Lynn, J., Schuster, J. L., & Kabcenell, A. (2000). *Improving care for the end of life: A sourcebook for health care managers and clinicians*. New York, NY: Oxford University Press.

Lyons, J. S., Howard, K. I., O'Mahoney, M. T., & Lish, J. D. (1997). *The measurement and management of clinical outcomes in mental health*. New York, NY: John Wiley & Sons.

Malvey, D., & Fottler, M. D. (2006). The retail revolution in health care. *Health Care Management, 31*(3), 168–178.

Maramba, P., Richards, S., Meyers, A. L., & Larrabee, J. H., (2004). Discharge planning process: Applying a model for evidence-based practice. *Journal of Nursing Quality Care, 19*(2), 123–129.

Marder, R., & Linsk, N. L. (1995). Addressing AIDS long-term care issues through education and advocacy. *Health & Social Work, 20*(1), 75–80.

Marengoni, A., Angleman, S., Melis, R., Mangialasche, F., Karp, A., Garmen, A., … Fratiglioni, L. (2011). Aging with multimorbidity: A systematic review of the literature. *Aging Research Reviews, 10*, 430–439.

Marinac, J. S., Buchinger, C. L., Godfrey, L. A., Wooten, J. M., Sun, C., & Willsie, S. K. (2007). Herbal products and dietary supplements: A survey of use, attitudes, and knowledge among older adults. *Journal of the American Osteopath Association, 107*(1), 13–23.

Marshall, J. W., Ruth, B. J., Sisco, S., Bethke, C., Piper, T. M., Cohen, M., & Bachman, S. (2011). Social work interest in prevention: A content analysis of the professional literature. *Social Work, 56*(3), 201–211.

Maruish, M. E. (2002). *Essentials of treatment planning*. New York, NY: John Wiley & Sons.

Masi, C. (2012). Community and health. In S. Gehlert & T. Browne (Eds.), *Handbook of health social work* (2nd ed., pp. 143–163). Hoboken, NJ: John Wiley & Sons.

Mathews, A. W. (2012, August 2). Medical care time warp. Remember managed care? It's quietly coming back. *Wall Street Journal* (U.S. Edition), B1. http://online.wsj.com/article/SB10000872396390444840104577552823507551472.html

Maus, S. (2010). Geriatric social work in a community hospital: High-touch, low-tech work in a high-tech, low-touch environment. In T. Kerson & J McCoyd's (Eds.), *Social work in health settings* (Chapter 19, 3rd ed.). Retrieved from www.amazon.com/Social-Work-Health-Settings-ebook/dp/B0035LG9UQ/ref=kinw_dp_ke

McAlynn, M., & McLaughlin, J. (2008). Key factors impeding discharge planning in hospital social work: An exploratory study. *Social Work in Health Care, 46*(3), 1–27.

McCall, M. D. (1998, May 12). *Alternative medicine: Is it for you?* Orlando, FL: *Orlando Sentinel*.

McEvoy, P. M., & Perini, S. J. (2009). Cognitive behavioral group therapy for social phobia with or without attention training: A controlled trial. *Journal of Anxiety Disorders, 23*, 519–528.

McLeod, E., & Bywaters, P. (2000). *Social work, health and equality*. New York, NY: Routledge.

McLeod, P. L., & Poole, M. S. (2010). Introduction to special section: Advances in interdisciplinary perspectives on small groups. *Small Group Research, 41*(60), 661–663.

McMullin, R. E. (2000). *The new handbook of cognitive therapy techniques*. New York, NY: W. W. Norton.

McSkimming, S., Myrick, M., & Wasinger, M. (2000). Supportive care of the dying: A coalition for compassionate care—conducting an organizational assessment. *American Journal of Hospice & Palliative Care, 17*(4), 245–252.

McWilliam, C. L., Ward-Griffin, C., Sweetland, D., Sutherland, C., & O'Halloran, L. (2001). The experience of empowerment in home care services delivery. *Home Health Care Services Quarterly, 20*(4), 49–71.

MedicineNet. (2012). Definition of chronic illness. Retrieved from www.medterms .com/script/main/art.asp?articlekey=2731.

Medigovich, K., Porock, D., Kristjanson, L. J., & Smith, M. (1999). Predictors of family satisfaction with an Australian palliative home care service: A test of discrepancy theory. *The Journal of Palliative Care, 15*(4), 48–56.

Meeks, S., Jones, M. W., Tikhtman, V., & Latourette, T. R. (2000). Mental health services in Kentucky nursing homes: A survey of administrators. *Journal of Clinical Geropsychology, 6*(3), 223–232.

Meenaghan, T. M. (2001). Exploring possible relations among social sciences, social work and health interventions. In G. Rosenberg & A. Weissman (Eds.), *Behavioral and social sciences in 21st century health care* (pp. 43–50). New York, NY: Haworth Social Work Practice Press.

Meikle, J. C. E. (2002). In defense of the biopsychosocial model (letter). *Clinical Psychology, 11*, 3–5.

Merriam-Webster Online Dictionary. (2012). Spirituality. Retrieved September 1, 2012, from www.merriam-webster.com/dictionary/spirituality.

Merriman, M. P. (1999). Documenting the impact of hospice. *The Hospice Journal, 14*(3–4), 177–192.

Miller, E. A., & Weissert, W. G. (2001). Incidence of four adverse outcomes in the elderly population: Implications for home care policy and research. *Home Health Care Quarterly, 20*(4), 17–47

Miller, N., Pinet-Peralta, L., & Elder, K. (2012). A profile of middle-aged and older adults admitted to nursing homes: 2000–2008. *Journal of Aging and Social Policy, 24*, 271–290.

Miller, P. J. (2008). Health-care policy: Should change be small or large? In K. M. Sowers & C. N. Dulmus (Series Eds.) & I. C. Colby (Vol. Ed.), *Comprehensive handbook of social work and social welfare: Social policy and policy practice* (Vol. 4, pp. 219–236). Hoboken, NJ: John Wiley & Sons.

Mizrahi, T. (1995). Health care: Reform initiatives. In R. L. Edwards (Ed.), *Encyclopedia of social work* (19th ed., Vol. 2, pp. 1185–1198). Silver Spring, MD: National Association of Social Workers.

Mizrahi, T., & Berger, C. (2005). A longitudinal look at social work leadership in hospitals: The impact of a changing health care system. *Health & Social Work, 30*(2), 155–165.

Molina, D. K., Clarkson, A., Farley, K. L., & Farley, N. J. (2012). A review of blunt force injury homicides of children aged 0 to 5 years in Bexar County, Texas, from 1988 to 2009. *American Journal of Forensic Medical Pathology 33*(4), 344–348.

Monette, D. R., Sullivan, T. J., & DeJong, C. R. (2005). *Applied social research: A tool for human services*. Belmont, CA: Books/Cole-Thompson Learning.

Moniz, C. (2010). Social work and the social determinants of health perspective: A good fit. *Health & Social Work, 35*(4), 310–313.

Moore, M. (2000). PPS takes effect in home health care. *American Speech-Language-Hearing Association Leader, 5*(19), 1.

Moore-Greene, G. (2000). Standardizing social indicators to enhance medical case management. *Social Work in Health Care, 30*(3), 39–53.

Mor, V., Intrator, O., Feng, Z., & Grabowski, D. C. (2010). The revolving door of re-hospitalization from skilled nursing facilities. *Health Affairs, 29*(1), 57–64.

Morales, A. T., Sheafor, B. W., & Scott, M. E. (2009). *Social work: A profession of many faces.* Boston, MA: Allyn & Bacon.

Morgan, D. (2012). *One in four Americans without health coverage: Study.* New York, NY: Thomson Reuters. Retrieved from www.reuters.com/article/2012/04/19/us-usa-healthcare-insurance-idUSBRE83I17420120419

Moses, T. (2009). Stigma and self-concept among adolescents receiving mental health treatment. *American Journal of Orthopsychiatry, 79*(2), 264–274.

Mpofu, E., & Oakland, T. (2009). *Rehabilitation and health assessment: Applying ICF guidelines.* New York, NY: Springer Publishing Company.

Multi-Society Taskforce on PVS, The. (1994). Medical aspects of the persistent vegetative state: First of two parts. *New England Journal of Medicine, 330*(21), 1499–1508.

Muni, R. H., Kohly, R. P., Sohn, E. C., & Lee, T. C. (2010). Hand-held spectral domain optical coherence tomography finding in shaken-baby syndrome. *Retina, 30*(4), 45–50.

Munson, C. E. (2002). The techniques and practice of supervisory practice. In A. R. Roberts & G. J. Greene (Eds.), *Social workers' desk reference* (pp. 38–44). New York, NY: Oxford University Press.

Murphy, J. J. (2008, March). *Solution-focused counseling in schools.* Based on a program presented at the ACA Annual Conference & Exhibition, Honolulu, HI. Retrieved June 27, 2008, from www.counselingoutfitters.com/vistas/vistas08/Murphy.htm

Murray Alzheimer Research and Education Program (MAREP). (2007). *Perceptions of the transition process to long-term care.* University of Waterloo, Ontario, Canada: Author. PDF retrieved September 1, 2012, from www.marep.uwaterloo.ca/research/STAFFResultsSummary-Newsletter_000.pdf.pdf

Myers, J. E., Sweeney, T. J., & Witmer, J. M. (2000, Summer). The wheel of wellness counseling for wellness: A holistic model for treatment planning. *Journal of Counseling and Development, 78*(3), 251–266.

Nacman, M. (1977). Social work in health settings: A historical review. *Social Work in Health Care, 2*(4), 407–418.

Nahin, R. L., Barnes, P. M., Stussman, B. J., & Bloom, B. (2009). National Health Statistics Report Number 18: Costs of complementary and alternative medicine (CAM) and Frequency of Visits to CAM Practitioners: Untied States, 2007. Retrieved from www.nccam.nih.gov/sites/nccam.nih.gov/files/nhsrn18.pdf

Narayanasamy, A. (2007). Palliative care and spirituality. *Indian Journal of Palliative Care, 13*(2), 32–41.

National Alliance on Mental Illness. (2012). Retrieved from www.nami.org/Template.cfm?Section=By_Illness

National Association for Home Care & Hospice. (2010). Basic statistics about home care: Update 2010. Retrieved September 10, 2012, from www.nahc.org/facts/08hc_stats.pdf

National Association of Social Workers. (1996, August). *Code of ethics* (Adopted by NASW Delegate Assembly, August 1996). Washington, DC: Author.

National Association of Social Workers. (2001). *NASW standards for cultural competence in social work practice.* Retrieved from www.naswdc.org/pubs/standards/cultural.htm

National Association of Social Workers. (2003a). *NASW standards for social work services in long-term care facilities*. Washington, DC: Author. Retrieved from www.socialworkers.org/practice/standards/NASWLongTermStandards.pdf

National Association of Social Workers. (2003b). Supervision and the clinical social worker [Practice Update]. *Clinical Social Work, 3*(2), 1–4.

National Association of Social Workers. (2005). *NASW standards for social work practice in health care settings*. Washington, DC: Author.

National Association of Social Workers. (2008a). *Code of ethics* (Revised by NASW Delegate Assembly, 2008). Washington, DC: Author.

National Association of Social Workers. (2008b). Social work in long-term care and aging: Decreased health care costs, increased quality of life. Retrieved from www.naswdc.org/practice/aging/2008/swLTChandout0808.pdf

National Association of Social Workers. (2011). NASW law notes: Client confidentiality and privileged communications. Washington, DC: Author.

National Association of Social Workers. (2012a). Health Care Policy. In *Social work speaks: NASW Policy Statements, 2012–2014* (9th ed.). Washington, DC: Author.

National Association of Social Workers. (2012b). Long-term care. In *Social work speaks: NASW Policy Statements, 2012–2014* (9th ed.). Washington, DC: Author.

National Center for Complementary and Alternative Medicine. (2011). What is complementary and alternative medicine? National Centers for Disease Control, NCCAM Pub. No. D347. Retrieved from www.nccam.nih.gov/health/whatiscam

National Center for Complementary and Alternative Medicine. (2012a). NCCAM: Funding appropriations history. National Centers for Disease Control. Retrieved from nccam.nih.gov/about/budget/appropriations.htm

National Center for Complementary and Alternative Medicine. (2012b). Terms related to complementary and alternative medicine. NIH. Retrieved from www.nccam.nih.gov/health/providers/camterms.htm

National Center for Workforce Studies & Social Work Practice. (2010). *Social workers in hospice and palliative care* [Brochure]. Washington, DC: National Association of Social Workers.

National Center for Workforce Studies & Social Work Practice. (2011a). *Social workers in hospitals and medical centers* [Brochure]. Washington, DC: National Association of Social Workers.

National Center for Workforce Studies & Social Work Practice. (2011b). *Social workers in psychiatric hospitals* [Brochure]. Washington, DC: National Association of Social Workers.

National Consensus Project for Quality Care. (2009). *Clinical practice guidelines for quality care* (2nd ed.). Retrieved August 12, 2012, from www.nationalconsensusproject.org

National Council on Practice of Clinical Social Work. (1994). *Guidelines for clinical social work supervision*. Washington, DC: NASW.

National Hospice and Palliative Care Organization. (2011). *Compliance tip sheet*. Retrieved August 13, 2012, from www.nhpco.org/files/public/regulatory/Tip_Sheet.pdf

National Hospice and Palliative Care Organization. (2012). *Facts and figures: Hospice care in America*. Alexandria, VA: Author. Retrieved from: www.nhpco.org/sites/default/files/.../Statistics.../2012_Facts_Figures

National Hospice and Palliative Care Organization. (n.d.). *Live without pain*. Retrieved May 30, 2012, from www.caringinfo.org/i4a/pages/index .cfm?pageid=3348

National Kidney Foundation. (2012). Retrieved from www.kidney.org/

Naylor, M. D., Kurtzman, E. T., Grabowski, D. C., Harrington, C., McClellan, M., & Reinhard, S. C. (2012). Unintended consequences of steps to cut readmission and reform payment may threaten care of vulnerable older adults. *Health Affairs, 31*(7), 1623–1632.

Nelson, J., & Powers, P. (2001). Community case management for frail, elderly clients: The nurse case manager's role. *Journal of Nursing Administration, 31*(9), 444–450.

Netting, F. N., & Williams, F. G. (1996). Case manager–physician collaboration: Implications for professional identity, roles and relationships. *Health & Social Work, 21*, 216–224.

Neuman, K. (2000). Understanding organizational reengineering in health care: Strategies for social work's survival. *Social Work in Health Care, 31*(1), 19–32.

Newman, B. M., & Newman, P. R. (2003). *Development through life: A psychosocial approach*. Belmont, CA: Wadswoth.

Noetscher, C., & Morreale, G. (2001). Length of stay reduction: Two innovative hospital approaches. *Journal of Nursing Administration, 16*(1), 1–14.

Nolen-Hoeksema, S., Larson, S., & Bishop, M. (2000). Predictors of family members' satisfaction with hospice. *The Hospice Journal, 15*(2), 29–48.

Norris-Shortle, C., & Cohen, R. R. (1987). Home visits revisited. *Social Casework, 68*, 54–58.

Nursing Times.net. (Practice Comment). (2012). Expand HCA role to focus on older people's rehabilitation. Retrieved September 5, 2012, from www .nursingtimes.net/nursing-practice/clinical-zones/older-people/expand-hca-role-to-focus-on-older-peoples-rehabilitation/5048850.article?blocktitle= Practice-comment&contentID=6854

O'Donnell, P., Farrar, A., Brintzenhofeszoc, K., Conrad, A. P., Danis, M., Grady, C., & Ullrich, C. M. (2008). Predictors of ethical stress, moral action and job dissatisfaction in health care social workers. *Social Work in Health Care, 46*(3), 29–51.

O'Hanlon, B., & Weiner-Davis, M. (2003). *In search of solutions: A new direction in psychotherapy* (Rev. ed.). New York, NY: W. W. Norton.

Ofosu, A. (2011). Implications for health care reform. *Health & Social Work, 36*(3), 229–231.

Ontario Association of Social Workers. (2009). Social workers: Addressing the needs of patients and families in a changing health care system. *News Magazine, 35*(1). Retrieved May 19, 2012, from www.newsmagazine.oasw.org/magazine.cfm? magazineid=5&articleid=80

Pack, M. J. (2012). Critical incident stress management: A review of the literature with implications for social work. *International Social Work*. [Published online before print March 28, 2012]. doi:10.1177/0020872811435371

Parsons, M., Senior, H., Kerse, N., Chen, M., Jacobs, S., Vanderhoorn, S., & Anderson, C. (2012). Should care managers for older adults be located in primary care? A randomized controlled trial. *Journal of American Geriatrics Society, 60*(1), 86–92.

Patrini, S. A. (2002). A window of opportunity: Preventing shaken baby syndrome in A&E. *Pediatric Nursing, 14*(7), 32–35.

Pearlman, H. H. (1957). *Social casework: A problem solving process*. Chicago, IL: University of Chicago Press Books.

Pearson, G. S. (2008). Advocating for the full-frame approach [Editorial]. *Perspectives in Psychiatric Care, 44*(1), 1–2.

Peleg-Oren, N., Aran, O., Even-Zahav, R., Molina, O., & Stanger, V. (2008). Supplementary educational model (SEM) in social work education from health care settings. *Social Work in Health Care, 47*, 306–319. doi:10.1080/00981380802174457

Penrod, J. D., Kane, R. A., & Kane, R. L. (2000). Effects of post-hospital informal care on nursing home discharge. *Research on Aging, 22*(1), 66–82.

Perk, S. (2012). Private practice: When it's not right for you. *Social Worker Today*, Retrieved August 12, 2012, from http://www.socialworker.com/home/Feature_Articles/Professional_Development_%26_Advancement/Private_Practice%3A_When_It%92s_Not_Right_For_You/

Pham, H. H., Schrag, D., Hargraves, J. L., & Bach, P. B. (July 27, 2005). Delivery of preventive services to older adults by primary care physicians. *The Journal of the American Medical Association, 294*(4), 473–481. doi:10.1001/jama.294.4.473

Physician's Desk Reference (PDR) (1995). Hearing impairment (1st ed.). Oradell, NJ: Medical Economics.

Plescia, M., Koontz, S., & Laurent, S. (2001, May). Community assessment in a vertically integrated health care system. *American Journal of Public Health, 91*(5), 811–814.

Pollak, J., Levy, S., & Breitholtz, T. (1999). Screening for medical and neurodevelopmental disorders for the professional counselor. *Journal of Counseling Development, 77*(Summer), 350–357.

Pomerantz, A. D., & Segrist, D. J. (2006). The influence of payment method on psychologists' diagnostic decisions regarding minimally impaired clients. *Ethics and Behavior, 16*(3), 253–263.

Pomeroy, E. C. (2011). On grief and loss. *Social Work, 56*(2), 101–105.

Poole, D. (1995). Health care: Direct practice. In *Encyclopedia of social work* (19th ed., Vol. 2, pp. 1156–1167). Washington, DC: NASW Press.

Power, C., Bahnisch, L., & McCarthy, D. (2011). Social work in the emergency department: Implementation of a domestic and family violence screening program. *Australian Social Work, 64*(4), 537–554.

Power, K. (2009). Social determinants of health: An opportunity for social work to showcase our skills. *OASW News Magazine, 35*(1), Retrieved from www.newsmagazine.oasw.org/magazine.cfm?magazineid=5&articleid=79

Prevention and Wellness. (2007). Retrieved from www.jnj.com/wps/wcm/connect/ab3b3c004f5567fd9f9dbf1bb31559c7/prevention-and-wellness.pdf?MOD=AJPERES

Pulido, M. L. (2012). The ripple effect: Lessons learned about secondary traumatic stress among clinicians responding to the September 11th terrorist attacks. *Clinical Social Work, 40*, 307–315.

Quinless, F. W., & Elliot, N. L. (2000). The future in health care delivery. *Nursing and Health Care Perspectives, 21*(2), 84.

Rabiee, P., & Glendinning, C. (2011). Organisation and delivery of home care re-ablement: What makes a difference? *Health care and social care in the community, 19*(5), 495–503.

Rankin, E. A. (1996). Patient and family education. In V. B. Carson & E. N. Arnold (Eds.), *Mental health nursing: The nurse patient journey* (pp. 503–516). Philadelphia, PA: Saunders.

Reamer, F. G. (2002a). Ethical issues in social work. In A. R. Roberts & G. J. Greene (Eds.), *Social workers' desk reference* (pp. 44–51). New York, NY: Oxford University Press.

Reamer, F. G. (2002b). Risk management. In A. R. Roberts & G. J. Greene (Eds.), *Social workers' desk reference* (pp. 44–51). New York, NY: Oxford University Press.

Reamer, F. G. (2009). Ethical issues in social work. In A. R. Roberts (Ed.), *Social workers' desk reference* (2nd ed., pp. 115–120). New York, NY: Oxford University Press.

Regensburg, J. (1978). *Toward education of the health professions.* New York, NY: Harper & Row.

Rehr, H., & Rosenberg, G., (2006). *The social work–medicine relationship.* Binghampton, NY: Hawthworth Press.

Reid, W. J., & Fortune, A. E. (2002). The task-centered model. In A. R. Roberts & G. J. Greene (Eds.), *Social workers' desk reference* (pp. 101–104). New York, NY: Oxford University Press.

Reinhard, S. C., Kassner, E., & Houser, A. (2011). How the Affordable Health Care Act can help move states toward a high-performing system of long-term services and supports. *Health Affairs, 30*(3), 447–453.

Resnick, B., Gruber-Baldini, A. L., Galik, E., Pretzer-Aboff, I., Russ, K., Hebel, J. R., & Zimmerman, S. (2009). Changing the philosophy of care in long-term care: Testing of the restorative care intervention. *The Gerontologist, 49*(2), 175–184.

Resnick, C., & Dziegielewski, S. F. (1996). The relationship between therapeutic termination and job satisfaction among medical social workers. *Social Work in Health Care, 23,* 17–35.

Respite Conference Notes. (2000, September). *Chicago gathering for respite care with the homeless.* Conference conducted at the Egan Conference Center, DePaul University, Chicago, IL.

Reuters Health Information. (2002). US Senate subcommittee approves health spending bill. *Reuters Medical News.* http:www.medscape.com/viewarticle/43860

Richardson, M. (1988). Mental health services: Growth and development of a system. In S. J. Williams & P. R. Torrens (Eds.), *Introduction to health services* (3rd ed., pp. 255–277). Albany, NY: Delmar.

Risley, M. (1961). *The house of healing.* London: Hale.

Rivers, P. A., McCleary, K. J., & Glover, S. H. (2000). Long-term care financing: Are current methods enough? *Journal of Health and Human Services Administration, 22*(4), 472–494.

Roberts, A.R. (1991). Conceptualizing crisis theory and the crisis intervention model. In A.R. Roberts (Ed.), *Contemporary perspectives on crisis intervention and prevention* (pp. 3–17). Englewood Cliffs, NJ: Prentice Hall.

Roberts, A.R. (1995). *Crisis intervention and time-limited cognitive treatment.* Thousand Oaks, CA: Sage.

Roberts, A. R. (2000). *Crisis intervention handbook: Assessment, treatment and research* (2nd ed.). New York, NY: Oxford University Press.

Roberts, A. R., & Dziegielewski, S. F. (1995). Foundation skills and applications of crisis intervention and cognitive therapy. In A. R. Roberts (Ed.), *Crisis intervention and time-limited cognitive treatment* (pp. 3–27). Thousand Oaks, CA: Sage.

Robinson, B. E., Barry, P. P., Renick, N., Bergen, M. R., & Stratos, G. A. (2001). Physician confidence and interest in learning more about common geriatric topics: A needs assessment. *Journal of American Geriatrics Society, 49,* 963–967.

Robison, J., Fortinsky, R., Kleppinger, A., Shugrue, N., & Porter, M. (2009). A broader view of family caregiving: Effects of caregiving and caregiver conditions on depressive symptoms, health, work, and social isolation. *Journals of Gerontology, 64B*(6), 788–798.

Rocha, D. (2010). Rewards and challenges in dialysis social work. *The New Social Worker, 17*(3), 20–21.

Rock, B. (2002). Social work in health care in the 21st century: The biopsychosocial model. In A. R. Roberts & G. J. Greene (Eds.), *Social workers' desk reference* (pp. 10–15). New York, NY: Oxford University Press.

Rogers, A. T. (2006). *Human behavior in the social environment.* New York, NY: McGraw-Hill.

Roland, D., Lyons, B., Salganicoff, A., & Long, P. (1994). A profile of the uninsured in America. *Health Affairs, 13,* 283–287.

Rolland, J. (2012). Families, health, and illness. In S. Gehlert & T. Browne (Eds.), *Handbook of health social work* (2nd ed., pp. 318–342). Hoboken, NJ: John Wiley & Sons.

Rosen, A., & Proctor, E. K. (2002). Standards for evidence based social work practice: The role of replicable and appropriate interventions, outcomes and practice guidelines. In A. R. Roberts & G. J. Greene (Eds.), *Social workers' desk reference* (pp. 743–747). New York, NY: Oxford University Press.

Rosenthal, H. (2011). Transformative impact and initiatives of the mental health consumer/survivor movement. In S. A. Estrine, R. T. Hettenbach, H. Authur, & M. Messina (Eds.), *Service delivery for vulnerable populations* (pp. 415–430). New York, NY: Springer Publishing Company.

Ross, C. E., & Mirowsky, J. (2000). Does medical insurance contribute to socioeconomic differentials in health? *The Milbank Quarterly, 78*(2), 291–321.

Ross, J. W. (1993). Redefining hospital social work: An embattled professional domain. *Health & Social Work, 18*(4), 243–247.

Rossi, P. (1999). *Case management in healthcare.* Philadelphia, PA: W.B. Saunders.

Rothman, J. (2002). An overview of case management. In A. R. Roberts & G. J. Greene (Eds.), *Social workers' desk reference* (pp. 467–472). New York, NY: Oxford University Press.

Rounsaville, B. J., O'Malley, S., Foley, S., & Weissman, M. M. (1988). Role of manual-guided training in the conduct and efficacy of interpersonal psychotherapy for depression. *Journal of Consulting and Clinical Psychology, 56,* 681–688.

Rubin, A. (2008). *Practitioner's guide to using research for evidence-based practice.* Hoboken, NJ: John Wiley & Sons.

Rudolph, C. S. (2000). Educational challenges facing health care social workers in the twenty-first century. *Professional Development, 3*(1), 31–41.

Ruth, B., & Sisco, S. (in press). Public health social work. In T. Mizrahi & L. Davis (Eds.), *Encyclopedia of social work* (21st ed.). New York, NY: National Association of Social Workers, Oxford University Press.

Sable, M. R., Schild, D. R., & Hipp, J. A. (2012). Public health and social work. In S. Gehlert & T. Browne (Eds.), *Handbook of health social work* (2nd ed., pp. 64–99). Hoboken, NJ: John Wiley & Sons.

Saleeby, P. W. (2011). Using international classification of functioning, disability and health in social work settings. *Health & Social Work, 36*(4), 303–305.

Saleh, S. S., Freire, C., Morris-Dickinson, G., & Shannon, T. (2012). An effectiveness and cost–benefit analysis of a hospital-based discharge transition program for elderly Medicare recipients. *Journal of the American Geriatric Society, 60*(6), 1051–1056.

Sample Living Will Form. (2012). Retrieved August 13, 2012, from www.estate.findlaw.com/living-will/sample-living-will-form.html

Sargent, P., Pickard, S., Sheaff, R., & Boaden, R. (2007). Patient and career perceptions of case management for long-term care conditions. *Health & Social Care in the Community, 15*(6), 511–519.

Satterly, B. A. (2007). The alternative lenses of assessment: Educating social workers about psychopathology. *Teaching in Social Work, 27*(3–4), 241–257.

Saxon, C., Dziegielewski, S. F., & Jacinto, G. A. (2006). Self-determination and confidentiality: The ambiguous nature of decision-making in social work practice. *Journal of Human Behavior in the Social Environment, 13*(4), 55–72.

Scaife, J. (2010). *Supervising the reflective practitioner: An essential guide to theory and practice*. New York, NY: Taylor & Francis.

Schalowitz, J. I. (1995). Total quality management at Motorola: A successful blueprint for manufacturing and service organizations. *Health Administration Education, 13*, 15–24.

Schiavo case highlights eating disorders (2005, February 26). *USA Today*. Retrieved from www.usatoday.com/news/health/2005-02-25-schiavo-eating-disorder _x.ht

Schoenwald, S. K., Kelleher, K., & Weisz, J. R. (2008). Building bridges to evidence-based practice: The MacArthur foundation child system and treatment enhancement projects (Child STEPs). *Administration and Policy in Mental Health and Mental Health Service Research, 35*, 66–72.

Schroeder, L. O. (1995). *The legal environment of social work* (Rev. ed.). Washington, DC: NASW Press.

Schuetze, K. (2006). Shining the light on the "800 lb" gorilla of professional rivalry in case management. *Lippincott's Case Management, 11*(6), 289–290.

Schutte, N. S., & Malouff, J. M. (1995). *Sourcebook of adult assessment strategies*. New York, NY: Plenum Press.

Sedgwick, T. W. (2012). Early hospital social work practice: The life and times of Janice Thornton. *Affilia: Journal of Women and Social Work, 27*(2), 212–221.

Seligson, S. V. (1998, May/June). Melding medicines. *Health*, 64–70.

Sheafor, B. W., & Horejsi, C. R. (2008). *Techniques and guidelines for social work practice* (8th ed.). Boston, MA: Allyn & Bacon.

Sheffield, A. E. (1920). *The social case history: Its construction and content*. New York, NY: Russell Sage.

Sheppard, M. (1992). Contact and collaboration with general practitioners: A comparison of social workers and community psychiatric nurses. *The British Journal of Social Work, 22*(4), 419–436.

Shortell, S. M., & Kaluzny, A. D. (Ed.). (1983). *Health care management: A text in organization theory and behavior*. New York, NY: John Wiley & Sons.

Shortell, S. M., & Kaluzny, A. D. (1994). Forward. In S. M. Shortell & A. D. Kaluzny (Eds.), *Health care management: Organizational behavior and design* (3rd ed., p. XI). Albany, NY: Delmar.

Shulman, L. (2002). Developing successful therapeutic relationships. In A. R. Roberts & G. J. Greene (Eds.), *Social workers' desk reference* (pp. 375–378). New York, NY: Oxford University Press.

Sidell, N. L. (2011). *Social work documentation: A guide to strengthening your case recording*. Washington, DC: NASW Press.

Siev, J., & Chambless, D. L. (2007/2008). Specificity of treatment effects: Cognitive therapy and relaxation for generalized anxiety and panic disorder. *Journal of Consulting and Clinical Psychology, 75*(4), 513–522.

Silveira, M. J., Kim, S. Y. H., & Langa, K. M. (2010). Advance directives and outcomes of surrogate decision making before death. *New England Journal of Medicine, 362*(13), 1211–1218.

Silverstone, B. (1981). Long-term care. *Health & Social Work, 6*, 285–345.

Simons, K., Shepherd, N., & Munn, J. (2008). Advancing the evidence base for social work in long term care: The disconnect between practice and research. *Social Work in Health Care, 47*(4), 392–415.

Siple, J. (1994). Drug therapy and the interdisciplinary team: A clinical pharmacist's perspective. *Generations Quarterly, 18*, 49–55.

Skelton, J. K., & Janosi, J. M. (1992). Unhealthy health care costs. *Journal of Medicine and Philosophy, 17*, 7–19.

Skinner, B. F. (1953). *Science and human behavior*. New York, NY: MacMillian.

Sledge, R., Aebel-Groesch, K., McCool, M., Johnstone, S., Witten, B., Contillo, M., & Hafner, J. (2011, June). Part 2: The promise of symptom-targeted intervention to manage depression in dialysis patients. *Nephrology News and Issues, 25*(7), 24–28, 30–31.

Smith, E., & Stark, C. (2012, June 28). By the numbers: Health insurance. *CNN Politics*. Retrieved from www.cnn.com/2012/06/27/politics/btn-health-care/index.html

Smith, S. A. (2011). Health literacy and human services delivery. In S. A. Estrine, R. T. Hettenbach, H. Arthur, & M. Messina (Eds.), *Service delivery for vulnerable populations* (pp. 395–415). New York, NY: Springer Publishing Company.

Smith, S. L., Myers, J. E., & Hensley, L. G. (2002, Spring). Putting more life into life career courses: The benefits of a holistic wellness model. *Jounral of College Counseling, 5*(1), 90–95.

Snow, J. (2001). Looking beyond nursing for clues to effective leadership. *Journal of Nursing Administration, 31*(9), 440–443.

Snowdon, J. (2001). Psychiatric care in nursing homes: More must be done. *Australasian Psychiatry, 9*(2), 108–115.

Sochalski, J. (2002). Nursing shortage redux: Turning the corner on an enduring problem. *Health Affairs, 21*(5), 157–164.

Solomon, P., Schmidt, L., Swarbrick, P., & Mannion, E. (2011). Innovative programs for consumers with psychiatric disabilities. In E. Estrine, R. T. Hettenbach, H. Authur, & M. Messina (Eds.), *Service delivery for vulnerable populations* (pp. 39–69). New York, NY: Springer Publishing Company.

Span, P. (2012, August 25). What the health care ruling means for Medicare. *The New York Times*. New York.

Sparks, J. (2012). Ethics and social work in health care. In S. Gehlert & T. Browne (Eds.), *Handbook of health social work* (2nd ed., pp. 41–63). Hoboken, NJ: John Wiley & Sons.

Specht, H., & Courtney, M. (1995). *Unfaithful angels: How social work has abandoned its mission*. New York, NY: The Free Press, Simon and Schuster.

Sperry, L. (1988). Biopsychosocial therapy: An integrative approach for tailoring treatment. *Individual Psychology, 44*, 225–235.

Squier, W. (2011). The shaken baby syndrome. Pathology and mechanisms. *ACTA NeuroPathologica, 122*(5), 519–542.

Statit Quality Software. (2007). *Statit quality control first aid kit*. Oregon: Statit Software. Retrieved from www.statit.com/services/CQIOverview.pdf

Stehlin, I. B. (1995). An FDA guide to choosing medical treatments. *FDA Consumer, 29*(5), 10–14.

Steps taken to watchdog managed care. (1997, January). *NASW NEWS, 42*, 12.

Stolee, P., Hillier, L. M., Webster, F., & O'Callaghan, C. (2006). Stroke care in long-term care facilities in Southwestern Ontario. *Topics in Stroke Rehabilitation, 13*(4), 97–108.

Straub, R. O. (2012). *Health psychology: A biopsychosocial approach.* New York, NY: Worth Publishers.

Sudore, R. L., & Fried, T. R. (2010). Redefining the "planning" in advance care planning: Prepare for end-of-life decision making. *Annals of Internal Medicine, 153*(4), 256–262.

Sunier, B. (2011). The devil is in the details: Managed care and the unforeseen costs of utilization review as a cost containment mechanism. *Issues in the Law & Medicine, 27*(1), 21–48.

Tahan, H. A. (1998). Case management: A heritage more than a century old. *Nursing Case Management, 3*(2), 55–62.

Tanner, C. A., & Bellack, J. P. (2001). Resolving the nursing shortage: Replacement plus one! *Journal of Nursing Education, 40*(3), 99–100.

Tarasoff v. Regents of the University of California, 551 p.2d 344 (1976).

Taylor, C. (2002). Assessing patients needs: Does the same information guide expert and novice nurses? *International Nursing Review, 49*(1), 11–19.

Temkin, M. (2009). Aging and developmental disabilities strategic issues for service agencies. *Garth Homer Society.* PDF retrieved from www.garthhomersociety .org/content/file/Publications/Final%20Aging%20Report%20external .pdf

Teno, J. M. (1999). Putting the patient and family voice back into measuring quality care for the dying. *The Hospice Journal, 14*(3–4), 167–176.

The Center for Workforce Studies and Practice. (2011a). Social workers in hospitals and medical centers (Brochure). Washington, DC: National Association of Social Workers. http://workforce.socialworkers.org/studies/profiles/Hospitals.pdf

The Center for Workforce Studies. (2011b). Social workers in Psychiatric Hospitals (Brochure). Washington, DC: National Association of Social Workers. http:// workforce.socialworkers.org/studies/profiles/Psychiatric%20Hospitals.pdf

The Joint Commission. (2012). About us. Retrieved September 10, 2012, from www .jointcommission.org/mobile/about_us.aspx

Thompson, S., Bott, M. J., Boyle, D., Gajewski, B., & Tilden, V. P. (2011). A Measure of Palliative Care in Nursing Homes. *Journal of Pain and Symptom Management, 41*, 57–67.

Thompson, S. A., Bott, M., Gajewski, B., & Tilden, V. P. (2012). Quality of care and quality of dying in nursing homes: Two measurement models. *Journal of Palliative Medicine, 15*(6), 690–695.

Thorpe, J. H., & Cascio, T. (2011, October). Medicare hospital readmissions reduction program. *Legal Notes, 3*(4), 1–4. Retrieved from www.rwjf.org/files/research/73455.legalnotes.pdf.

Thrall, J. H. (2005). Prevalence and costs of chronic disease in a health care system structured for treatment of acute illness. *Radiology, 235*, 9–12.

Thyer, B. A. (2002). Developing Discipline specific knowledge for social work: Is it possible? *Council on Social Work Education, 38*(1), 101–114.

Timms, N. (1972). *Recording in social work.* Boston, MA: Routledge & Kegan Paul.

Tinetti, M. E., Charpentier, P., Gottschalk, M., & Baker, D. I. (2012). Effect of restorative model of posthospital home care on hospital readmissions. *Journal of the American Geriatrics Society, 60*(8), 1521–1526.

Turner-Stokes, L. (2009). Goal attainment scaling (GAS) in rehabilitation: A practical guide. *Clinical Rehabilitation, 23*(4), 362–370.

Tuzman, L. (1993). Clinical decision making for discharge planner in psychiatric settings. *DAI, 50*(09), 320. (University Microfilms No. AAC9000681)

UNC Kidney Center. (2012). *Nephrology social workers*. Chapel Hill, NC: Author. Retrieved from www.unckidneycenter.org/hcprofessionals/nephsocialworkers .html#guidelines

Unger, J., & Cunningham, M. (2002). Case management and the BSW Curriculum. *Journal of Baccalaureate Social Work, 8*(1), 69–82.

U.S. Census Bureau (1984). *Current population survey*. Washington, DC: Government Printing Office.

U.S. Census Bureau, Statistical Abstract of the United States: 2012. Washington, DC. Retrieved from www.census.gov/compendia/statab/2012/tables/12s0162.pdf

U.S. Department of Health and Human Services (IIHS), Assistant Secretary for Planning and Evaluation, Office of Disability, Aging and Long-Term Care Policy. (2006). *The supply and demand of professional social workers providing long-term care services: Report to Congress*. Retrieved June 13, 2008, from aspe.hhs.gov/daltcp/reports/2006/SWsupply.htm

U.S. Department of Health and Human Services. (2009). Developing healthy people 2020 Public Meetings (2009 Draft Objectives). Retrieved from www.pdpciowa .org/Meetings/Appendices/JanuaryMaterials2010/Appendix7_Combined PDFHP2020Objectives.pdf

U.S. Department of Health and Human Services (Health Reform.Gov). (2012). *Fact Sheet: The Affordable Care Act's New Patient's Bill of Rights*. Retrieved from www .healthreform.gov/newsroom/new_patients_bill_of_rights.html

Van Dijk-de Vries, A., Moser, A., Mertens, V., van der Linden, J., van der Weijden, T., & van Eijk, J. (2012). The ideal of biopsychosocial chronic care: How to make it real? A qualitative study among Dutch stakeholders. *BMC Family Practice*. doi:10.1186/1471-2296-13-14

Vlaeyen, J. W., Morley, S. J., Linton, S. J., Boersma, K., & de Jong, J. (2012). *Pain related fear: Exposure-based treatment for chronic pain*. Seattle, WA: IASP.

Vonk, M. E., & Early, T. J. (2002). Cognitive-behavioral therapy. In A. R. Roberts & G. J. Greene (Eds.), *Social workers' desk reference* (pp. 116–120). New York, NY: Oxford University.

Waananen, L. (2012). How the number of uninsured may change with and without the health care law. *The New York Times*. Retrieved from www.nytimes.com/ interactive/2012/06/27/us/how-the-number-of-uninsured-may-change-with-and-without-the-health-care-law.html

Wagner, E. R. (1993). Types of managed care organizations. In P. R. Kongstvedt (Ed.), *The managed health care handbook* (2nd ed., pp. 12–21). Rockville, MD: Aspen.

Walls, C. (2006). Shaken baby syndrome education: A role for nurse practitioners working with small children. *Journal of Pediatric Health Care, 20*(5), 304–310.

Walter, J. L., & Peller, J. E. (1992). *Becoming solution-focused in brief therapy*. New York, NY: Brunner/Mazel.

Walter, J. L., & Peller, J. E. (2000). *Recreating brief therapy: Preferences and possibilities*. New York, NY: W. W. Norton.

Wandrei, K. M., & Karls, J. M. (1996). Structure of the PIE system. In J. M. Karls & K. M. Wandrei (Eds.), *Person-in-environment system: The PIE classification system for social functioning problems* (pp. 23–40). Washington, DC: NASW Press.

Wang, W. Y., Shyu, Y. I. L., Chen M. C., & Yang P. S. (2011). Reconciling work and family caregiving among adult–child family caregivers of older people with dementia: Effects on role strain and depressive symptoms. *Journal of Advanced Nursing, 67*(4), 829–840.

Ward, J. (2012). The nurse's role in discharge planning. *Nurse Together*. Retrieved May 19, 2012, from www.nursetogether.com/Career/Career-Article/itemId/2177/The-Nurse%E2%80%99s-Role-in-Discharge-Planning.aspx

Wasabi, G. (2012). Acceptance, fear, or denial. Perception of death and dying throughout history. *HubPages*. Retrieved from www.greenwasabi.hubpages.com/hub/Death-and-Dying-Throughout-History

Watt, H. M. (2001). Community-based case management: A model for outcome-based research for non-institutionalized elderly. *Home Health care Services Quarterly*, *20*(1), 39–65.

Watts, R. J., Gardner, H., & Pierson, J. (2005). Factors that enhance or impede critical care nurses' discharge planning practices. *Intensive Critical Care Nursing*, *21*(5), 302–313.

Webb, N., & Bartone, R. (2012). Social work with children and adolescents with medical conditions. In S. Gehlert & T. Browne (Eds.), *Handbook of health social work* (2nd ed., pp. 373–391). Hoboken, NJ: John Wiley & Sons.

Wheeler, D. P., & Dodd, S. (2011). LGBTQ capacity building in health care systems: A social work imperative. *Health & Social Work*, *36*(4), 307–309.

Whitaker, T., Weismiller, T., Clark, E., & Wilson, M. (2006). *Assuring the Sufficiency of a Front Line Workforce: A National Study of Licensed Social Workers* (Special Report: Social Work Services in Health Care Settings). Washington, DC: National Association of Social Workers.

White House Domestic Policy Council. (1993). *President's health security plan: The Clinton blueprint*, New York, NY: Times Books/Random House.

Whiting, L. (1996). Forward. In J. M. Karls & K. M. Wandrei (Eds.), *Person-in-environment system: The PIE classification system for social functioning problems* (pp. xiii–xv). Washington, DC: NASW Press.

Wilson, A. (2012). Improving life satisfaction for the elderly living independently in the community: Care recipients' perspective of volunteers. *Social Work in Health Care*, *51*, 125–139.

Winslow, L. C., & Shapiro, H. (2002, May). Physicians want education about complementary and alternative medicine to enhance communication with their patients. *Archives of Internal Medicine*, *162*(10), 1176–1181. doi:10-1001/pubs0AarchInternMed-ISSN-0003-9926-10-10110405

Wise, T. N. (1997). Psychiatric diagnoses in primary care: The biopsychosocial perspective. In H. Leigh (Ed.), *Biopsychosocial approaches in primary care: State of the art and challenges for the 21st century* (pp. 9–27). New York, NY: Springer Science + Business Media.

Wodarski, J., & Dziegielewski, S.F. (2002). *Human growth and development: Integrating theory and empirical practice*. New York: Springer Publishing.

Woody, R. (2012). *Legal self-defense for mental health practitioners: Quality care and risk management strategies*. New York, NY: Springer Publishing Company.

Wu, C., Wang, C., & Kennedy, J. (2007). Changes in herb and dietary supplements use in the US adult population: A comparison of the 2002 and 2007 National Health Interview Surveys. *Clinical Therapeutics*, *33*(11), 1749–1758.

Xie, C., Hughes, J., Sutcliffe, C., Chester, H., & Challis, D. (2012). Promoting personalization in social care services for older people. *Journal of Gerontological Social Work*, *55*, 218–232. doi: 10.1080/01634372.2011.639437

Zabora, J. R. (2011). How can social work affect health care reform? *Health & Social Work*, *36*(3), 231–232.

Index

CPSIA information can be obtained
at www.ICGtesting.com
Printed in the USA
LVOW10s2142131117

556119LV00022B/367/P